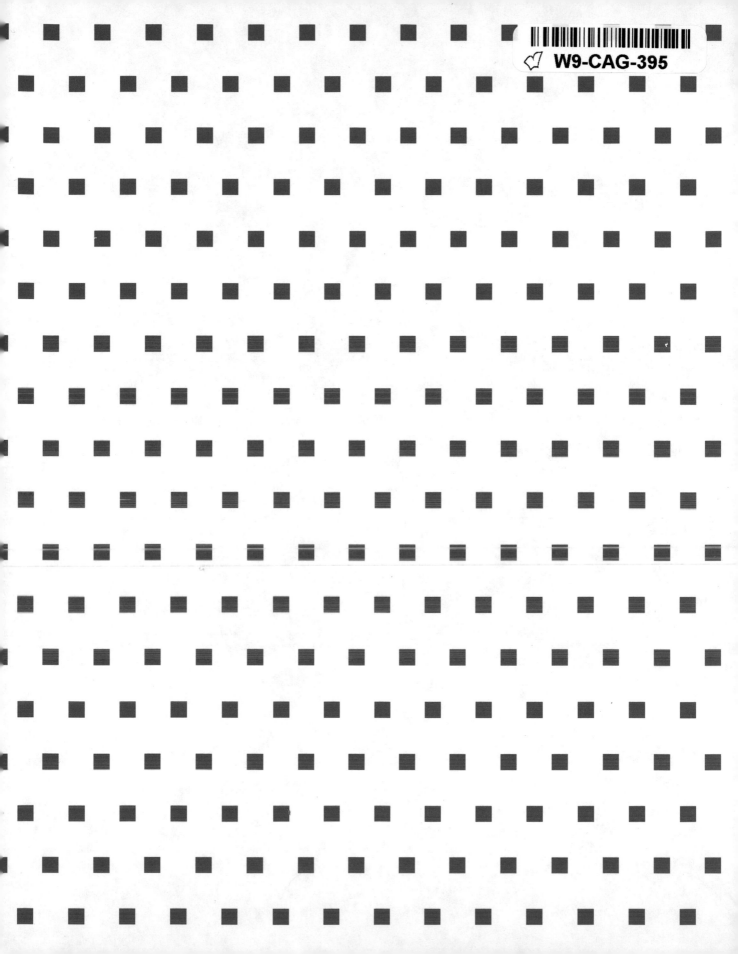

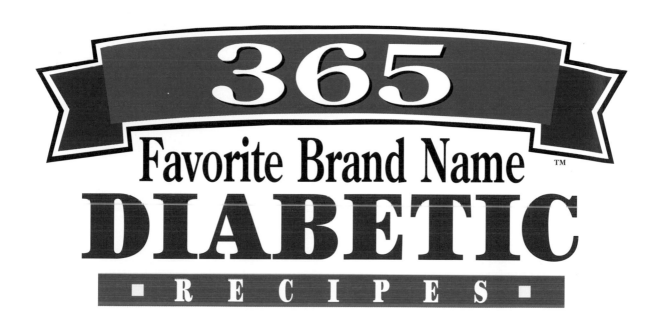

365 Favorite Brand Name™ DIABETIC · RECIPES ·

PUBLICATIONS INTERNATIONAL, LTD.

Nutritional Analysis: The nutritional information that appears with each recipe was submitted in part by the participating companies and associations. Every effort has been made to check the accuracy of these numbers. However, because numerous variables account for a wide range of values for certain foods, nutritive analyses in this book should be considered approximate.

Microwave Cooking: Microwave ovens vary in wattage. Use the cooking times as guidelines and check for doneness before adding more time.

The HEALTHY CHOICE® recipes contained in this book have been tested by the manufacturers and have been carefully edited by the publisher. The publisher and the manufacturers cannot be held responsible for any ill effects caused by the errors in the recipes, or by spoiled ingredients, unsanitary conditions, incorrect preparation procedures or any other cause.

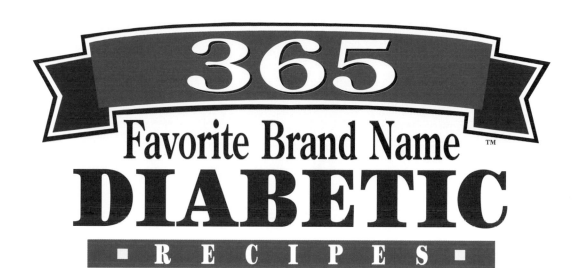

365 Favorite Brand Name™ DIABETIC ▪ R E C I P E S ▪

Facts About
Diabetes

FACTS ABOUT THE DISEASE

Diabetes is a disease that affects the body's ability to use glucose as a source of fuel. When glucose is utilized improperly, it can build up in the bloodstream, creating higher than normal blood sugar levels. Left unchecked, elevated blood sugar levels may lead to the development of more serious long-term complications like blindness and heart and kidney disease.

Not all cases of diabetes are alike. In fact, the disease presents itself in two very distinct forms—Type I and Type II. Development of diabetes during childhood or adolescence is typical of Type I, or juvenile-onset, diabetes. These individuals are unable to make insulin, a hormone produced by the pancreas that moves glucose from the bloodstream into the body's cells, where it is used as a source of fuel. Daily injections of insulin, coupled with a balanced meal plan, are the focus of treatment.

People who develop Type II diabetes, the more common form of the disease, are typically over the age of 40 and obese. These individuals produce insulin but the amount is insufficient to meet their needs, or their excess weight renders the hormone incapable of adequately performing its functions. Treatment includes balanced eating, moderate weight loss, exercise and, in extreme cases, oral hypoglycemic agents or insulin injections.

RISK FACTORS

Diabetes increases one's risk of developing high blood pressure and high blood cholesterol levels. Over time, elevated levels may progress to more serious complications, including heart and kidney disease, stroke and hypertension. In fact, research shows that individuals with diabetes are nineteen times more likely to develop kidney disease and four times more likely to suffer from heart disease or a stroke than people who do not have diabetes. While heredity plays a major role in the development of these complications, regular check-ups with your physician and registered dietitian to fine-tune treatment strategies are good ways to help minimize complications. Strategies for treatment vary among individuals, yet overall goals remain the same: achieving and maintaining near-normal blood sugar levels by balancing food intake, insulin and activity; achieving optimal blood cholesterol levels; and improving overall health through good nutrition.

BALANCE IS THE KEY

Achieving optimal nutrition often requires lifestyle changes to balance the intake of nutrients. The United States Department of Agriculture and the United States Department of Health and Human Services developed the Dietary Guidelines to simplify the basics of

FACTS ABOUT DIABETES

balanced eating and to help all individuals develop healthful eating plans. Several of the guidelines which follow were adjusted to include the revised 1994 American Diabetes Association's Nutrition Recommendations. Because these recommendations are broad, work with your physician and registered dietitian to personalize the guidelines to meet your specific needs.

Eat a variety of foods. Energy, protein, vitamins, minerals and fiber are essential for optimal health, but no one food contains them all. Including a wide range of foods in your diet and using fats sparingly are easy ways to consume all the nutrients your body needs. Carbohydrate should comprise between 45 and 55 percent of total calories and protein should contribute between 10 and 20 percent.

Maintain a healthy weight. Excess weight can worsen your diabetes and encourages the development of more severe complications. Research shows that shedding 10 to 20 pounds is enough to initiate positive results for obese individuals. Combining a healthful eating plan with physical activity outlined by your health care team is the best medicine for maintaining a healthy weight.

Choose a diet low in fat, saturated fat and cholesterol. Fat has more than double the calories of an equal amount of protein or carbohydrate. Thus, diets low in fat make it easier to maintain a desirable weight and decrease the likelihood of developing high blood cholesterol levels. Limit fat to no more than 30 percent of total calories, saturated fat to no more than 10 percent of total calories and daily cholesterol to no more than 300 mg. The 30 percent of calories from fat goal applies to a total diet over time, not to a single food, serving of a recipe or meal.

Choose a diet with plenty of vegetables, fruits and grain products. Vitamins, minerals, fiber and complex carbohydrates abound in these low fat food choices. Filling up on fiber leaves less room for fat and may produce a slight decrease in blood cholesterol levels.

Use sugars in moderation. The ban on sugar has been lifted for people with diabetes but it is not altogether gone. The new guidelines for simple sugar intake are based on research that indicates that carbohydrate in the form of simple sugars does not raise blood sugar levels more rapidly than any other type of carbohydrate food. What is more important is the total amount of carbohydrate consumed, not the source. It is a good idea to limit your intake of simple sugars to no more than 25 percent of total carbohydrate.

Use salt and sodium in moderation. Some people with diabetes may be more sensitive to sodium than others, making them more susceptible to high blood pressure. Minimize this risk by limiting sodium intake to no more than 2,400 mg a day and choosing single food items with less than 400 mg of sodium and entrées with less than 800 mg of sodium per serving.

FACTS ABOUT THE FOODS

The recipes in this publication were designed for people with diabetes in mind. All are based on the principles of sound nutrition as outlined by the Dietary Guidelines, making them perfect for the entire family. Though the recipes in this publication are not intended as a medically therapeutic program, nor as a substitute for medically approved meal plans for individuals with diabetes, they are low in calories, fat, sodium and cholesterol and will fit easily into an individualized meal plan designed by your physician, registered dietitian and you

FACTS ABOUT THE EXCHANGES

The nutrition information that appears with each recipe was submitted in part by the participating companies and associations. The Dietary Exchanges are based on the Exchange Lists for Meal Planning developed by American Diabetes Association/The American Dietetic Association. Every effort has been made to check the accuracy of these numbers. However, because numerous variables account for a wide range of values in certain foods, all analyses that appear in this book should be considered approximate.

Bountiful Brunches

1 WESTERN OMELET

½ cup finely chopped red or green bell
　pepper
⅓ cup cubed cooked potato
2 slices turkey bacon, diced
¼ teaspoon dried oregano leaves
2 teaspoons FLEISCHMANN'S® 70% Corn
　Oil Spread, divided
1 cup EGG BEATERS® Healthy Real Egg
　Substitute
　Fresh oregano sprig, for garnish

In 8-inch nonstick skillet, over medium heat,
sauté bell pepper, potato, turkey bacon and
dried oregano in 1 teaspoon spread until
tender.* Remove from skillet; keep warm.

In same skillet, over medium heat, melt
remaining spread. Pour Egg Beaters into
skillet. Cook, lifting edges to allow
uncooked portion to flow underneath. When
almost set, spoon vegetable mixture over
half of omelet. Fold other half over
vegetable mixture; slide onto serving plate.
Garnish with fresh oregano.

Makes 2 servings

**For frittata, sauté vegetables, turkey bacon and
dried oregano in 2 teaspoons spread. Pour Egg
Beaters evenly into skillet over vegetable mixture.
Cook without stirring for 4 to 5 minutes or until
cooked on bottom and almost set on top. Carefully
turn frittata; cook for 1 to 2 minutes more or until
done. Slide onto serving platter; cut into wedges to
serve.*

Prep Time: 15 minutes
Cook Time: 10 minutes

Nutrients per Serving: Calories: 147,
Total Fat: 6 g, Saturated Fat: 1 g,
Cholesterol: 10 mg, Sodium: 384 mg, Fiber: 1 g

Dietary Exchanges: 1 Starch/Bread,
2 Lean Meat

Western Omelet

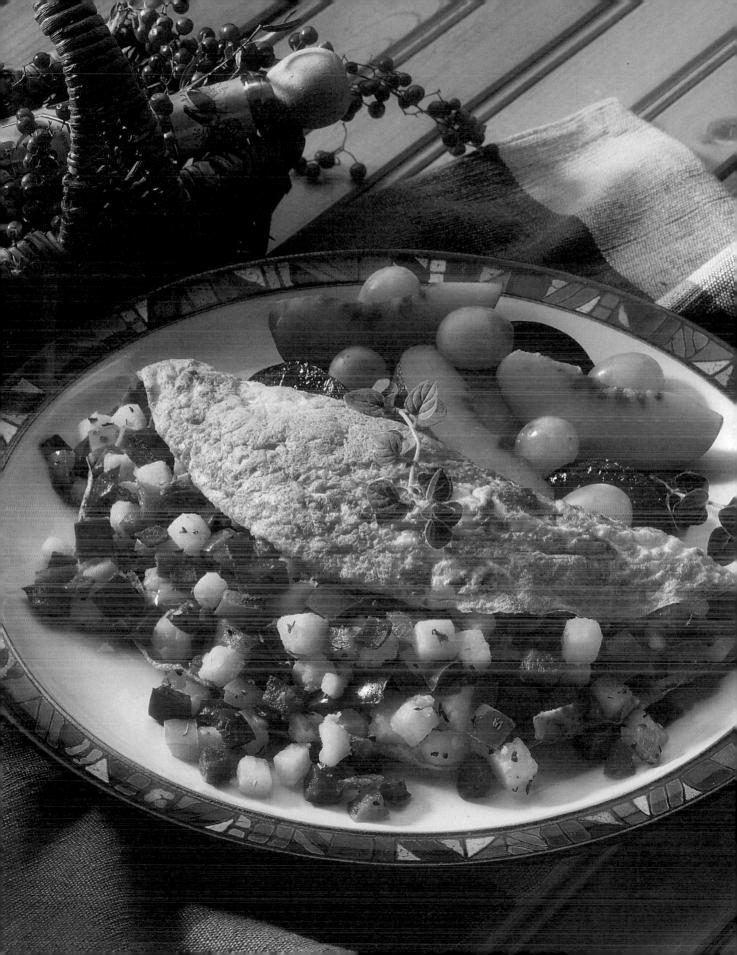

BOUNTIFUL BRUNCHES

2 TRIPLE–DECKER VEGETABLE OMELET

1 cup finely chopped broccoli
½ cup diced red bell pepper
½ cup shredded carrot
⅓ cup sliced green onions
1 clove garlic, minced
2½ teaspoons FLEISCHMANN'S® 70% Corn Oil Spread, divided
¾ cup low fat cottage cheese (1% milkfat), divided
1 tablespoon plain dry bread crumbs
1 tablespoon grated Parmesan cheese
½ teaspoon Italian seasoning
1½ cups EGG BEATERS® Healthy Real Egg Substitute, divided
⅓ cup chopped tomato
Chopped fresh parsley, for garnish

In 8-inch nonstick skillet, over medium-high heat, sauté broccoli, bell pepper, carrot, green onions and garlic in 1 teaspoon spread until tender. Remove from skillet; stir in ½ cup cottage cheese. Keep warm. Combine bread crumbs, Parmesan cheese and Italian seasoning; set aside.

In same skillet, over medium heat, melt ½ teaspoon spread. Pour ½ cup Egg Beaters into skillet. Cook, lifting edges to allow uncooked portion to flow underneath. When almost set, slide unfolded omelet onto ovenproof serving platter. Top with half each of the vegetable mixture and bread crumb mixture; set aside.

Prepare 2 more omelets with remaining Egg Beaters and spread. Layer 1 omelet onto serving platter over vegetable and bread crumb mixture; top with remaining vegetable mixture and bread crumb mixture. Layer with remaining omelet. Top omelet with remaining cottage cheese and tomato.

Bake at 425°F for 5 to 7 minutes or until heated through. Garnish with parsley. Cut into wedges to serve. *Makes 4 servings*

Prep Time: 20 minutes
Cook Time: 30 minutes

Nutrients per Serving: Calories: 124, Total Fat: 3 g, Saturated Fat: 1 g, Cholesterol: 3 mg, Sodium: 363 mg, Fiber: 2 g

Dietary Exchanges: 2 Lean Meat, 2 Vegetable

3 ITALIAN OMELET

¼ cup chopped tomato
¼ cup (1 ounce) shredded part-skim mozzarella cheese
¼ teaspoon dried basil leaves
¼ teaspoon dried oregano leaves
1 teaspoon FLEISCHMANN'S® 70% Corn Oil Spread
1 cup EGG BEATERS® Healthy Real Egg Substitute
Chopped fresh parsley, for garnish

In small bowl, combine tomato, cheese, basil and oregano; set aside.

In 8-inch nonstick skillet, over medium heat, melt spread. Pour Egg Beaters into skillet. Cook, lifting edges to allow uncooked portion to flow underneath. When almost set, spoon tomato mixture over half of omelet. Fold other half over tomato mixture; cover and continue to cook for 1 to 2 minutes. Slide onto serving plate. Garnish with parsley. *Makes 2 servings*

Prep Time: 10 minutes
Cook Time: 10 minutes

Nutrients per Serving: Calories: 119, Total Fat: 4 g, Saturated Fat: 2 g, Cholesterol: 8 mg, Sodium: 286 mg, Fiber: 0 g

Dietary Exchanges: 2 Lean Meat

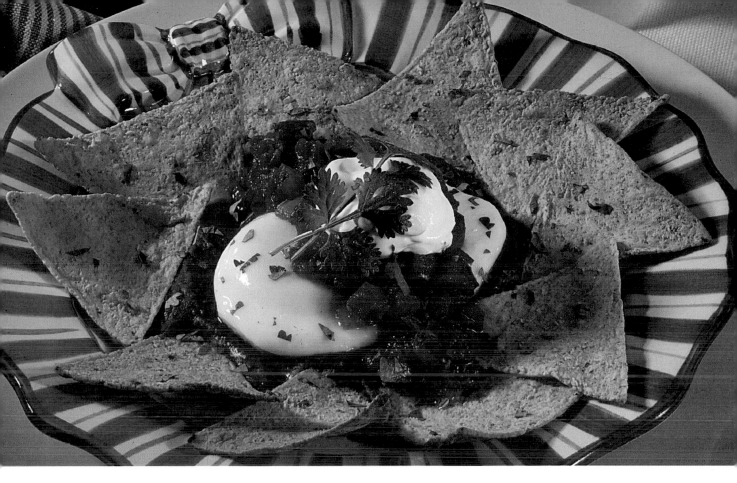

Eggs Santa Fe

4 EGGS SANTA FE

2 eggs
½ cup GUILTLESS GOURMET® Black Bean Dip (mild or spicy)
¼ cup GUILTLESS GOURMET® Salsa (medium)
1 ounce (about 18) GUILTLESS GOURMET® Unsalted Baked Tortilla Chips
2 tablespoons low fat sour cream
1 teaspoon chopped fresh cilantro Fresh cilantro sprigs (optional)

To poach eggs, bring water to a boil in small skillet over high heat; reduce heat to medium-low and maintain a simmer. Gently break eggs into water, being careful not to break yolks. Cover and simmer 5 minutes or until desired firmness.

Meanwhile, place bean dip in small microwave-safe bowl or small saucepan. Microwave bean dip on HIGH (100% power) 2 to 3 minutes or heat over medium heat until warm. To serve, spread ¼ cup warm bean dip in center of serving plate; top with 1 poached egg and 2 tablespoons salsa. Arrange 10 tortilla chips around egg. Dollop with 1 tablespoon sour cream and sprinkle with ½ teaspoon chopped cilantro. Repeat with remaining ingredients. Garnish with cilantro sprigs, if desired.

Makes 2 servings

Nutrients per Serving: Calories: 217 (28% Calories from Fat), Total Fat: 7 g, Saturated Fat: 2 g, Protein: 12 g, Carbohydrate: 24 g, Cholesterol: 218 mg, Sodium: 430 mg, Fiber: 3 g

Dietary Exchanges: 1½ Starch/Bread, 1 Lean Meat, ½ Vegetable, ½ Fat

BOUNTIFUL BRUNCHES

5 CHILE SCRAMBLE

2 tablespoons minced onion
1 teaspoon FLEISCHMANN'S® 70% Corn Oil Spread
1 cup EGG BEATERS® Healthy Real Egg Substitute
1 (4-ounce) can diced green chiles, drained
¼ cup whole kernel corn
2 tablespoons diced pimientos

In 10-inch nonstick skillet, over medium-high heat, sauté onion in spread for 2 to 3 minutes or until onion is translucent. Pour Egg Beaters into skillet; cook, stirring occasionally until mixture is set. Stir in chiles, corn and pimientos; cook 1 minute more or until heated through.

Makes 2 servings

Prep Time: 5 minutes
Cook Time: 10 minutes

Nutrients per Serving: Calories: 118, Total Fat: 2 g, Saturated Fat: 0 g, Cholesterol: 0 mg, Sodium: 254 mg, Fiber: 1 g

Dietary Exchanges: ½ Starch/Bread, 1 Lean Meat

6 EGGS BENEDICT

Mock Hollandaise Sauce (recipe follows)
4 eggs, divided
2 English muffins, halved
Fresh spinach leaves
8 ounces sliced lean Canadian bacon
4 tomato slices, cut ¼ inch thick
Paprika

1. Prepare Mock Hollandaise Sauce. Set aside.

2. Bring 6 cups water to a boil in large saucepan over high heat. Reduce heat to simmer. Carefully break 1 egg into small dish and slide egg into water. Repeat with remaining 3 eggs. Simmer, uncovered, about 5 minutes or until yolks are just set.

3. Meanwhile, toast muffin halves; place on serving plates. Top each muffin half with spinach leaves, 2 ounces Canadian bacon, 1 tomato slice and 1 egg. Spoon Mock Hollandaise Sauce over eggs; sprinkle with paprika.
Makes 4 servings

MOCK HOLLANDAISE SAUCE

4 ounces fat-free cream cheese
3 tablespoons plain nonfat yogurt
1 tablespoon lemon juice
1 teaspoon Dijon-style mustard

1. Process all ingredients in food processor or blender until smooth. Heat in small saucepan over medium-high heat until hot.
Makes about ¾ cup sauce

Nutrients per Serving: Calories: 237 (25% Calories from Fat), Total Fat: 6 g, Saturated Fat: 2 g, Protein: 24 g, Carbohydrate: 19 g, Cholesterol: 248 mg, Sodium: 1209 mg, Fiber: 1 g, Sugar: 2 g

Dietary Exchanges: 1 Starch/Bread, 2½ Lean Meat, ½ Vegetable

Eggs Benedict

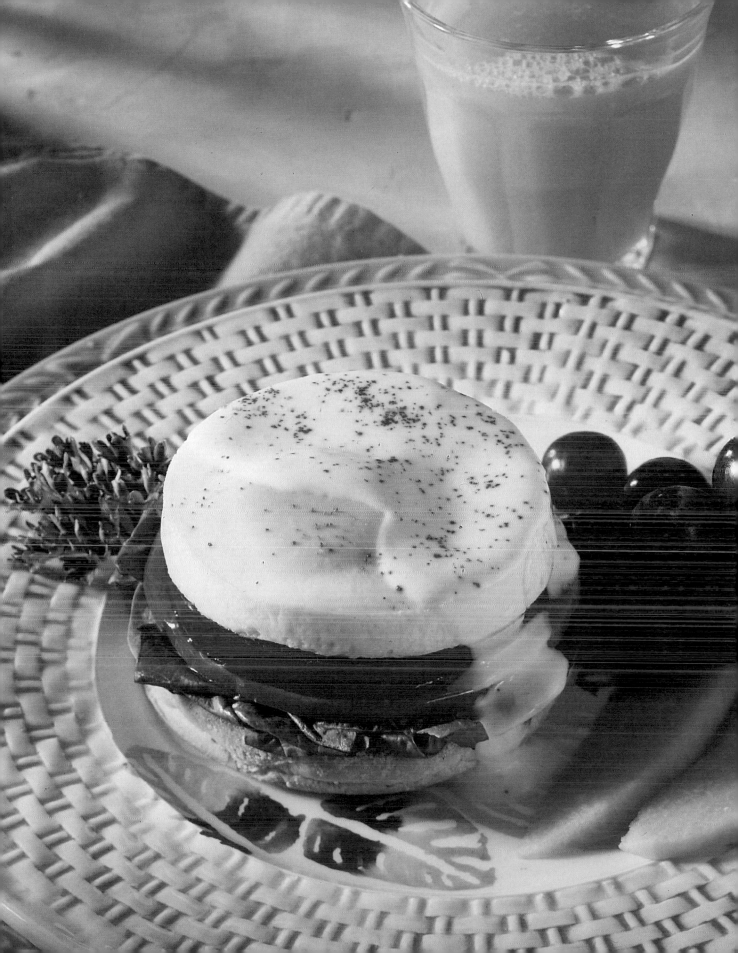

BOUNTIFUL BRUNCHES

7 SCRAMBLED EGG BURRITOS

Nonstick cooking spray
1 red bell pepper, chopped
5 green onions, sliced
½ teaspoon red pepper flakes
1 cup cholesterol-free egg substitute
1 tablespoon chopped fresh cilantro or parsley
4 (8-inch) flour tortillas
½ cup (2 ounces) shredded low-sodium, reduced-fat Monterey Jack cheese
⅓ cup salsa

1. Spray medium nonstick skillet with cooking spray. Heat over medium heat until hot. Add red pepper, onions and red pepper flakes. Cook and stir 3 minutes or until vegetables are crisp-tender.

2. Add egg substitute to vegetables. Reduce heat to low. Cook and stir 3 minutes or until set. Sprinkle with cilantro.

3. Stack tortillas and wrap in paper towels. Microwave at HIGH 1 minute or until tortillas are hot.

4. Place one fourth of egg mixture on each tortilla. Sprinkle with cheese. Fold sides over to enclose filling. Serve with salsa.

Makes 4 servings

Nutrients per Serving: Calories: 186 (20% Calories from Fat), Total Fat: 4 g, Saturated Fat: 1 g, Protein: 14 g, Carbohydrate: 23 g, Cholesterol: 6 mg, Sodium: 425 mg, Fiber: 1 g, Sugar: 1 g

Dietary Exchanges: 1 Starch/Bread, 1½ Lean Meat, 1 Vegetable

8 BREAKFAST BURRITOS WITH TOMATO–BASIL TOPPING

1 large tomato, diced
2 teaspoons finely chopped basil (or ½ teaspoon dried basil leaves)
1 medium potato, peeled and shredded (about 1 cup)
¼ cup chopped onion
2 teaspoons FLEISCHMANN'S® 70% Corn Oil Spread
1 cup EGG BEATERS® Healthy Real Egg Substitute
⅛ teaspoon ground black pepper
4 (8-inch) flour tortillas, warmed
⅓ cup shredded reduced-fat Cheddar cheese

In small bowl, combine tomato and basil; set aside.

In large nonstick skillet, over medium heat, sauté potato and onion in spread until tender. Pour Egg Beaters into skillet; sprinkle with pepper. Cook, stirring occasionally until mixture is set.

Divide egg mixture evenly between tortillas; top with cheese. Fold tortillas over egg mixture. Top with tomato mixture.

Makes 4 servings

Prep Time: 15 minutes
Cook Time: 25 minutes

Nutrients per Serving: Calories: 226, Total Fat: 6 g, Saturated Fat: 1 g, Cholesterol: 5 mg, Sodium: 364 mg, Fiber: 2 g

Dietary Exchanges: 2½ Starch/Bread, 1 Lean Meat, ½ Fat

Breakfast Burritos with Tomato-Basil Topping

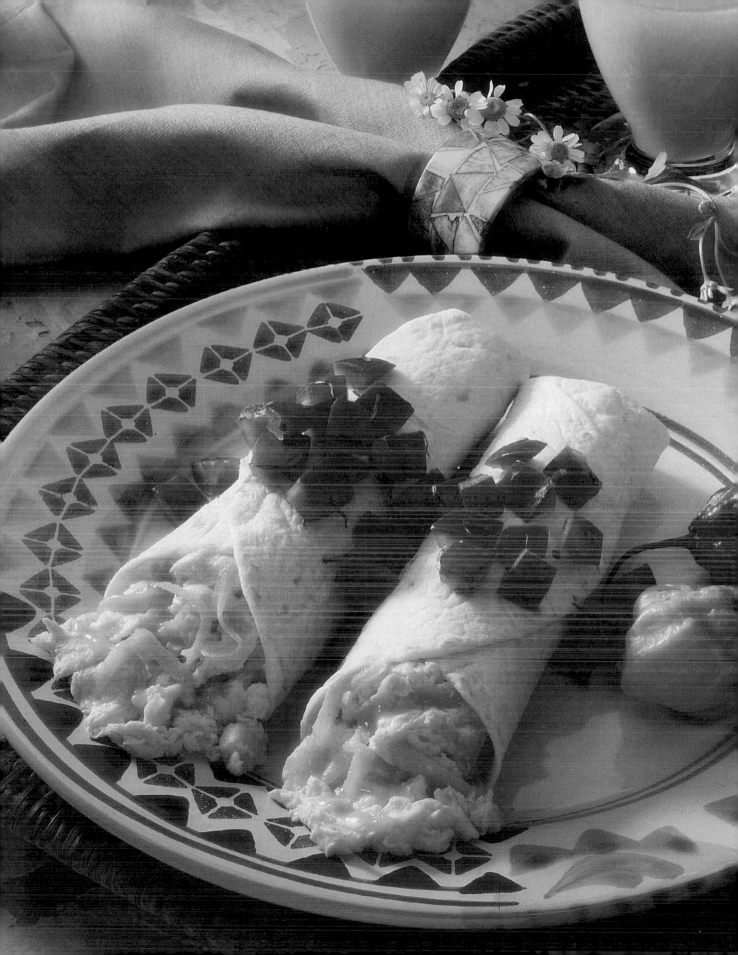

BOUNTIFUL BRUNCHES

9 MEXICAN STRATA OLÉ

4 (6-inch) corn tortillas, halved, divided
1 cup chopped onion
½ cup chopped green bell pepper
1 clove garlic, crushed
1 teaspoon dried oregano leaves
½ teaspoon ground cumin
1 teaspoon FLEISCHMANN'S® 70% Corn Oil Spread
1 cup dried kidney beans, cooked in unsalted water according to package directions
½ cup (2 ounces) shredded reduced-fat Cheddar cheese
1½ cups skim milk
1 cup EGG BEATERS® Healthy Real Egg Substitute
1 cup thick and chunky salsa

Arrange half the tortilla pieces in bottom of greased 12×8×2-inch baking dish; set aside.

In large nonstick skillet, over medium-high heat, sauté onion, bell pepper, garlic, oregano and cumin in spread until tender; stir in beans. Spoon half the mixture over tortillas; repeat layers once. Sprinkle with cheese.

In medium bowl, combine milk and Egg Beaters; pour evenly over cheese. Bake at 350°F for 40 minutes or until puffed and golden brown. Let stand 10 minutes before serving. Serve topped with salsa.

Makes 8 servings

Prep Time: 25 minutes
Cook Time: 50 minutes

Nutrients per Serving: Calories: 142, Total Fat: 3 g, Saturated Fat: 0 g, Cholesterol: 1 mg, Sodium: 293 mg, Fiber: 0 g

Dietary Exchanges: 1 Starch/Bread, 1 Lean Meat, 1 Vegetable

10 VEGETABLE STRATA

2 slices white bread, cubed
¼ cup shredded reduced-fat Swiss cheese
½ cup sliced carrots
½ cup sliced mushrooms
¼ cup chopped onion
1 clove garlic, crushed
1 teaspoon FLEISCHMANN'S® 70% Corn Oil Spread
½ cup chopped tomato
½ cup snow peas
1 cup EGG BEATERS® Healthy Real Egg Substitute
¾ cup skim milk

Place bread cubes evenly into bottom of greased 1½-quart casserole dish. Sprinkle with cheese; set aside.

In medium nonstick skillet, over medium heat, sauté carrots, mushrooms, onion and garlic in spread until tender. Stir in tomato and snow peas; cook 1 to 2 minutes more. Spoon over cheese. In small bowl, combine Egg Beaters and milk; pour over vegetable mixture. Bake at 375°F for 45 to 50 minutes or until knife inserted in center comes out clean. Let stand 10 minutes before serving.

Makes 6 servings

Prep Time: 15 minutes
Cook Time: 55 minutes

Nutrients per Serving: Calories: 94, Total Fat: 2 g, Saturated Fat: 1 g, Cholesterol: 3 mg, Sodium: 161 mg, Fiber: 1 g

Dietary Exchanges: 1 Lean Meat, 1 Vegetable

Vegetable Strata

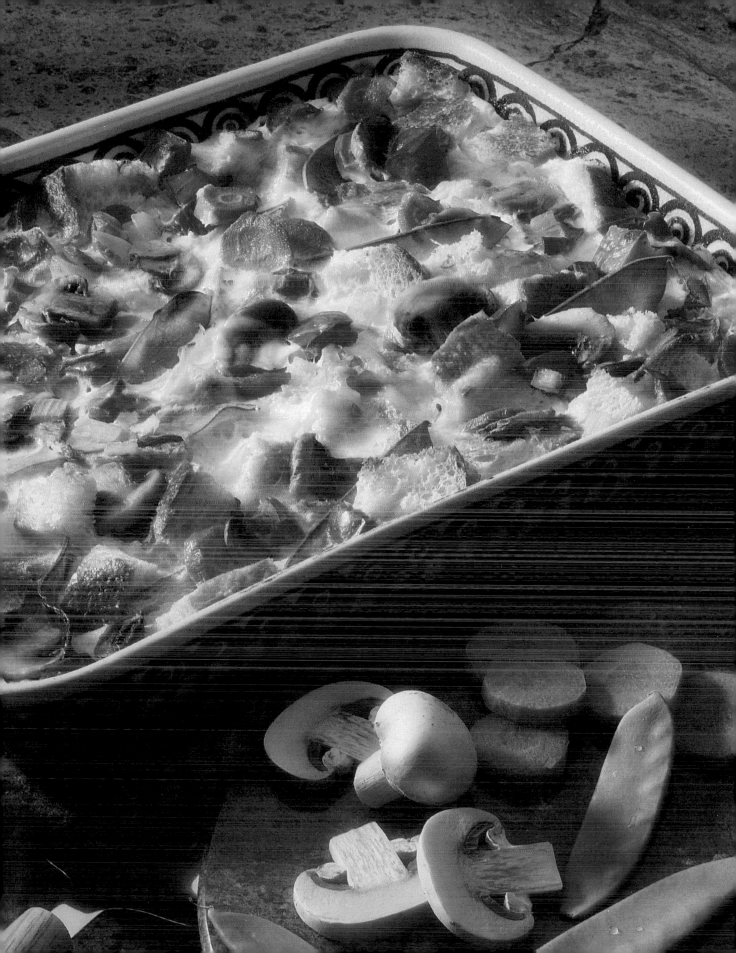

BOUNTIFUL BRUNCHES

11 EASY BRUNCH FRITTATA

1 cup small broccoli florets
2½ cups (12 ounces) frozen hash brown potatoes with onions and peppers (O'Brien style), thawed
1½ cups cholesterol-free egg substitute, thawed
2 tablespoons 2% low-fat milk
¾ teaspoon salt
¼ teaspoon black pepper
½ cup (2 ounces) shredded reduced-fat Cheddar cheese

1. Preheat oven to 450°F. Coat medium nonstick ovenproof skillet with nonstick cooking spray. Heat skillet over medium heat until hot. Add broccoli; cook and stir 2 minutes. Add potatoes; cook and stir 5 minutes.

2. Beat together egg substitute, milk, salt and pepper in small bowl; pour over potato mixture. Cook 5 minutes or until edges are set (center will still be wet).

3. Transfer skillet to oven; bake 6 minutes or until center is set. Sprinkle with cheese; let stand 2 to 3 minutes or until cheese is melted.

4. Cut into wedges; serve with low-fat sour cream, if desired.   *Makes 6 servings*

Nutrients per Serving: Calories: 102 (20% Calories from Fat), Total Fat: 2 g, Saturated Fat: 1 g, Protein: 9 g, Carbohydrate: 11 g, Cholesterol: 7 mg, Sodium: 627 mg, Fiber: 1 g, Sugar: 1 g

Dietary Exchanges: ½ Starch/Bread, 1 Lean Meat

Easy Brunch Frittata

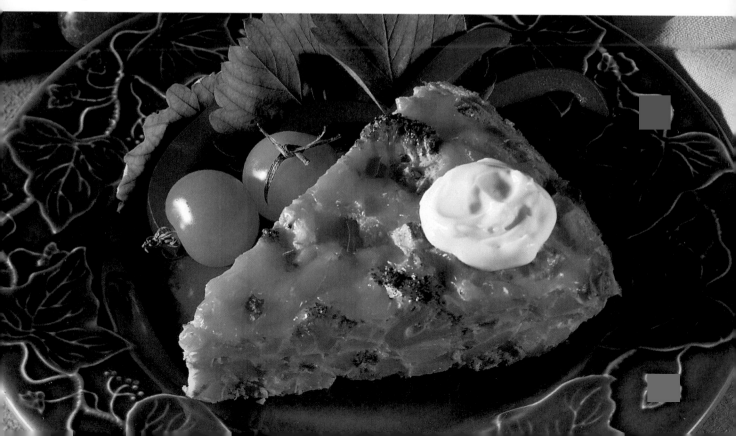

BOUNTIFUL BRUNCHES

12 ZUCCHINI MUSHROOM FRITTATA

1½ cups EGG BEATERS® Healthy Real Egg
      Substitute
½ cup (2 ounces) shredded reduced-fat
      Swiss cheese
¼ cup skim milk
½ teaspoon garlic powder
¼ teaspoon seasoned pepper
      Nonstick cooking spray
1 medium zucchini, shredded (1 cup)
1 medium tomato, chopped
1 (4-ounce) can sliced mushrooms,
      drained
      Tomato slices and fresh basil leaves, for
      garnish

In medium bowl, combine Egg Beaters, cheese, milk, garlic powder and seasoned pepper; set aside.

Spray 10-inch ovenproof nonstick skillet lightly with nonstick cooking spray. Over medium-high heat, sauté zucchini, tomato and mushrooms in skillet until tender. Pour egg mixture into skillet, stirring well. Cover; cook over low heat for 15 minutes or until cooked on bottom and almost set on top. Remove lid and place skillet under broiler for 2 to 3 minutes or until desired doneness. Slide onto serving platter; cut into wedges to serve. Garnish with tomato slices and basil.

Makes 6 servings

Prep Time: 20 minutes
Cook Time: 20 minutes

Nutrients per Serving: Calories: 71,
Total Fat: 2 g, Saturated Fat: 1 g,
Cholesterol: 7 mg, Sodium: 147 mg, Fiber: 0 g

Dietary Exchanges: 1 Lean Meat, 1 Vegetable

13 SPINACH QUICHE

½ cup chopped onion
1 clove garlic, crushed
1 teaspoon FLEISCHMANN'S® 70% Corn
      Oil Spread
1 (10-ounce) package frozen chopped
      spinach, thawed and well drained
1 (9-inch) pastry crust, unbaked
1 cup EGG BEATERS® Healthy Real Egg
      Substitute
1 cup skim milk
1 tablespoon all-purpose flour
1 teaspoon dried basil leaves
¾ teaspoon liquid hot pepper seasoning

In medium nonstick skillet, over medium-high heat, sauté onion and garlic in spread until tender; add spinach. Spoon into bottom of pie crust; set aside.

In small bowl, combine Egg Beaters, milk, flour, basil and liquid hot pepper seasoning; pour evenly over spinach mixture. Bake at 350°F for 45 to 50 minutes or until knife inserted in center comes out clean. Let stand 10 minutes before serving.

Makes 8 servings

Prep Time: 30 minutes
Cook Time: 50 minutes

Nutrients per Serving: Calories: 156,
Total Fat: 8 g, Saturated Fat: 2 g,
Cholesterol: 1 mg, Sodium: 234 mg, Fiber: 0 g

Dietary Exchanges: 1 Starch/Bread,
1 Lean Meat

BOUNTIFUL BRUNCHES

14 VEGETABLE QUICHE

Vegetable cooking spray
2 cups frozen diced potatoes with onions and peppers, thawed
1 can HEALTHY CHOICE® RECIPE CREATIONS™ Cream of Mushroom with Cracked Pepper & Herbs Condensed Soup, divided
1 (16-ounce) package frozen mixed vegetables (such as zucchini, carrots and beans), thawed and drained
1 cup fat free egg substitute (equivalent to 4 eggs)
½ cup fat free shredded Parmesan cheese, divided
¼ cup nonfat milk
¼ teaspoon dried dill weed

In 9-inch pie plate sprayed with vegetable cooking spray, press potatoes onto bottom and side to form crust. Spray potatoes lightly with vegetable cooking spray. Bake at 400°F 15 minutes.

In small bowl, combine half the soup, mixed vegetables, egg substitute and half the cheese; mix well. Pour egg mixture into potato shell; sprinkle with remaining cheese. Bake at 375°F 35 to 40 minutes or until set.

In small saucepan, combine remaining soup, milk and dill; mix well. Simmer 5 minutes until heated through. Serve sauce with quiche.   *Makes 6 servings*

Nutrients per Serving: Calories: 113 (3% Calories from Fat), Fat: 1 g, Protein: 9 g, Sodium: 436 mg

Dietary Exchanges: 1½ Starch/Bread, 1 Lean Meat, 1 Vegetable

15 MINI VEGETABLE QUICHES

2 cups cut-up vegetables (bell peppers, broccoli, zucchini and/or carrots)
2 tablespoons chopped green onions
2 tablespoons FLEISCHMANN'S® 70% Corn Oil Spread
4 (8-inch) flour tortillas, each cut into 8 triangles
1 cup EGG BEATERS® Healthy Real Egg Substitute
1 cup skim milk
½ teaspoon dried basil leaves

In medium nonstick skillet, over medium-high heat, sauté vegetables and green onions in spread until tender.

Arrange 4 tortilla pieces in each of 8 (6-ounce) greased custard cups or ramekins, placing points of tortilla pieces at center of bottom of cup and pressing lightly to form shape of cup. Divide vegetable mixture evenly among cups. In small bowl, combine Egg Beaters, milk and basil. Pour evenly over vegetable mixture. Place cups on baking sheet. Bake at 375°F for 20 to 25 minutes or until puffed and knife inserted into centers comes out clean. Let stand 5 minutes before serving.

Makes 8 servings

Prep Time: 25 minutes
Cook Time: 30 minutes

Nutrients per Serving: Calories: 122, Total Fat: 4 g, Saturated Fat: 1 g, Cholesterol: 1 mg, Sodium: 198 mg, Fiber: 1 g

Dietary Exchanges: 1 Starch/Bread, 1 Lean Meat

Mini Vegetable Quiches

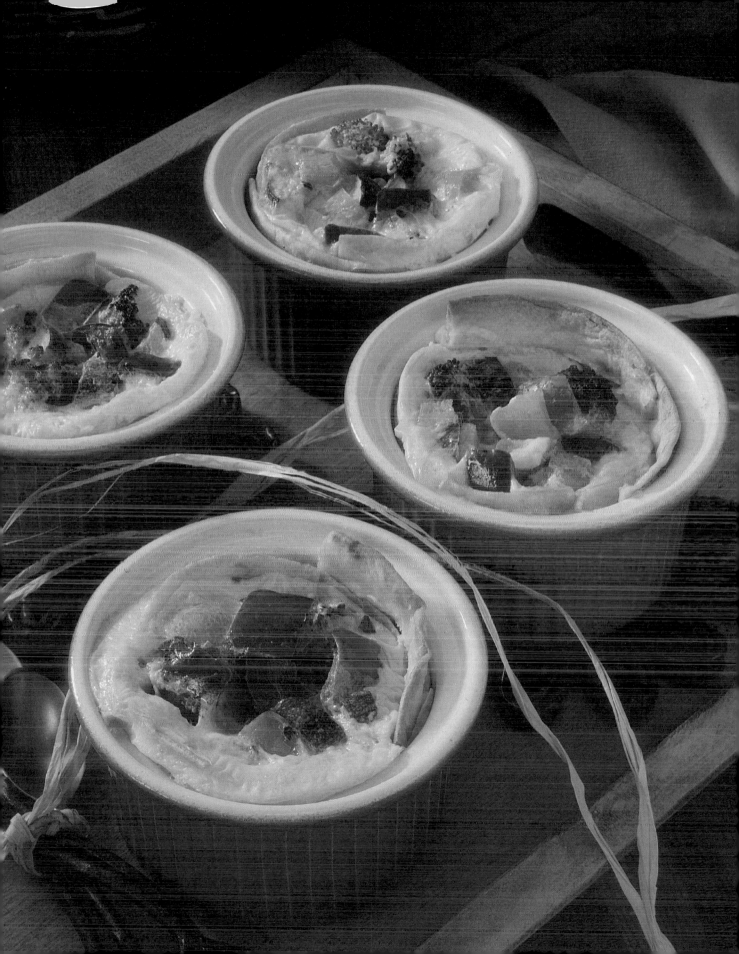

BOUNTIFUL BRUNCHES

16 BLUEBERRY MUFFINS WITH A TWIST OF LEMON

1 cup all-purpose flour
1 cup uncooked rolled oats
¼ cup packed brown sugar
1 teaspoon baking powder
1 teaspoon baking soda
¾ teaspoon cinnamon, divided
¼ teaspoon salt
8 ounces lemon-flavored low-fat yogurt
¼ cup cholesterol-free egg substitute
1 tablespoon vegetable oil
1 teaspoon grated lemon peel
1 teaspoon vanilla
1 cup fresh or frozen blueberries
1 tablespoon granulated sugar
1 tablespoon sliced almonds (optional)

1. Preheat oven to 400°F. Spray 12 (2½-inch) muffin cups with nonstick cooking spray.

2. Combine flour, oats, brown sugar, baking powder, baking soda, ½ teaspoon cinnamon and salt in large bowl.

3. Combine yogurt, egg substitute, oil, lemon peel and vanilla in small bowl; stir into flour mixture just until blended. Gently stir in blueberries. Spoon mixture into muffin cups.

4. Mix granulated sugar, remaining ¼ teaspoon cinnamon and almonds in small bowl. Sprinkle over muffin mixture.

5. Bake 18 to 20 minutes or until lightly browned and wooden pick inserted into centers comes out clean. Cool slightly on racks before serving.   *Makes 12 servings*

Nutrients per Serving: Calories: 125 (14% Calories from Fat), Total Fat: 2 g, Saturated Fat: 0 g, Protein: 3 g, Carbohydrate: 24 g, Cholesterol: 1 mg, Sodium: 198 mg, Fiber: 1 g, Sugar: 5 g

Dietary Exchanges: 1½ Starch/Bread, ½ Fat

17 DATE BRAN MUFFINS

1½ cups 100% bran cereal
1½ cups skim milk
⅓ cup margarine, melted
1 egg
1 teaspoon vanilla
1¼ cups all-purpose flour
4¼ teaspoons EQUAL® MEASURE™ or
        14 packets EQUAL® sweetener *or*
        ½ cup plus 4 teaspoons EQUAL®
        SPOONFUL™
1 tablespoon baking powder
2 teaspoons ground cinnamon
½ teaspoon salt
½ cup pitted dates, chopped

• Combine cereal and milk in medium bowl; let stand 5 minutes. Stir in margarine, egg and vanilla. Add combined flour, Equal®, baking powder, cinnamon and salt, stirring just until mixture is blended. Stir in dates.

• Spoon batter into greased muffin pans; bake in preheated 375°F oven until muffins are browned and toothpicks inserted in centers come out clean, 20 to 25 minutes. Cool in pans on wire rack 5 minutes; remove from pans and cool on wire rack.

Makes 1 dozen

Nutrients per Serving: (1 muffin), Calories: 164, Fat: 6 g, Protein: 5 g, Carbohydrates: 27 g, Cholesterol: 18 mg, Sodium: 390 mg

Dietary Exchanges: 2 Starch/Bread, 1 Fat

Blueberry Muffins with a Twist of Lemon

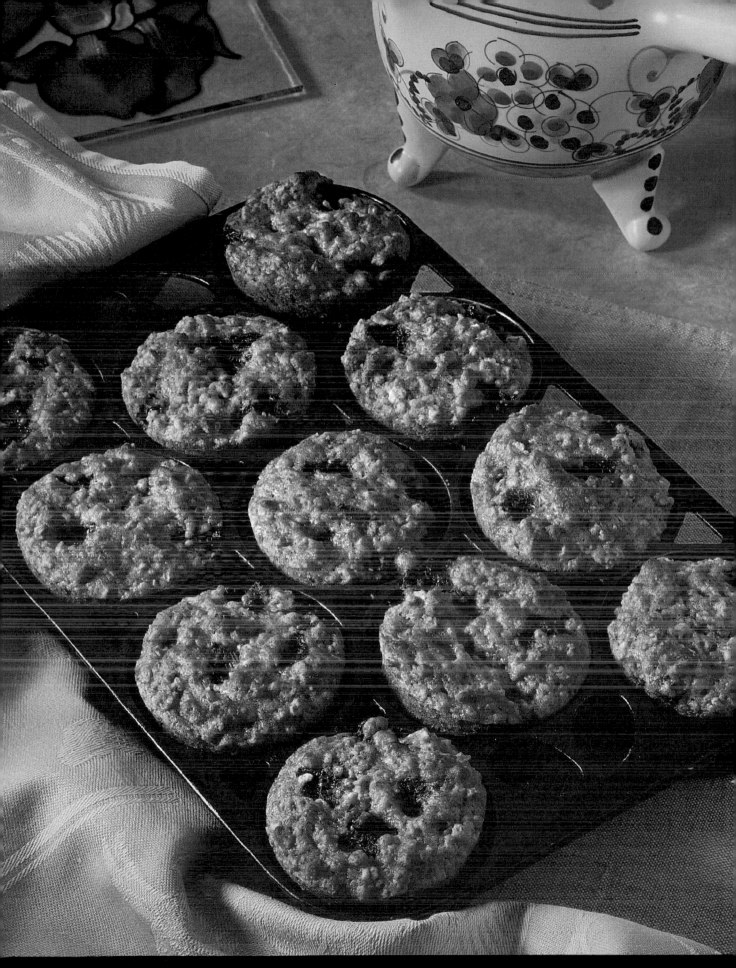

BOUNTIFUL BRUNCHES

18 MINIATURE FRUIT MUFFINS

1 cup whole wheat flour
¾ cup all-purpose flour
½ cup packed dark brown sugar
2 teaspoons baking powder
½ teaspoon baking soda
¼ teaspoon salt
1 cup buttermilk, divided
¾ cup frozen blueberries
1 small ripe banana, mashed
¼ teaspoon vanilla
⅓ cup unsweetened applesauce
2 tablespoons raisins
½ teaspoon ground cinnamon

1. Preheat oven to 400°F. Spray 36 miniature muffin cups with nonstick cooking spray.

2. Combine flours, sugar, baking powder, baking soda and salt in medium bowl. Place ⅓ cup dry ingredients in each of 2 small bowls.

3. To one portion flour mixture, add ⅓ cup buttermilk and blueberries. Stir just until blended; spoon into 12 prepared muffin cups. To second portion, add ⅓ cup buttermilk, banana and vanilla. Stir just until blended; spoon into 12 more prepared muffin cups. To final portion, add remaining ⅓ cup buttermilk, applesauce, raisins and cinnamon. Stir just until blended; spoon into remaining 12 prepared muffin cups.

4. Bake 18 minutes or until lightly browned and wooden pick inserted into centers comes out clean. Cool 10 minutes on wire racks. *Makes 12 servings*

Nutrients per Serving: (3 miniature muffins), Calories: 130 (4% Calories from Fat), Total Fat: 1 g, Saturated Fat: trace, Protein: 3 g, Carbohydrate: 29 g, Cholesterol: 1 mg, Sodium: 178 mg, Fiber: 2 g, Sugar: 13 g

Dietary Exchanges: 1 Starch/Bread, 1 Fruit

19 APRICOT OATMEAL MUFFINS

1 cup QUAKER® Oats (quick or old fashioned, uncooked)
1 cup low-fat buttermilk
¼ cup egg substitute *or* 2 egg whites
2 tablespoons margarine, melted
1 cup all-purpose flour
⅓ cup finely chopped dried apricots
¼ cup chopped nuts* (optional)
3 tablespoons granulated sugar *or*
    1¾ teaspoons EQUAL® MEASURE™
    (7 packets) *or* 2 tablespoons fructose
1 teaspoon baking powder
½ teaspoon baking soda
¼ teaspoon salt (optional)

* To toast nuts for extra flavor, spread evenly in small baking pan. Bake in 400°F oven 5 to 7 minutes or until light golden brown. Or, spread nuts on plate. Microwave on HIGH 1 minute; stir. Continue microwaving, checking every 30 seconds, until nuts are crunchy.

Heat oven to 400°F. Lightly spray 12 medium muffin cups with vegetable oil cooking spray. Combine oats and buttermilk; let stand 10 minutes. Add egg substitute and margarine; mix well. Add wet ingredients to dry ingredients; mix just until moistened. Fill muffin cups almost full. Bake 20 to 25 minutes or until golden brown. Let muffins stand a few minutes; remove from pan. *Makes 1 dozen*

Nutrients per Serving: 1 muffin without nuts (made with granulated sugar, Equal® or fructose), Calories: 110, Calories From Fat: 25, Total Fat: 3 g, Saturated Fat: 1 g, Protein: 4 g, Cholesterol: 0 mg, Sodium: 125 mg, Fiber: 1 g, Total Carbohydrates: 1 muffin made with granulated sugar: 19 g, made with Equal®: 16 g, made with fructose: 18 g, Sugar: 6 g (with granulated sugar)

Dietary Exchanges: 1 Bread/Starch, ½ Fat

BOUNTIFUL BRUNCHES

20 ORANGE–PECAN SCONES

2½ cups all-purpose flour
½ cup sugar
1 tablespoon baking powder
1 teaspoon baking soda
¾ teaspoon salt
¼ cup Prune Purée (page 25) or prepared prune butter
2 tablespoons cold margarine or butter
1 container (8 ounces) nonfat lemon yogurt
2 tablespoons frozen orange juice concentrate, thawed
Grated peel of 1 orange
¼ cup chopped toasted pecans

Preheat oven to 400°F. Coat baking sheet with vegetable cooking spray. In large bowl, combine flour, sugar, baking powder, baking soda and salt. Cut in prune purée and margarine with pastry blender until mixture resembles coarse crumbs. Add yogurt, juice concentrate and orange peel; mix just until blended. Stir in pecans. Turn dough out onto floured surface and knead two or three times. Pat into 8-inch circle and cut into 12 equal wedges. Place wedges on prepared baking sheet, spacing 2 inches apart. Bake in center of oven 15 to 20 minutes or until lightly browned and springy to the touch. Serve warm or at room temperature.

Makes 12 scones

Nutrients per Serving: (1 scone), Calories: 190, Fat: 4 g, Protein: 4 g, Carbohydrate: 36 g, Cholesterol: 5 mg, Sodium: 320 mg, Fiber: 1 g

Dietary Exchanges: 2 Starch/Bread, 1 Fat

*Favorite recipe from **California Prune Board***

21 BLUEBERRY LEMON SCONES

2⅔ cups all-purpose flour
½ cup plus 2 tablespoons sugar, divided
2½ teaspoons baking powder
1 teaspoon baking soda
½ teaspoon salt
½ cup dried blueberries
1 container (8 ounces) nonfat lemon yogurt
⅓ cup Prune Purée (page 25) or prepared prune butter
3 tablespoons butter or margarine, melted
1 tablespoon grated lemon peel
2 teaspoons vanilla
¼ teaspoon ground nutmeg

Preheat oven to 400°F. Coat baking sheet with vegetable cooking spray. In large bowl, combine flour, ½ cup sugar, baking powder, baking soda and salt. Add blueberries. In small bowl, mix yogurt, prune purée, butter, lemon peel and vanilla until blended. Add to flour mixture; mix just until mixture holds together. Turn dough out onto lightly floured surface and pat into 10-inch round. Combine the remaining 2 tablespoons sugar and nutmeg; sprinkle evenly over dough. Pat sugar mixture gently into dough; cut into 12 equal wedges. Place wedges on prepared baking sheet, spacing 1 inch apart. Bake in center of oven about 15 minutes until lightly browned and cracked on top. Remove to wire rack to cool slightly.

Makes 12 scones

VARIATION: Substitute currants, raisins or chopped dried cherries for the blueberries.

Nutrients per Serving: (1 scone), Calories: 211, Fat: 3 g, Protein: 4 g, Carbohydrate: 45 g, Cholesterol: 10 mg, Sodium: 280 mg, Fiber: 2 g

Dietary Exchanges: 3 Starch/Bread

*Favorite recipe from **California Prune Board***

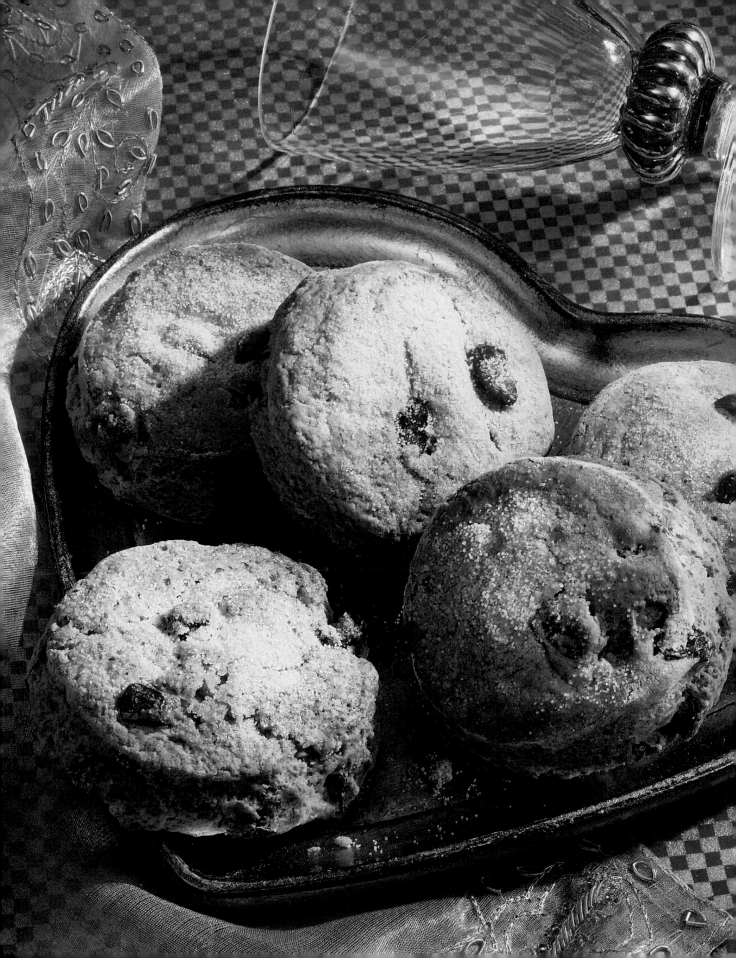

BOUNTIFUL BRUNCHES

22 CRANBERRY SCONES

2½ **cups all-purpose flour**
½ **cup packed brown sugar**
1 **tablespoon baking powder**
1 **teaspoon baking soda**
¾ **teaspoon salt**
½ **teaspoon ground cinnamon**
¼ **cup Prune Purée (recipe follows) or**
   prepared prune butter
2 **tablespoons cold margarine or butter**
1 **container (8 ounces) nonfat vanilla**
   yogurt
¾ **cup dried cranberries**
1 **egg white, lightly beaten**
1 **tablespoon granulated sugar**

Preheat oven to 400°F. Coat baking sheet
with vegetable cooking spray. In large bowl,
combine flour, brown sugar, baking powder,
baking soda, salt and cinnamon. Cut in
prune purée and margarine with pastry
blender until mixture resembles coarse
crumbs. Mix in yogurt just until blended. Stir
in cranberries. On floured surface, roll or pat
dough to ¾-inch thickness. Cut out with 2½
to 3-inch biscuit cutter, rerolling scraps as
needed. Arrange on prepared baking sheet,
spacing 2 inches apart. Brush with egg white
and sprinkle with granulated sugar. Bake in
center of oven about 15 minutes until golden
brown and springy to the touch.

Makes 12 scones

PRUNE PURÉE

1⅓ **cups (8 ounces) pitted prunes**
6 **tablespoons hot water**

Combine pitted prunes and hot water in
container of food processor or blender.
Pulse on and off until prunes are finely
chopped and smooth. Store leftovers in a
covered container in the refrigerator for up
to two months.   *Makes 1 cup*

Cranberry Scones

Nutrients per Serving: (1 scone),
Calories: 190, Fat: 2 g, Protein: 4 g,
Carbohydrate: 39 g, Cholesterol: 0 mg,
Sodium: 280 mg, Fiber: 1 g

Dietary Exchanges: 2½ Starch/Bread

Favorite recipe from **California Prune Board**

23 MAPLE–WALNUT BREAD

1 **cup packed brown sugar**
¼ **cup Prune Purée (page 25) or prepared**
   prune butter
2 **egg whites**
1½ **teaspoons maple flavoring**
¾ **cup low fat buttermilk**
2 **cups all-purpose flour**
2 **teaspoons baking powder**
½ **teaspoon baking soda**
½ **teaspoon salt**
⅓ **cup finely chopped, toasted walnuts**

Preheat oven to 350°F. Coat 8½×4½×2¾-
inch loaf pan with vegetable cooking spray.
In bowl, beat sugar, prune purée, egg whites
and maple flavoring until well blended. Mix
in buttermilk. In medium bowl, combine
flour, baking powder, baking soda and salt;
stir into sugar mixture. Stir in walnuts.
Spoon batter into prepared pan. Bake in
center of oven 50 minutes or until pick
inserted into center comes out clean. Cool in
pan 5 minutes; remove from pan to wire
rack. Cool completely.

Makes 1 loaf (12 slices)

Nutrients per Serving: (1 slice), Calories: 190,
Fat: 2 g, Protein: 4 g, Carbohydrate: 38 g,
Cholesterol: 1 mg, Sodium: 160 mg, Fiber: 1 g

Dietary Exchanges: 2½ Starch/Bread

Favorite recipe from **California Prune Board**

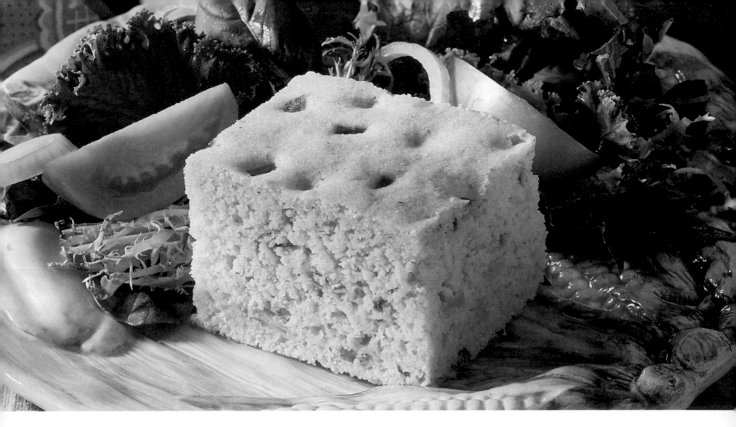

Chili Cornbread

24 CHILI CORNBREAD

Nonstick cooking spray
¼ **cup chopped red bell pepper**
¼ **cup chopped green bell pepper**
2 **small jalapeño peppers,* minced**
2 **cloves garlic, minced**
¾ **cup corn**
1½ **cups yellow cornmeal**
½ **cup all-purpose flour**
2 **tablespoons sugar**
2 **teaspoons baking powder**
½ **teaspoon baking soda**
½ **teaspoon ground cumin**
½ **teaspoon salt**
1½ **cups buttermilk**
1 **whole egg**
2 **egg whites**
4 **tablespoons margarine, melted**

*Jalapeño peppers can sting and irritate the skin; wear rubber gloves when handling peppers and do not touch eyes. Wash hands after handling.

1. Preheat oven to 425°F. Spray 8×8-inch square baking pan with cooking spray. Set aside.

2. Spray small skillet with cooking spray. Add bell and jalapeño peppers and garlic; cook and stir 3 to 4 minutes or until peppers are tender. Stir in corn; cook 1 to 2 minutes. Remove from heat.

3. Combine cornmeal, flour, sugar, baking powder, baking soda, cumin and salt in large bowl. Add buttermilk, whole egg, egg whites and margarine; mix until smooth. Stir in corn mixture.

4. Pour batter into prepared baking pan. Bake 25 to 30 minutes or until golden brown. Cool on wire rack.   *Makes 12 servings*

Nutrients per Serving: Calories: 151 (30% Calories from Fat), Total Fat: 5 g, Saturated Fat: 1 g, Protein: 4 g, Carbohydrate: 22 g, Cholesterol: 19 mg, Sodium: 304 mg, Fiber: 3 g, Sugar: 4 g

Dietary Exchanges: 1½ Starch/Bread, 1 Fat

BOUNTIFUL BRUNCHES

25 PINEAPPLE ZUCCHINI BREAD

1 cup vegetable oil
3 eggs
3½ teaspoons EQUAL® MEASURE™ or
    12 packets EQUAL® sweetener or
    ½ cup EQUAL® SPOONFUL™
1 teaspoon vanilla
2 cups shredded zucchini
1 can (8½ ounces) unsweetened crushed
    pineapple in juice, drained
3 cups all-purpose flour
1½ teaspoons ground cinnamon
1 teaspoon baking soda
¾ teaspoon ground nutmeg
¾ teaspoon salt
1 cup raisins
½ cup chopped walnuts, optional

• Mix oil, eggs, Equal® and vanilla in large bowl; stir in zucchini and pineapple. Combine flour, cinnamon, baking soda, nutmeg and salt in medium bowl; stir into oil mixture. Stir in raisins and walnuts, if desired. Spread batter evenly in 2 greased and floured 8½×4½×2½-inch loaf pans.

• Bake in preheated 350°F oven until breads are golden and toothpick inserted in centers comes out clean, 50 to 60 minutes. Cool in pans on wire rack 10 minutes; remove from pans and cool completely on wire rack.

Makes 2 loaves (about 16 slices each)

Nutrients per Serving: (1 slice), Calories: 134, Fat: 7 g, Protein: 2 g, Carbohydrates: 14 g, Cholesterol: 20 mg, Sodium: 97 mg

Dietary Exchanges: 1 Starch/Bread, 1 Fat

26 APPLE–CINNAMON BREAD

⅓ cup packed brown sugar
⅓ cup granulated sugar
3 egg whites
¼ cup Prune Purée (page 25) or prepared
    prune butter
⅔ cup buttermilk
1¾ cups all-purpose flour
1 teaspoon ground cinnamon
¾ teaspoon baking powder
¾ teaspoon baking soda
½ teaspoon salt
¼ teaspoon ground nutmeg
¼ teaspoon ground cloves
¾ cup peeled and finely chopped apple
    (spooned, not packed, into cup)

Preheat oven to 375°F. Coat 8½×4½×2¾-inch loaf pan with vegetable cooking spray. In mixer bowl, beat sugars, egg whites and prune purée until well blended. Mix in buttermilk until blended. In medium bowl, combine flour, cinnamon, baking powder, baking soda, salt, nutmeg and cloves; stir into sugar mixture just until blended. Stir in apple. Spoon batter into prepared pan. Bake in center of oven 45 to 50 minutes until pick inserted into center comes out clean. Cool in pan 5 minutes; remove from pan to wire rack. Cool completely before slicing.

Makes 1 loaf (12 slices)

Nutrients per Serving: (1 slice), Calories: 140, Fat: 0 g, Protein: 3 g, Carbohydrate: 30 g, Cholesterol: 0 mg, Sodium: 180 mg, Fiber: 1 g

Dietary Exchanges: 2 Starch/Bread

Favorite recipe from **California Prune Board**

BOUNTIFUL BRUNCHES

27 BANANA WALNUT BREAD

½ **cup skim milk**
2 **eggs**
4 **tablespoons margarine, softened**
7¼ **teaspoons EQUAL® MEASURE™ or**
    24 **packets EQUAL® sweetener or**
    1 **cup EQUAL® SPOONFUL™**
1 **teaspoon vanilla**
½ **teaspoon banana extract**
1¼ **cups mashed ripe bananas (about**
    2 **large)**
1¾ **cups all-purpose flour**
1 **teaspoon baking soda**
1 **teaspoon ground cinnamon**
½ **teaspoon salt**
¼ **teaspoon baking powder**
⅓ **cup coarsely chopped walnuts**

• Beat milk, eggs, margarine, Equal®, vanilla and banana extract in large bowl with electric mixer 30 seconds; add bananas and beat on high speed 1 minute.

• Add combined flour, baking soda, cinnamon, salt and baking powder, mixing just until blended. Stir in walnuts. Spread mixture evenly in greased 8½×4½×2½-inch loaf pan.

• Bake in preheated 350°F oven until bread is golden and toothpick inserted in center comes out clean, about 60 minutes. Cool in pan on wire rack 5 minutes; remove from pan and cool on wire rack.

Makes 1 loaf (about 16 slices)

Nutrients per Serving: (1 slice), Calories: 127, Fat: 5 g, Protein: 3 g, Carbohydrates: 17 g, Cholesterol: 27 mg, Sodium: 199 mg

Dietary Exchanges: 1 Starch/Bread, 1 Fat

28 ORANGE FRUIT BREAD

2 **cups all-purpose flour**
¼ **cup sugar**
1½ **teaspoons baking powder**
½ **teaspoon baking soda**
½ **teaspoon salt**
¼ **cup Prune Purée (page 25) or prepared**
    prune butter
¾ **cup orange juice**
½ **cup orange marmalade**
    Grated peel of 1 orange
1 **package (6 ounces) mixed dried**
    fruit bits
¼ **cup chopped toasted pecans**

Preheat oven to 350°F. Coat 8½×4½×2¾-inch loaf pan with vegetable cooking spray. In mixer bowl, combine flour, sugar, baking powder, baking soda and salt. Add prune purée; beat at low speed until blended. Add juice, marmalade and orange peel. Beat at low speed just until blended. Stir in fruit bits and pecans. Spoon batter into prepared pan. Bake in center of oven about 1 hour until pick inserted into center comes out clean. Cool in pan 5 minutes; remove from pan to wire rack. Cool completely. For best flavor, wrap securely and store overnight before slicing. Serve with orange marmalade, if desired. *Makes 1 loaf (12 slices)*

Nutrients per Serving: (1 slice), Calories: 200, Fat: 2 g, Protein: 3 g, Carbohydrate: 44 g, Cholesterol: 0 mg, Sodium: 170 mg, Fiber: 3 g

Dietary Exchanges: 3 Starch/Bread

*Favorite recipe from **California Prune Board***

Orange Fruit Bread

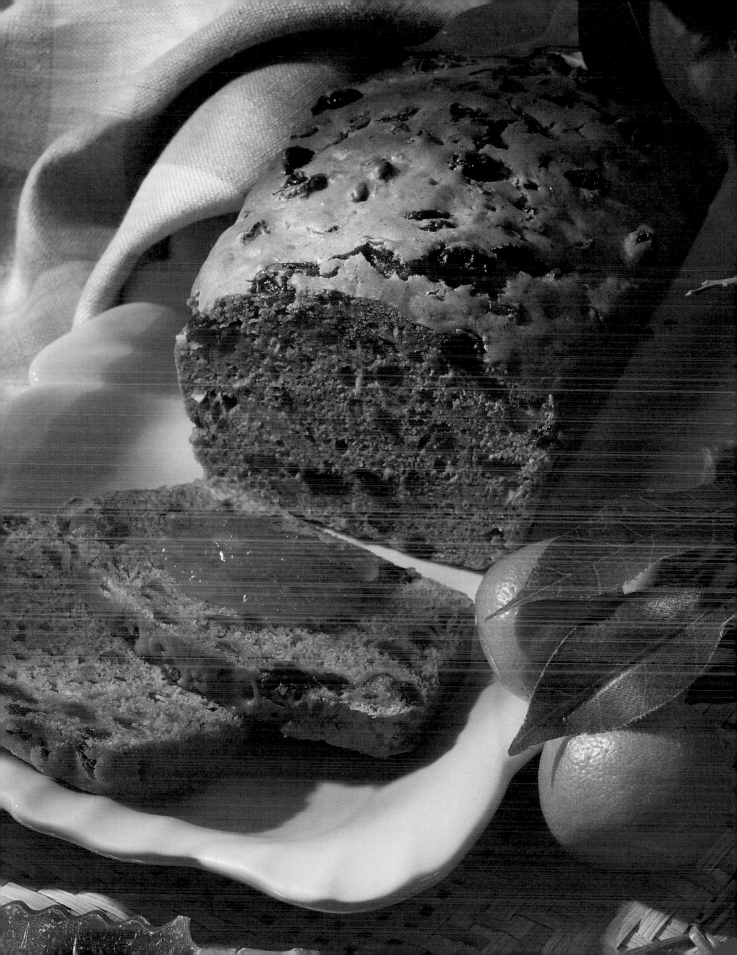

BOUNTIFUL BRUNCHES

29 APRICOT–ALMOND COFFEE RING

1 cup dried apricots, sliced
1 cup water
3½ teaspoons EQUAL® MEASURE™ or
    12 packets EQUAL® sweetener or
    ½ cup EQUAL® SPOONFUL™
⅛ teaspoon ground mace
1 loaf (16 ounces) frozen Italian bread
    dough, thawed
⅓ cup sliced or slivered almonds
    Skim milk
1 teaspoon EQUAL® MEASURE™ or
    3 packets EQUAL® sweetener or
    2 tablespoons EQUAL® SPOONFUL™

• Heat apricots, water, 3½ teaspoons Equal® Measure™ *or* 12 packets Equal® sweetener *or* ½ cup Equal® Spoonful™ and mace to boiling in small saucepan; reduce heat and simmer, covered, until apricots are tender and water is absorbed, about 10 minutes. Simmer, uncovered, until no water remains, 2 to 3 minutes. Cool.

• Roll dough on floured surface into 14×8-inch rectangle. Spread apricot mixture on dough to within 1 inch of edges; sprinkle with ¼ cup almonds. Roll dough up jelly-roll style, beginning with long edge; pinch edge of dough to seal. Place dough seam side down on greased cookie sheet, forming circle; pinch ends to seal.

Apricot-Almond Coffee Ring

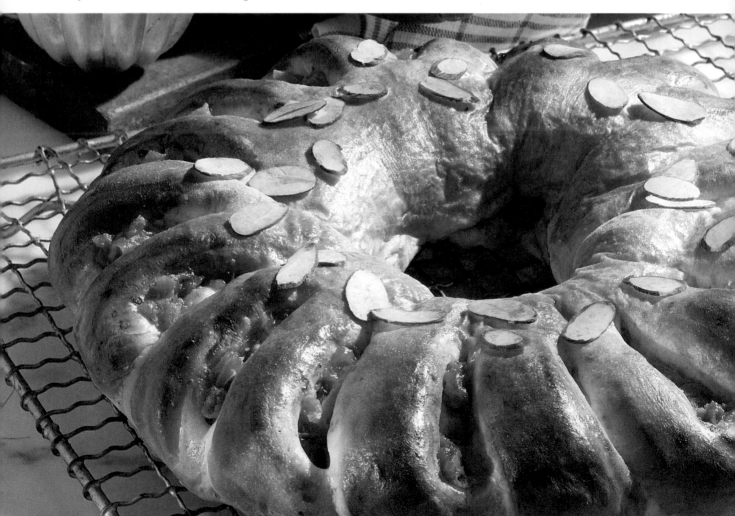

BOUNTIFUL BRUNCHES

• Using scissors, cut dough from outside edge almost to center, making cuts 1 inch apart. Turn each section cut side up so filling shows. Let rise, covered, in warm place until dough is double in size, about 1 hour.

• Brush top of dough lightly with milk; sprinkle with remaining almonds and 1 teaspoon Equal® Measure™ *or* 3 packets Equal® sweetener *or* 2 tablespoons Equal® Spoonful™. Bake coffee cake in preheated 375°F oven until golden, 25 to 30 minutes. Cool on wire rack.

Makes about 12 servings

Nutrients per Serving: Calories: 154, Fat: 3 g, Protein: 4 g, Carbohydrates: 27 g, Cholesterol: 0 mg, Sodium: 180 mg

Dietary Exchanges: 1 Starch/Bread, ½ Fruit, ½ Fat

30 HERB BISCUITS

¼ **cup hot water (130°F)**
1½ **teaspoons (½ package) fast-rising active dry yeast**
2½ **cups all-purpose flour**
3 **tablespoons sugar**
1½ **teaspoons baking powder**
½ **teaspoon baking soda**
½ **teaspoon salt**
5 **tablespoons cold margarine, cut into pieces**
2 **teaspoons finely chopped fresh parsley** *or* ½ **teaspoon dried parsley flakes**
2 **teaspoons finely chopped fresh basil** *or* ½ **teaspoon dried basil leaves**
2 **teaspoons finely chopped fresh chives** *or* ½ **teaspoon dried chives**
¾ **cup buttermilk**

1. Preheat oven to 425°F. Spray cookie sheet with nonstick cooking spray.

2. Combine hot water and yeast in small cup; let stand 2 to 3 minutes. Combine flour, sugar, baking powder, baking soda and salt in medium bowl; cut in margarine using pastry blender or 2 knives until mixture resembles coarse crumbs. Mix in parsley, basil and chives. Stir in milk and yeast mixture to make soft dough. Turn dough out onto lightly floured surface. Knead 15 to 20 times.

3. Roll to ½-inch thickness. Cut hearts or other shapes with 2½-inch cookie cutter. Place biscuits on prepared cookie sheet. Bake 12 to 15 minutes or until browned. Cool on wire racks. Serve immediately.

Makes 18 biscuits

Nutrients per Serving: (1 biscuit), Calories: 156 (29% Calories from Fat), Total Fat: 5 g, Saturated Fat: 1 g, Protein: 3 g, Carbohydrate: 24 g, Cholesterol: 0 mg, Sodium: 254 mg, Fiber: 1 g, Sugar: 4 g

Dietary Exchanges: 1½ Starch/Bread, 1 Fat

BOUNTIFUL BRUNCHES

31 SILVER DOLLAR PANCAKES WITH MIXED BERRY TOPPING

1¼ cups all-purpose flour
2 tablespoons sugar
2 teaspoons baking soda
1½ cups buttermilk
½ cup EGG BEATERS® Healthy Real Egg Substitute
3 tablespoons FLEISCHMANN'S® 70% Corn Oil Spread, melted, divided
Mixed Berry Topping (recipe follows)

In large bowl, combine flour, sugar and baking soda. Stir in buttermilk, Egg Beaters and 2 tablespoons spread just until blended.

Brush large nonstick griddle or skillet with some of remaining spread; heat over medium-high heat. Using 1 heaping tablespoon batter for each pancake, spoon batter onto griddle. Cook until bubbly; turn and cook until lightly browned. Repeat with remaining batter using remaining spread as needed to make 28 pancakes. Serve hot with Mixed Berry Topping.

Makes 28 (2-inch) pancakes

Prep Time: 20 minutes
Cook Time: 20 minutes

MIXED BERRY TOPPING: In medium saucepan, over medium-low heat, combine 1 (12-ounce) package frozen mixed berries, thawed, ¼ cup honey and ½ teaspoon grated gingerroot (*or* ⅛ teaspoon ground ginger). Cook and stir just until hot.

Nutrients per Serving: (4 pancakes, ¼ cup topping), Calories: 228, Total Fat: 6 g, Saturated Fat: 1 g, Cholesterol: 2 mg, Sodium: 491 mg, Fiber: 1 g

Dietary Exchanges: 2 Starch/Bread, ½ Fruit, 1 Fat

32 APPLE RAISIN PANCAKES

2 cups all-purpose flour
2 tablespoons sugar
1 tablespoon baking powder
2 teaspoons ground cinnamon
1¾ cups skim milk
⅔ cup EGG BEATERS® Healthy Real Egg Substitute
5 tablespoons FLEISCHMANN'S® 70% Corn Oil Spread, melted, divided
¾ cup chopped apple
¾ cup seedless raisins

In large bowl, combine flour, sugar, baking powder and cinnamon. In medium bowl, combine milk, Egg Beaters and 4 tablespoons spread; stir into dry ingredients just until blended. Stir in apple and raisins.

Brush large nonstick griddle or skillet with some of remaining spread; heat over medium-high heat. Using ¼ cup batter for each pancake, pour batter onto griddle. Cook until bubbly; turn and cook until lightly browned. Repeat with remaining batter using remaining spread as needed to make 16 pancakes.

Makes 16 (4-inch) pancakes

Prep Time: 10 minutes
Cook Time: 15 minutes

Nutrients per Serving: (1 pancake), Calories: 134, Total Fat: 4 g, Saturated Fat: 1 g, Cholesterol: 1 mg, Sodium: 157 mg, Fiber: 1 g

Dietary Exchanges: 1 Starch/Bread, ½ Fruit, ½ Fat

*Silver Dollar Pancakes
with Mixed Berry Topping*

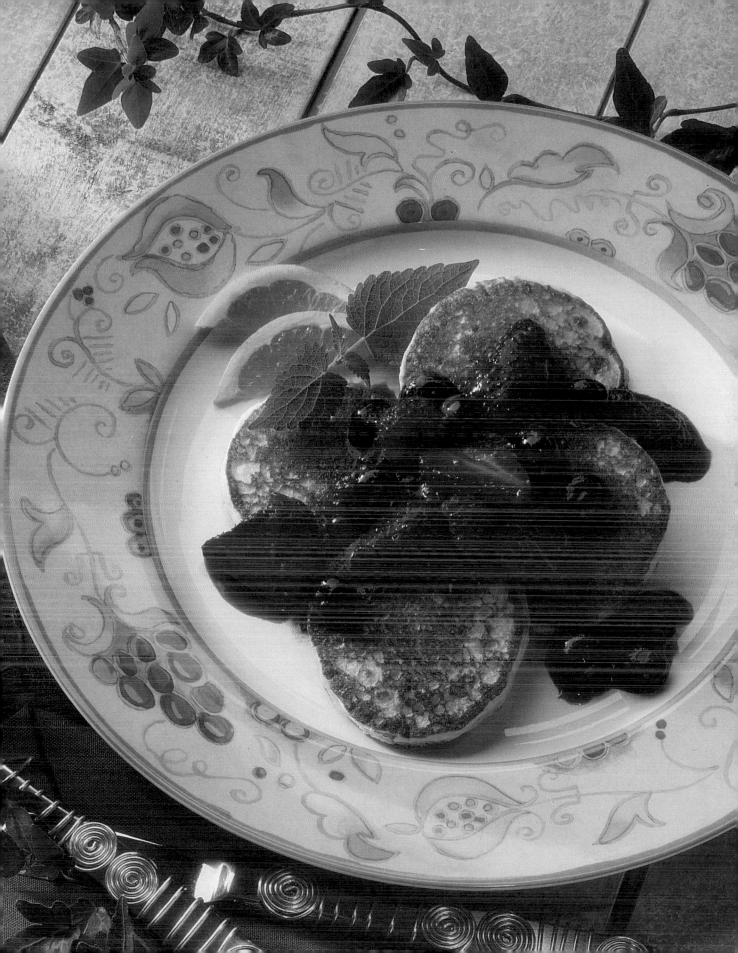

BOUNTIFUL BRUNCHES

33 BLACK BEAN PANCAKES & SALSA

1 cup GUILTLESS GOURMET® Black Bean Dip (mild or spicy)
2 egg whites
½ cup unbleached all-purpose flour
½ cup skim milk
1 tablespoon canola oil
   Nonstick cooking spray
½ cup fat free sour cream
½ cup GUILTLESS GOURMET® Salsa (medium)
   Yellow tomatoes and fresh mint leaves (optional)

For pancake batter, place bean dip, egg whites, flour, milk and oil in blender or food processor; blend until smooth. Refrigerate 2 hours or overnight.

Preheat oven to 350°F. Coat large nonstick skillet with cooking spray; heat over medium heat until hot. For each pancake, spoon 2 tablespoons batter into skillet; cook until bubbles form and break on pancake surface. Turn pancakes over; cook until lightly browned on other side. Place on baking sheet; keep warm in oven. Repeat to make 16 small pancakes. (If batter becomes too thick, thin with more milk.) Serve hot with sour cream and salsa. Garnish with tomatoes and mint, if desired.

Makes 4 servings

Nutrients per Serving: (4 pancakes, 2 tablespoons sour cream and 2 tablespoons salsa), Calories: 192 (18% Calories from Fat), Total Fat: 4 g, Saturated Fat: 0 g, Protein: 12 g, Carbohydrate: 27 g, Cholesterol: 0 mg, Sodium: 403 mg, Fiber: 2 g

Dietary Exchanges: 1½ Starch/Bread, 1 Lean Meat

34 POTATO LATKES

⅔ cup EGG BEATERS® Healthy Real Egg Substitute
⅓ cup all-purpose flour
¼ cup grated onion
¼ teaspoon ground black pepper
4 large potatoes, peeled and shredded (about 4 cups)
3 tablespoons FLEISCHMANN'S® 70% Corn Oil Spread, divided
1½ cups sweetened applesauce
   Fresh chives, for garnish

In large bowl, combine Egg Beaters, flour, onion and pepper; set aside.

Pat shredded potatoes dry with paper towels. Stir into egg mixture. In large nonstick skillet, over medium-high heat, melt 1½ tablespoons spread. For each pancake, spoon about ⅓ cup potato mixture into skillet, spreading into a 4-inch circle. Cook for 3 minutes on each side or until golden; remove and keep warm. Repeat with remaining mixture, using remaining spread as needed to make 12 pancakes. Serve hot with applesauce. Garnish with chives.

Makes 4 servings

Prep Time: 20 minutes
Cook Time: 18 minutes

Nutrients per Serving: Calories: 460, Total Fat: 12 g, Saturated Fat: 4 g, Cholesterol: 0 mg, Sodium: 208 mg, Fiber: 4 g

Dietary Exchanges: 4 Starch/Bread, 1 Fruit, 1½ Fat

Potato Latkes

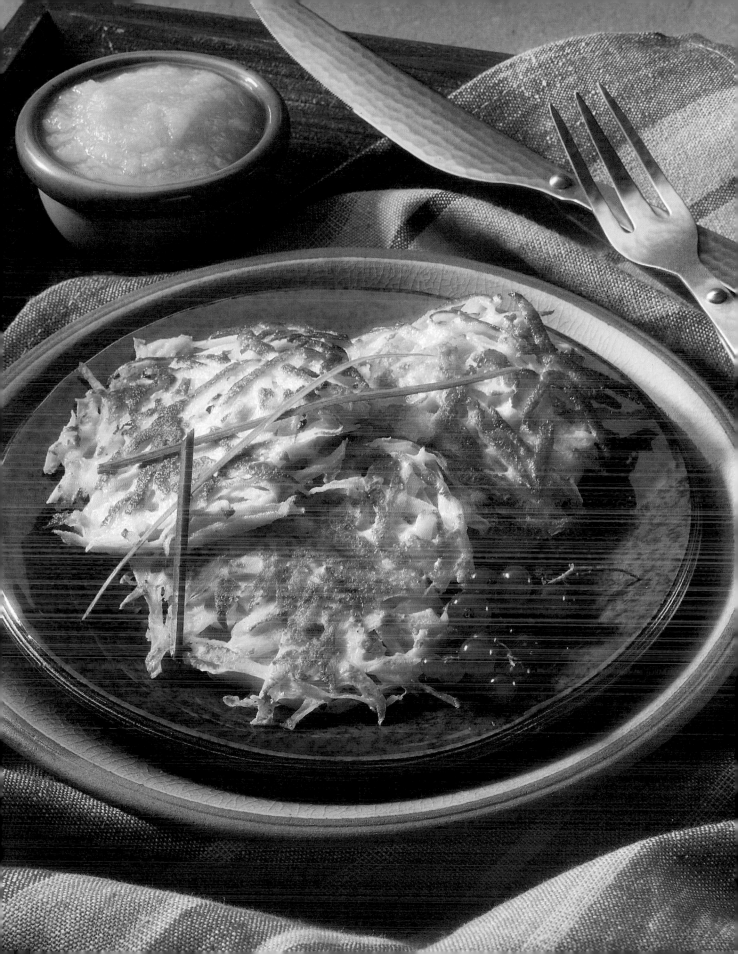

BOUNTIFUL BRUNCHES

35 BLINTZES WITH RASPBERRY SAUCE

1 (16-ounce) container low fat cottage
    cheese (1% milkfat)
3 tablespoons EGG BEATERS® Healthy
    Real Egg Substitute
½ teaspoon sugar
10 prepared French Breakfast Crêpes
    (recipe follows)
    Raspberry Sauce (recipe follows)

In small bowl, combine cottage cheese, Egg
Beaters and sugar; spread 2 tablespoonfuls
mixture down center of each crêpe. Fold
two opposite ends of each crêpe over filling,
then fold in sides like an envelope. In lightly
greased large nonstick skillet, over medium
heat, place blintzes seam-side down. Cook
for 4 minutes on each side or until golden
brown. Serve hot with Raspberry Sauce.

Makes 10 servings

Prep Time: 30 minutes
Cook Time: 45 minutes

RASPBERRY SAUCE: In electric blender
container or food processor, purée 1 (16-
ounce) package frozen raspberries, thawed;
strain. Stir in 2 tablespoons sugar. Serve
over blintzes.

Nutrients per Serving: Calories: 161,
Total Fat: 2 g, Saturated Fat: 1 g,
Cholesterol: 2 mg, Sodium: 231 mg,
Fiber: 0 g

Dietary Exchanges: 1½ Starch/Bread,
1 Lean Meat

FRENCH BREAKFAST CRÊPES
1 cup all-purpose flour
1 cup skim milk
⅔ cup EGG BEATERS® Healthy Real Egg
    Substitute
1 tablespoon FLEISCHMANN'S® 70%
    Corn Oil Spread, melted

In medium bowl, combine flour, milk, Egg
Beaters and spread; let stand 30 minutes.

Heat lightly greased 8-inch nonstick skillet
or crêpe pan over medium-high heat. Pour in
scant ¼ cup batter, tilting pan to cover
bottom. Cook for 1 to 2 minutes; turn and
cook for 30 seconds to 1 minute more. Place
on waxed paper. Stir batter and repeat to
make 10 crêpes. Fill with desired fillings or
use in recipes calling for prepared crêpes.

Makes 10 crêpes

Prep Time: 10 minutes
Cook Time: 40 minutes

36 PB & J FRENCH TOAST

¼ cup blueberry preserves, or any flavor
6 slices whole wheat bread, divided
¼ cup creamy peanut butter
½ cup EGG BEATERS® Healthy Real Egg
    Substitute
¼ cup skim milk
2 tablespoons FLEISCHMANN'S® 70%
    Corn Oil Spread
1 large banana, sliced
1 tablespoon honey
1 tablespoon orange juice
1 tablespoon dry roasted unsalted
    peanuts, chopped
    Low fat vanilla yogurt, optional

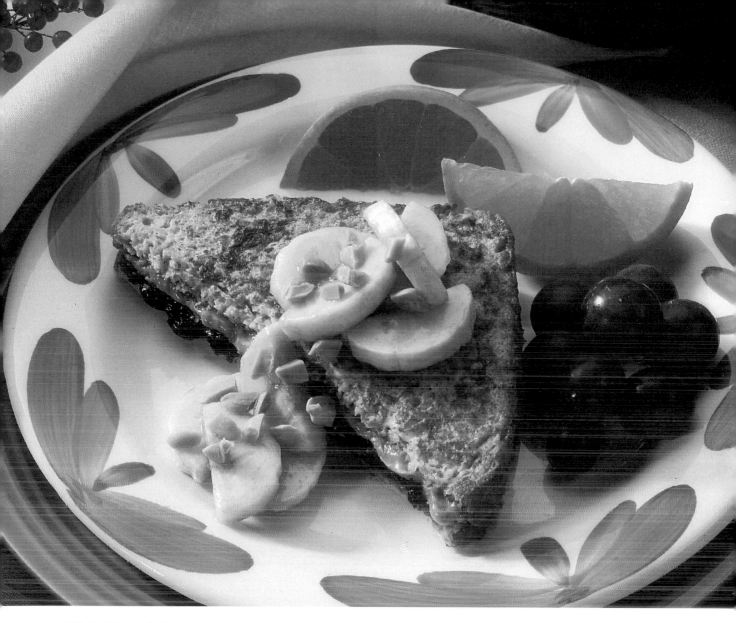

PB & J French Toast

Spread preserves evenly over 3 bread slices. Spread peanut butter evenly over remaining bread slices. Press preserves and peanut butter slices together to form 3 sandwiches; cut each diagonally in half. In shallow bowl, combine Egg Beaters and milk. In large nonstick griddle or skillet, over medium-high heat, melt spread. Dip each sandwich in egg mixture to coat; transfer to griddle. Cook sandwiches for 2 minutes on each side or until golden. Keep warm.

In small bowl, combine banana slices, honey, orange juice and peanuts. Arrange sandwiches on platter; top with banana mixture. Serve warm with a dollop of yogurt if desired.   *Makes 6 servings*

Prep Time: 25 minutes
Cook Time: 10 minutes

Nutrients per Serving: (without yogurt), Calories: 242, Total Fat: 11 g, Saturated Fat: 2 g, Cholesterol: 1 mg, Sodium: 262 mg, Fiber: 3 g
Dietary Exchanges: 2 Starch/Bread, 2 Fat

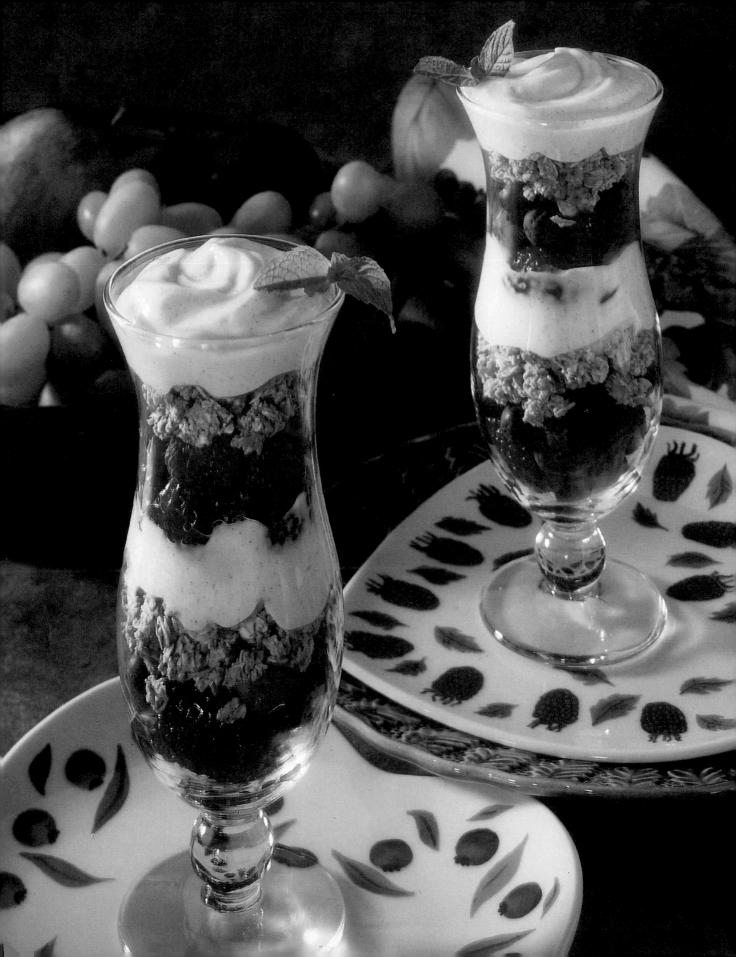

BOUNTIFUL BRUNCHES

37 TRIPLE BERRY BREAKFAST PARFAIT

  2 cups vanilla sugar-free nonfat yogurt
  ¼ teaspoon ground cinnamon
  1 cup sliced strawberries
  ½ cup blueberries
  ½ cup raspberries
  1 cup low-fat granola without raisins

1. Combine yogurt and cinnamon in small bowl. Combine strawberries, blueberries and raspberries in medium bowl.

2. For each parfait, layer ¼ cup fruit mixture, 2 tablespoons granola and ¼ cup yogurt mixture in parfait glass. Repeat layers. Garnish with mint leaves, if desired.

Makes 4 servings

Nutrients per Serving: Calories: 236 (9% Calories from Fat), Total Fat: 2 g, Saturated Fat: trace, Protein: 9 g, Carbohydrate: 49 g, Cholesterol: 0 mg, Sodium: 101 mg, Fiber: 2 g, Sugar: 5 g

Dietary Exchanges: 2 Starch/Bread, ½ Milk, 1 Fruit, ½ Fat

38 BANANA–ORANGE DATE OATMEAL

  2 cups orange juice
  1 cup water
  ¼ teaspoon salt (optional)
  ⅛ teaspoon ground nutmeg
  1½ cups QUAKER® Oats (quick or old fashioned, uncooked)
  ¾ cup chopped dates or raisins
  1 medium ripe banana, mashed

In medium saucepan, bring juice, water, salt and nutmeg to a boil; stir in oats and dates. Return to a boil; reduce heat. Cook 1 minute for quick oats or 5 minutes for old fashioned oats, stirring occasionally. Stir in banana. Let stand until of desired consistency.

Makes 4 servings

MICROWAVE DIRECTIONS: In 3-quart microwaveable bowl, combine all ingredients except banana. Microwave at HIGH 6 to 7 minutes for quick oats or 9 to 10 minutes for old fashioned oats or until most of juice is absorbed; stir. Stir in banana. Let stand until of desired consistency.

Nutrients per Serving: 1 serving (with dates), Calories: 290 (7% Calories from Fat), Total Fat: 2 g, Saturated Fat: 0 g, Protein: 6 g, Carbohydrate: 65 g, Cholesterol: 0 mg, Sodium: 5 mg, Fiber: 5 g, Sugar: 35 g

Exchanges: 2 Bread/Starch, 2½ Fruit

Triple Berry Breakfast Parfait

BOUNTIFUL BRUNCHES

39 STRAWBERRY SMOOTHIE

1 carton (8 ounces) plain nonfat yogurt
$\frac{1}{4}$ cup skim milk
1 teaspoon EQUAL® MEASURE™ or
    3 packets EQUAL® sweetener or
    2 tablespoons EQUAL® SPOONFUL™
3 cups frozen strawberries
1 cup ice cubes

• Combine yogurt, milk and Equal® in blender container. With blender running, add berries, a few at a time, through opening in lid. Blend until smooth; add ice cubes one at a time through opening in lid, blending until slushy. Pour into glasses.

Makes 4 (6-ounce) servings

Nutrients per Serving: Calories: 82, Fat: 0 g, Protein: 4 g, Carbohydrates: 17 g, Cholesterol: 1 mg, Sodium: 58 mg

Dietary Exchanges: ½ Milk, 1 Fruit

40 ORANGE JUBILEE

1 small can (6 ounces) frozen orange juice
    concentrate
2$\frac{1}{4}$ cups skim milk
½ teaspoon vanilla
1$\frac{3}{4}$ teaspoons EQUAL® MEASURE™ or
    6 packets EQUAL® sweetener or
    ¼ cup EQUAL® SPOONFUL™
8 ice cubes
    Ground nutmeg or cinnamon (optional)

• Process orange juice concentrate, milk, vanilla and Equal® in food processor or blender until smooth; add ice cubes and process again until smooth. Serve in small glasses; sprinkle with nutmeg or cinnamon, if desired. *Makes 6 (4-ounce) servings*

Nutrients per Serving: Calories: 94, Fat: 0 g, Protein: 4 g, Carbohydrates: 19 g, Cholesterol: 2 mg, Sodium: 49 mg

Dietary Exchanges: ½ Milk, 1 Fruit

41 FITNESS SHAKE

2 cups skim milk
2 medium-size ripe bananas, cut into
    1-inch pieces
½ cup plain or banana nonfat yogurt
½ cup nonfat dry milk powder
⅓ cup wheat germ
1 teaspoon vanilla
2½ teaspoons EQUAL® MEASURE™ or
    8 packets EQUAL® sweetener or
    ⅓ cup EQUAL® SPOONFUL™
    Ground cinnamon (optional)

• Blend all ingredients except cinnamon in blender or food processor until smooth. Pour into glasses and sprinkle with cinnamon, if desired.

Makes 4 (8-ounce) servings

Nutrients per Serving: Calories: 190, Fat: 2 g, Protein: 12 g, Carbohydrates: 33 g, Cholesterol: 4 mg, Sodium: 134 mg

Dietary Exchanges: 1½ Milk, 1 Fruit, ½ Fat

Strawberry Smoothie and Orange Jubilee

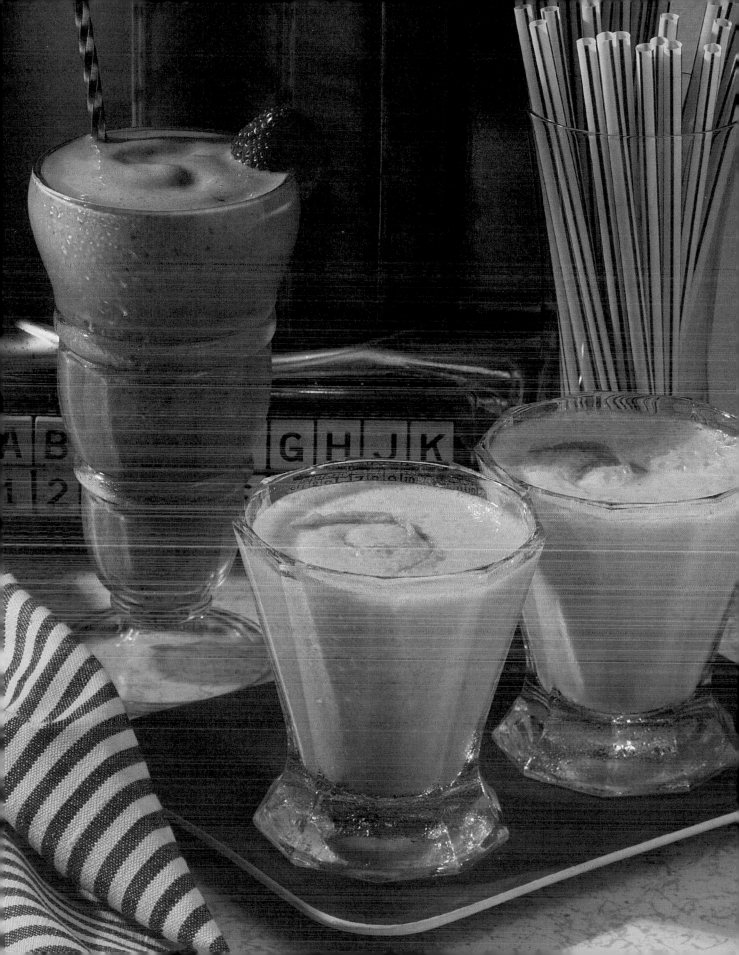

BOUNTIFUL BRUNCHES

42 HOLIDAY EGGNOG

2 cups skim milk
2 tablespoons cornstarch
3½ teaspoons EQUAL® MEASURE™ or
     12 packets EQUAL® sweetener or
     ½ cup EQUAL® SPOONFUL™
2 eggs, beaten
2 teaspoons vanilla
¼ teaspoon ground cinnamon
2 cups skim milk, chilled
⅛ teaspoon ground nutmeg

• Mix 2 cups milk, cornstarch and Equal® in small saucepan; heat to boiling. Boil 1 minute, stirring constantly. Mix about half of milk mixture into eggs; return egg mixture to remaining milk in saucepan. Cook over low heat until slightly thickened, stirring constantly. Remove from heat; stir in vanilla and cinnamon. Cool to room temperature; refrigerate until chilled. Stir 2 cups chilled milk into custard mixture; serve in small glasses. Sprinkle with nutmeg.

Makes 8 (4-ounce) servings

VARIATION: Stir 1 to 1½ teaspoons rum or brandy extract into eggnog, if desired.

Nutrients per Serving: Calories: 79, Fat: 1 g, Protein: 6 g, Carbohydrates: 10 g, Cholesterol: 55 mg, Sodium: 79 mg

Dietary Exchanges: 1 Milk

43 COFFEE LATTE

1¼ cups regular grind espresso or other
     dark roast coffee
1 cinnamon stick, broken into pieces
6 cups water
2½ teaspoons EQUAL® MEASURE™ or
     8 packets EQUAL® sweetener or
     ⅓ cup EQUAL® SPOONFUL™
2½ cups skim milk
     Ground cinnamon or nutmeg

• Place espresso and cinnamon stick in filter basket of drip coffee pot; brew coffee with water. Stir Equal® into coffee; pour into 8 mugs or cups.

• Heat milk in small saucepan until steaming. Process half of milk in blender at high speed until foamy, about 15 seconds; pour milk into 4 mugs of coffee, spooning foam on top. Repeat with remaining milk and coffee. Sprinkle with cinnamon or nutmeg before serving.

Makes about 8 (8-ounce) servings

Nutrients per Serving: Calories: 31, Fat: 0 g, Protein: 3 g, Carbohydrates: 5 g, Cholesterol: 1 mg, Sodium: 46 mg

Dietary Exchanges: ½ Milk

Coffee Latte

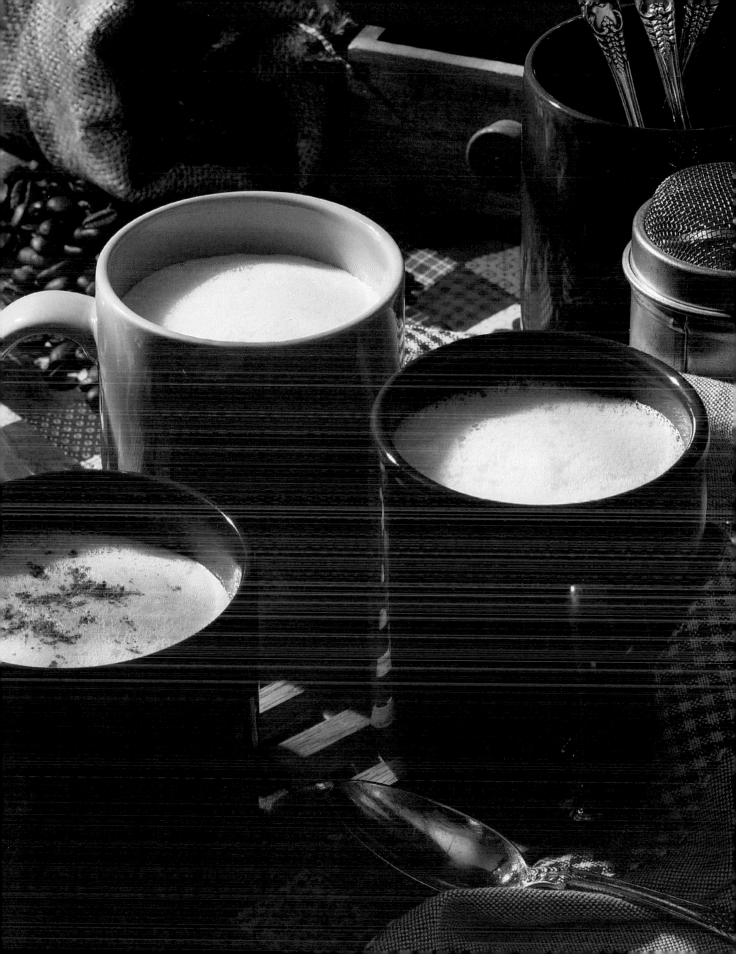

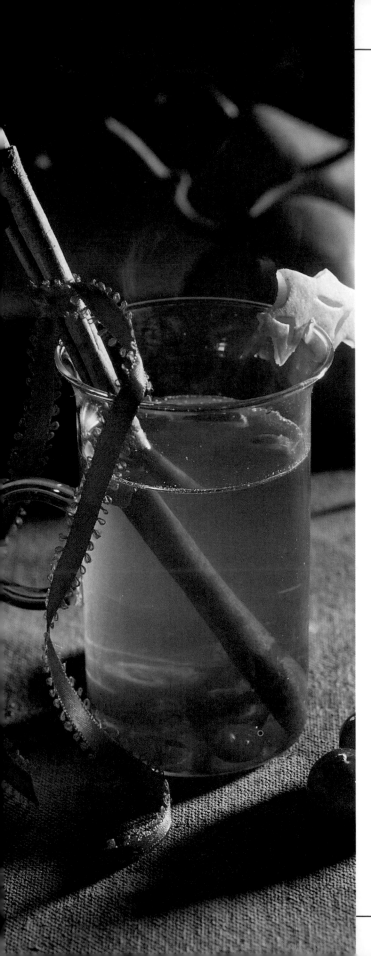

44 OREGON HOT APPLE CIDER

8 whole cloves
8 cups apple cider
½ cup dried cherries
½ cup dried cranberries
3 cinnamon sticks, broken in half
1 pear, quartered, cored, sliced

1. Bundle cloves in small piece of cheesecloth. Tie cheesecloth to form small sack.

2. Combine cider, cherries, cranberries, cinnamon and cheesecloth sack in large saucepan. Heat just to a simmer; do not boil. Remove cheesecloth sack and discard.

3. Add pear before serving.

Makes 8 servings

Nutrients per Serving: Calories: 180 (3% Calories from Fat), Total Fat: 1 g, Saturated Fat: trace, Protein: 1 g, Carbohydrate: 48 g, Cholesterol: 0 mg, Sodium: 10 mg, Fiber: 2 g, Sugar: 2 g

Dietary Exchanges: 3 Fruit

45 CRANBERRY–LIME MARGARITA PUNCH

6 cups water
1 container (12 ounces) frozen cranberry juice cocktail
½ cup lime juice
¼ cup sugar
2 cups ice cubes
1 cup ginger ale or tequila
1 lime, sliced

Oregon Hot Apple Cider

BOUNTIFUL BRUNCHES

1. Combine water, cranberry juice, lime juice and sugar in punch bowl; stir until sugar dissolves.

2. Stir in ice cubes, ginger ale and lime; garnish with fresh cranberries, if desired.

Makes 10 servings

Nutrients per Serving: Calories: 97 (0% Calories from Fat), Total Fat: trace, Saturated Fat: trace, Carbohydrate: 25 g, Protein: trace, Cholesterol: 0 mg, Sodium: 3 mg, Fiber: trace, Sugar: 7 g

Dietary Exchanges: 1½ Fruit

46 TRIPLE–BERRY JAM

4 cups fresh strawberries or thawed frozen
　　unsweetened strawberries
2 cups fresh raspberries or thawed frozen
　　unsweetened raspberries
1 cup fresh blueberries or thawed frozen
　　unsweetened blueberries
1 package (1¾ ounces) no-sugar-needed
　　pectin
2 tablespoons EQUAL® MEASURE™ or
　　20 packets EQUAL® sweetener or
　　¾ cup plus 4 teaspoons EQUAL®
　　SPOONFUL™

• Mash strawberries, raspberries and blueberries, by hand or with food processor, to make 4 cups pulp. Stir in pectin; let mixture stand 10 minutes, stirring frequently. Transfer to large saucepan. Cook and stir over medium heat until mixture comes to a boil. Cook and stir 1 minute more. Remove from heat; stir in Equal®. Skim off foam, if necessary.

• Immediately fill containers, leaving ½-inch headspace. Seal and let stand at room temperature until firm (several hours). Store up to 2 weeks in refrigerator or 6 months in freezer.

Makes 8 (½-pint) jars

Nutrients per Serving: (1 tablespoon), Calories: 9, Fat: 0 g, Protein: 0 g, Carbohydrate: 2 g, Cholesterol: 0 mg, Sodium: 3 mg

Dietary Exchanges: Free Food

47 PEACH PRESERVES

2½ to 3 pounds ripe peaches (10 to 12)
2 tablespoons lemon juice
1 package (1¾ ounces) no-sugar-needed
　　pectin
7¼ teaspoons EQUAL® MEASURE™ or
　　24 packets EQUAL® sweetener or
　　1 cup EQUAL® SPOONFUL™

• Peel, pit and finely chop peaches; measure 4 cups into saucepan. Stir in lemon juice and pectin. Let stand 10 minutes, stirring frequently. Cook and stir until boiling. Cook and stir 1 minute more. Remove from heat; stir in Equal®. Skim off foam.

• Immediately ladle into freezer containers or jars, leaving ½-inch headspace. Seal and label containers. Let stand at room temperature several hours or until set. Store up to 2 weeks in refrigerator or 6 months in freezer.

Makes 8 (½-pint) jars

Nutrients per Serving: (1 tablespoon), Calories: 10, Fat: 0 g, Protein: 0 g, Carbohydrates: 3 g, Cholesterol: 0 mg, Sodium: 3 mg

Dietary Exchanges: Free Food

BOUNTIFUL BRUNCHES

48 ■ STRAWBERRY JAM

2 quarts fresh or frozen strawberries
1 package (1¾ ounces) no-sugar-needed
    pectin
4 tablespoons EQUAL® MEASURE™ or
    40 packets EQUAL® sweetener or
    1⅔ cup EQUAL® SPOONFUL™

• Mash strawberries to make 4 cups pulp. Combine strawberries and pectin in large saucepan. Let stand 10 minutes, stirring frequently. Cook and stir over medium heat until mixture comes to a boil. Cook and stir 1 minute more. Remove from heat; stir in Equal®. Skim off foam if necessary.

• Immediately fill containers, leaving ½-inch headspace. Seal and let stand at room temperature several hours or until set. Store up to 2 weeks in refrigerator or 6 months in freezer.   *Makes 4 (½-pint) jars*

Nutrients per Serving: (1 tablespoon), Calories: 8, Fat: 0 g, Protein: 0 g, Carbohydrates: 2 g, Cholesterol: 0 mg, Sodium: 0 mg

Dietary Exchanges: Free Food

49 ■ SPICED FRUIT BUTTER

3 pounds apples, pears or peaches
¾ cup apple juice, pear nectar or peach
    nectar
1 to 2 teaspoons ground cinnamon
½ teaspoon ground nutmeg
⅛ teaspoon ground cloves
5 teaspoons EQUAL® MEASURE™ or
    16 packets EQUAL® sweetener or
    ⅔ cup EQUAL® SPOONFUL™

• Peel and core or pit fruit; slice. Combine prepared fruit, fruit juice and spices in Dutch oven. Bring to boiling; cover and simmer until very tender, about 15 minutes. Cool slightly. Purée in batches in blender or food processor. Return to Dutch oven.

• Simmer, uncovered, over low heat until desired consistency, stirring frequently. (This may take up to 1 hour.) Remove from heat; stir in Equal®. Transfer to freezer containers or jars, leaving ½-inch headspace. Store up to 2 weeks in refrigerator or up to 3 months in freezer.   *Makes 6 (½-pint) jars*

Nutrients per Serving: (1 tablespoon), Calories: 16, Fat: 0 g, Protein: 0 g, Carbohydrates: 4 g, Cholesterol: 0 mg, Sodium: 0 mg

Dietary Exchanges: Free Food

50 ■ MAPLE–FLAVORED SYRUP

1 cup apple juice
2½ teaspoons cornstarch
1 tablespoon margarine
1¾ teaspoons EQUAL® MEASURE™ or
    6 packets EQUAL® sweetener or
    ¼ cup EQUAL® SPOONFUL™
1 teaspoon maple flavoring
1 teaspoon vanilla

• Combine apple juice and cornstarch in small saucepan. Cook and stir until thickened and bubbly. Cook and stir 2 minutes more. Remove from heat. Stir in margarine, Equal®, maple flavoring and vanilla. Serve over pancakes, waffles or French toast.   *Makes 1 cup*

Nutrients per Serving: (1 tablespoon), Calories: 18, Fat: 1 g, Protein: 0 g, Carbohydrates: 3 g, Cholesterol: 0 mg, Sodium: 9 mg

Dietary Exchanges: Free Food

Strawberry Jam and Spiced Fruit Butter

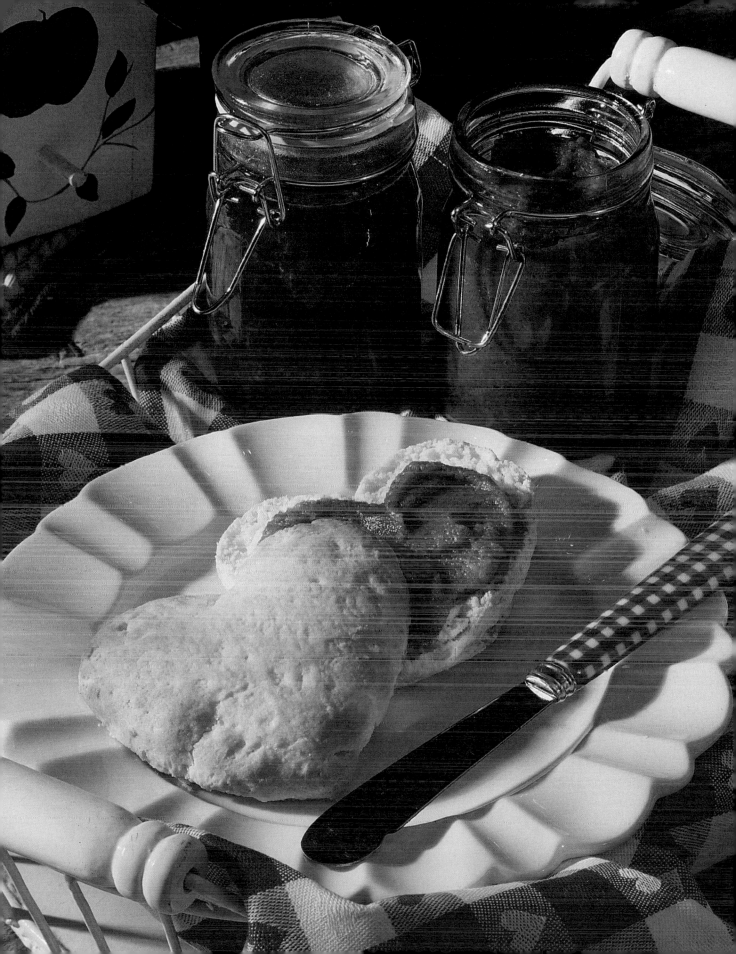

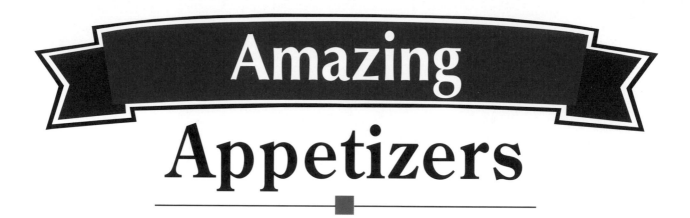

Amazing Appetizers

51 VENEZUELAN SALSA

1 mango, peeled, pitted and diced
½ medium papaya, peeled, seeded and diced
½ medium avocado, peeled, pitted and diced
1 carrot, finely chopped
1 small onion, finely chopped
1 rib celery, finely chopped
Juice of 1 lemon
3 cloves garlic, minced
2 tablespoons chopped cilantro
1 jalapeño pepper,* finely chopped
1½ teaspoons ground cumin
½ teaspoon salt

Jalapeño peppers can sting and irritate the skin; wear rubber gloves when handling peppers and do not touch eyes. Wash hands after handling.

Combine all ingredients in medium bowl. Refrigerate several hours to allow flavors to blend. Serve with baked tortilla chips, if desired.   *Makes 10 servings*

Nutrients per Serving: Calories: 52 (27% Calories from Fat), Total Fat: 2 g, Saturated Fat: trace, Protein: 1 g, Carbohydrates: 9 g, Cholesterol: 0 mg, Sodium: 117 mg, Fiber: 2 g, Sugar: 5 g

Dietary Exchanges: 1 Fruit

52 GREEN PEA MOCKAMOLE

1 package (16 ounces) frozen petit peas
4 green onions
½ cup lightly packed fresh cilantro
2 tablespoons lemon juice
½ cup GUILTLESS GOURMET® Salsa (medium)
   Fresh cilantro sprigs (optional)
1 large bag (7 ounces) GUILTLESS GOURMET® Baked Tortilla Chips (yellow, white or blue corn)

Cook peas according to package directions; drain. Place peas, onions, ½ cup cilantro and juice in food processor or blender; process until smooth. Transfer to serving bowl; gently stir in salsa to combine. Garnish with cilantro sprigs, if desired. Serve warm with tortilla chips or cover and refrigerate until ready to serve.   *Makes 12 servings*

Nutrients per Serving: (¼ cup dip and 12 chips), Calories: 96 (9% of Calories from Fat), Total Fat: 1 g, Saturated Fat: 0 g, Protein: 3 g, Carbohydrate: 18 g, Cholesterol: 0 mg, Sodium: 171 mg, Fiber: 2 g

Dietary Exchanges: 1 Starch/Bread, ½ Vegetable

Venezuelan Salsa

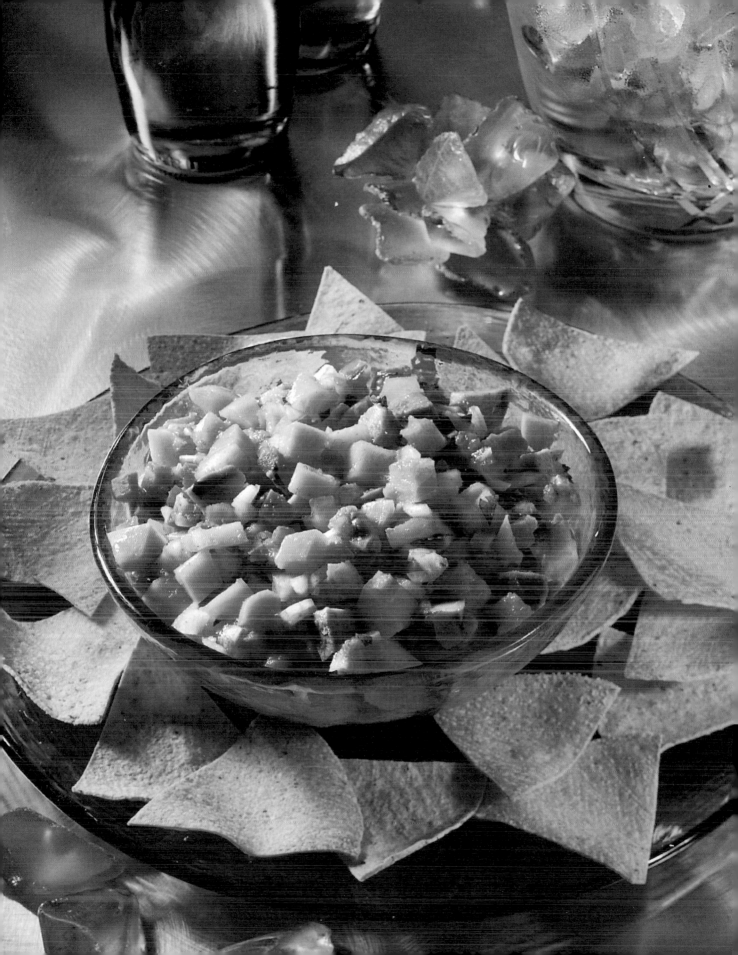

AMAZING APPETIZERS

53 COWBOY CAVIAR

Nonstick cooking spray
2 teaspoons olive oil
1 small eggplant (about ¾ pound), peeled and chopped
1 cup chopped onion
1 jalapeño pepper,* seeded and finely chopped (optional)
1 can (15 ounces) salsa-style chunky tomatoes, undrained
1 can (15 ounces) black-eyed peas, rinsed and drained
1 teaspoon ground cumin
½ cup minced fresh cilantro
Baked fat-free tortilla chips

Jalapeño peppers can sting and irritate the skin; wear rubber gloves when handling peppers and do not touch eyes. Wash hands after handling.

1. Coat large nonstick skillet with cooking spray. Add oil; heat over medium heat until hot. Add eggplant, onion and jalapeño pepper, if desired; cook and stir 10 minutes or until vegetables are tender.

2. Stir in tomatoes with juices, black-eyed peas and cumin. Cook 5 minutes, stirring frequently. Remove from heat; stir in cilantro.

3. Serve with tortilla chips.

Makes 16 servings

Nutrients per Serving: (4 chips, ¼ cup salsa), Calories: 107 (26% Calories from Fat), Total Fat: 3 g, Saturated Fat: 1 g, Protein: 3 g, Carbohydrate: 17 g, Cholesterol: 0 mg, Sodium: 272 mg, Fiber: 1 g, Sugar: 1 g

Dietary Exchanges: 1 Starch/Bread, ½ Fat

54 ROASTED EGGPLANT SPREAD

1 large eggplant
1 can (14½ ounces) diced tomatoes, drained
½ cup finely chopped green onions
½ cup chopped parsley
2 tablespoons red wine vinegar
1 tablespoon olive oil
3 cloves garlic, finely chopped
½ teaspoon salt
½ teaspoon dried oregano leaves
2 rounds pita bread

1. Preheat oven to 375°F.

2. Place eggplant on baking sheet. Bake 1 hour or until tender, turning occasionally. Remove eggplant from oven. Let stand 10 minutes or until cool enough to handle.

3. Cut eggplant lengthwise in half; remove pulp. Place pulp in medium bowl; mash with fork until smooth. Add tomatoes, onions, parsley, vinegar, oil, garlic, salt and oregano; blend well. Cover eggplant mixture; refrigerate 2 hours.

4. Preheat broiler. Split pitas horizontally in half to form 4 rounds. Stack rounds; cut into sixths to form 24 wedges. Place wedges on baking sheet. Broil 3 minutes or until crisp.

5. Serve eggplant mixture with warm pita wedges. Garnish with lemon and lime slices, if desired.   *Makes 4 servings*

Nutrients per Serving: (6 pita bread wedges, ½ cup eggplant spread), Calories: 134 (20 % Calories from Fat), Total Fat: 3 g, Saturated Fat: trace, Protein: 4 g, Carbohydrate: 23 g, Cholesterol: 0 mg, Sodium: 347 mg, Fiber 3 g, Sugar: 1 g

Dietary Exchanges: 1 Starch/Bread, 1 Vegetable, ½ Fat

Roasted Eggplant Spread

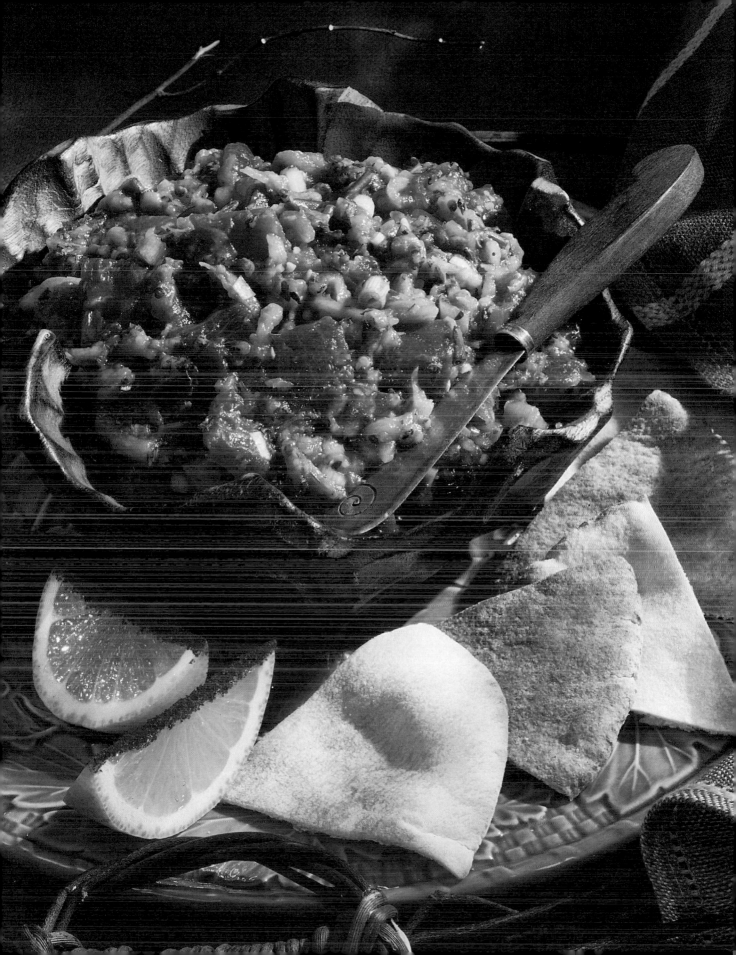

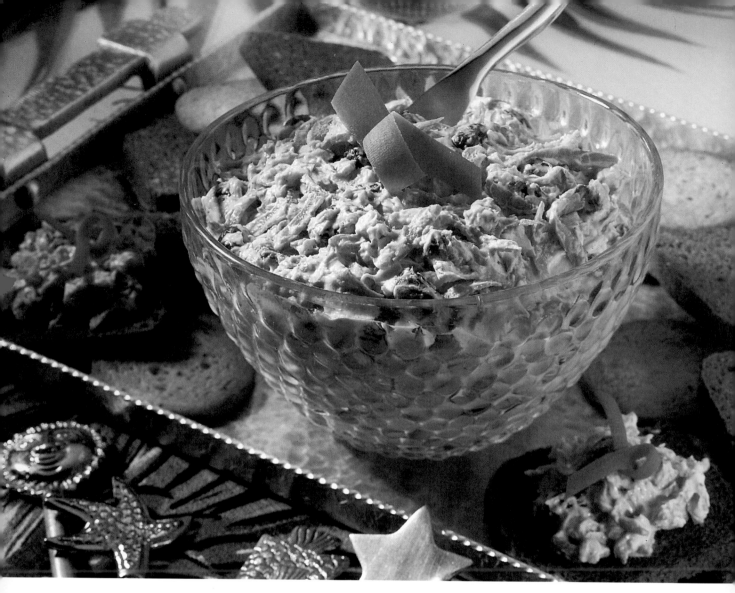

Nutty Carrot Spread

55 NUTTY CARROT SPREAD

6 ounces fat-free cream cheese, softened
2 tablespoons frozen orange juice
concentrate, thawed
¼ teaspoon ground cinnamon
1 cup shredded carrot
¼ cup finely chopped pecans, toasted
¼ cup raisins
36 party pumpernickel bread slices,
toasted, or melba toast rounds

1. Combine cream cheese, orange juice concentrate and cinnamon in small bowl; stir until well blended. Stir in carrot, pecans and raisins.

2. Spread about 1 tablespoon cream cheese mixture onto each bread slice.

Makes 18 servings

Nutrients per Serving: (2 pieces),
Calories: 68 (19% Calories from Fat),
Total Fat: 1 g, Saturated Fat: trace, Protein: 3 g,
Carbohydrate: 11 g, Cholesterol: 2 mg,
Sodium: 149 mg, Fiber: trace, Sugar: 2 g

Dietary Exchanges: 1 Starch/Bread

AMAZING APPETIZERS

56 BERRY GOOD DIP

**8 ounces fresh or thawed frozen
    strawberries
4 ounces fat-free cream cheese, softened
1/4 cup reduced-fat sour cream
1 tablespoon sugar**

1. Place strawberries in food processor or blender container; process until smooth.

2. Beat cream cheese in small bowl until smooth. Stir in sour cream, strawberry purée and sugar; cover. Refrigerate until ready to serve.

3. Spoon dip into small serving bowl. Serve with assorted fresh fruit dippers or angel food cake cubes.   *Makes 6 servings*

Nutrients per Serving: Calories: 47 (16% Calories from Fat), Total Fat: 1 g, Saturated Fat: trace, Protein: 3 g, Carbohydrate: 6 g, Cholesterol: 7 mg, Sodium: 120 mg, Fiber: 1 g, Sugar: 4

Dietary Exchanges: 1/2 Lean Meat, 1/2 Fruit

57 ARTICHOKE DIP

**1 (14-ounce) can non-marinated artichoke
    hearts, chopped
1 can HEALTHY CHOICE® RECIPE
    CREATIONS™ Cream of Roasted
    Garlic Condensed Soup
1 cup fat free cream cheese
1/2 cup *each* fat free shredded Parmesan
    cheese, HEALTHY CHOICE® Fat Free
    Shredded Mozzarella Cheese, sliced
    green onions and roasted red bell
    peppers
1/4 teaspoon black pepper
1/8 teaspoon crushed red pepper (optional)
    Salt (optional)
    Vegetable cooking spray**

In medium bowl, combine artichoke hearts, soup, cream cheese, Parmesan cheese, mozzarella cheese, green onions, roasted peppers, black pepper, red pepper and salt. Spread mixture in 2-quart baking dish sprayed with vegetable cooking spray.

Cover and bake at 400°F 20 minutes or until bubbly. Serve with pita or bagel chips for dipping.   *Makes 8 servings*

Nutrients per Serving: Calories: 80 (4% Calories from Fat), Total Fat: trace, Protein: 9 g, Sodium: 565 mg

Dietary Exchanges: 1 Lean Meat, 2 Vegetable

58 CHEESY BARBECUED BEAN DIP

**1/2 cup canned vegetarian baked beans
3 tablespoons pasteurized process cheese
    spread
2 tablespoons regular or hickory smoke-
    flavored barbecue sauce
2 large carrots, diagonally sliced
1 medium red or green bell pepper, cut
    into chunks**

1. Place beans in small microwavable bowl; mash slightly with fork. Stir in process cheese spread and barbecue sauce. Cover with plastic wrap; vent.

2. Microwave at HIGH 1 minute; stir. Microwave 30 seconds or until hot. Garnish with green onion and bell pepper cutouts, if desired. Serve with carrot and bell pepper dippers.   *Makes 4 servings*

Nutrients per Serving: Calories: 93 (25% Calories from Fat), Total Fat: 3 g, Saturated Fat: 1 g, Protein: 4 g, Carbohydrate: 15 g, Cholesterol: 10 mg, Sodium: 355 mg, Fiber: 4 g, Sugar: 3 g

Dietary Exchanges: 1 Starch/Bread, 1/2 Fat

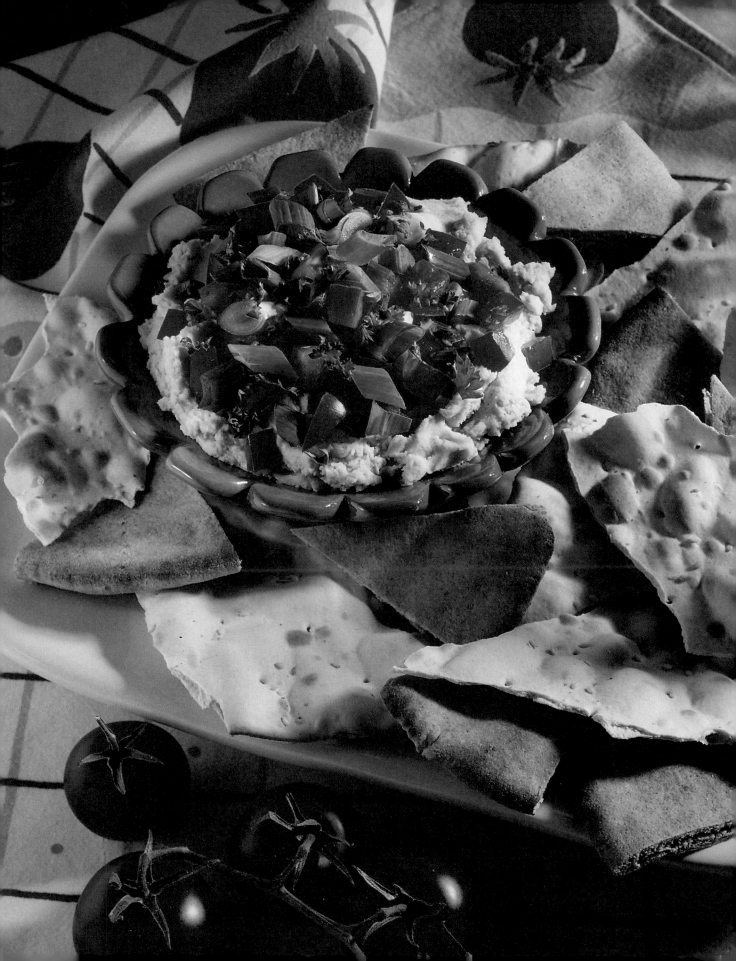

AMAZING APPETIZERS

59 VEGETABLE–TOPPED HUMMUS

1 can (about 15 ounces) chick-peas, rinsed
   and drained
2 tablespoons tahini
2 tablespoons lemon juice
1 clove garlic
¾ teaspoon salt
1 tomato, finely chopped
2 green onions, finely chopped
2 tablespoons chopped parsley

1. Combine chick-peas, tahini, lemon juice, garlic and salt in food processor; process until smooth.

2. Combine tomato, green onions and parsley in small bowl.

3. Place chick-pea mixture in medium serving bowl; spoon tomato mixture evenly over top. Serve with pita wedges or assorted crackers.   *Makes 8 servings*

Nutrients per Serving: Calories: 82 (31% Calories from Fat), Total Fat: 3 g, Saturated Fat: trace, Protein: 3 g, Carbohydrate: 11 g, Cholesterol: 0 mg, Sodium: 429 mg, Fiber: 3 g, Sugar: 1 g

Dietary Exchanges: ½ Starch/Bread, 1 Vegetable, ½ Fat

60 CONFETTI DIP

1 cup nonfat or reduced-fat sour cream
4 teaspoons dry Ranch dressing mix
¼ cup finely chopped carrot
¼ cup finely chopped cucumber
¼ cup finely chopped red bell pepper
¼ cup finely chopped zucchini

1. Combine sour cream and dressing mix in medium bowl; mix well. Stir in chopped vegetables; cover. Refrigerate 2 to 3 hours for flavors to blend.

2. Transfer dip to medium serving bowl. Serve with assorted fresh vegetable dippers.
         Makes 8 servings

Nutrients per Serving: Calories: 31 (26% Calories from Fat), Total Fat: 1 g, Saturated Fat: trace, Protein: 2 g, Carbohydrate: 4 g, Cholesterol: 1 g, Sodium: 37 mg, Fiber: trace, Sugar: trace

Dietary Exchanges: 1 Vegetable

61 SEÑOR NACHO DIP

4 ounces fat-free cream cheese
½ cup (2 ounces) shredded reduced-fat
   Cheddar cheese
¼ cup mild or medium chunky salsa
2 teaspoons 2% low-fat milk
4 ounces baked fat-free tortilla chips or
   assorted fresh vegetable dippers

1. Combine cheeses in small saucepan; stir over low heat until melted. Stir in salsa and milk; heat thoroughly, stirring occasionally.

2. Transfer dip to small serving bowl. Serve with tortilla chips.   *Makes 4 servings*

Nutrients per Serving: Calories: 181 (18% Calories from Fat), Total Fat: 4 g, Saturated Fat: 1 g, Protein: 11 g, Carbohydrate: 25 g, Cholesterol: 11 mg, Sodium: 629 mg, Fiber: 2 g, Sugar: trace

Dietary Exchanges: 1½ Starch/Bread, 1 Lean Meat

Vegetable-Topped Hummus

AMAZING APPETIZERS

62 OVEN–FRIED TEX–MEX ONION RINGS

½ cup plain dry bread crumbs
⅓ cup yellow cornmeal
1½ teaspoons chili powder
⅛ to ¼ teaspoon ground red pepper
⅛ teaspoon salt
1 tablespoon plus 1½ teaspoons margarine, melted
2 medium onions (about 10 ounces), sliced ⅜ inch thick
2 egg whites

1. Preheat oven to 450°F. Spray large nonstick baking sheet with nonstick cooking spray; set aside.

2. Combine bread crumbs, cornmeal, chili powder, pepper and salt in medium shallow dish; mix well. Stir in margarine and 1 teaspoon water.

3. Separate onion slices into rings. Place egg whites in large bowl; beat lightly. Add onions; toss lightly to coat evenly. Transfer to bread crumb mixture; toss to coat evenly. Place in single layer on prepared baking sheet.

4. Bake 12 to 15 minutes or until onions are tender and coating is crisp.

Makes 6 servings

Nutrients per Serving: Calories: 111 (30% Calories from Fat), Total Fat: 4 g, Saturated Fat: 1 g, Protein: 4 g, Carbohydrate: 16 g, Cholesterol: 0 mg, Sodium: 184 mg, Fiber: 2 g, Sugar: 1 g

Dietary Exchanges: 1 Starch/Bread, ½ Vegetable, ½ Fat

63 SAVORY ZUCCHINI STIX

Nonstick olive oil-flavored cooking spray
2 small zucchini (about 4 ounces each)
3 tablespoons seasoned dry bread crumbs
2 tablespoons grated Parmesan cheese
1 egg white
1 teaspoon 2% low-fat milk
⅓ cup spaghetti sauce, heated

1. Preheat oven to 400°F. Spray baking sheet with cooking spray; set aside.

2. Cut zucchini lengthwise into quarters; set aside.

3. Combine bread crumbs and Parmesan cheese in shallow dish. Combine egg white and milk in another shallow dish; beat with fork until well blended.

4. Dip each zucchini wedge first into crumb mixture, then into egg white mixture, letting excess drip back into dish. Roll in crumb mixture to coat again.

5. Place zucchini sticks on prepared baking sheet; coat well with cooking spray.

6. Bake 15 to 18 minutes or until golden brown. Serve with spaghetti sauce.

Makes 4 servings

Nutrients per Serving: Calories: 69 (26% Calories from Fat), Total Fat: 2 g, Saturated Fat: 1 g, Protein: 4 g, Carbohydrate: 9 g, Cholesterol: 6 mg, Sodium: 329 mg, Fiber: 1 g, Sugar: 1 g

Dietary Exchanges: ½ Starch/Bread, ½ Lean Meat, ½ Vegetable

Oven-Fried Tex-Mex Onion Rings

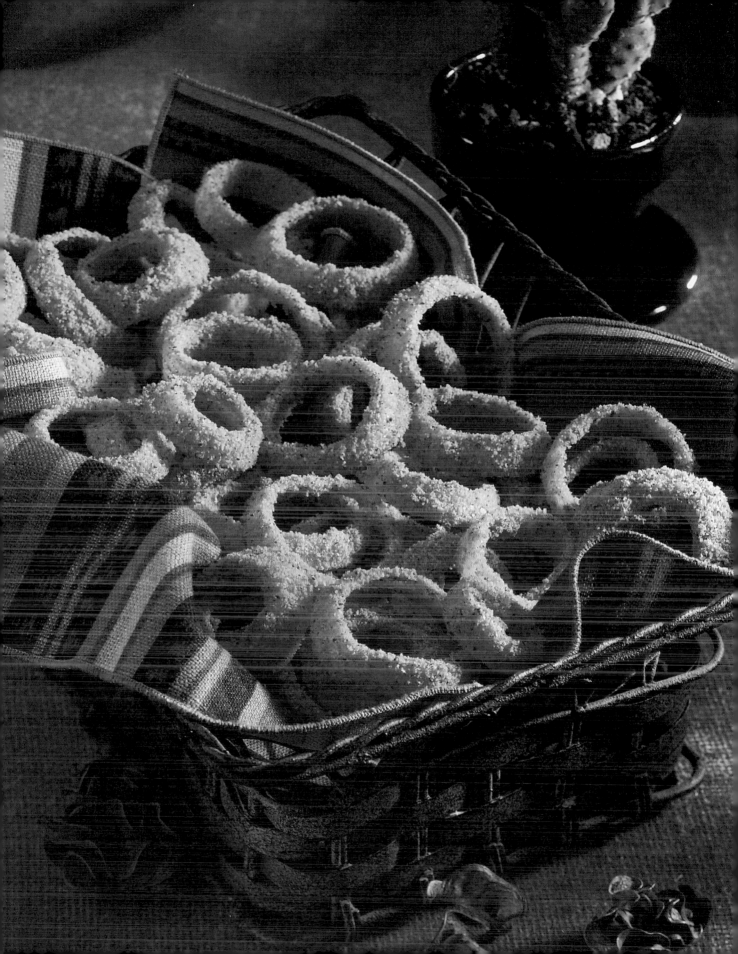

AMAZING APPETIZERS

64 SOFT PRETZELS

1 package (16 ounces) hot roll mix, plus
    ingredients to prepare mix
1 egg white
2 teaspoons water
2 tablespoons each assorted coatings:
    grated Parmesan cheese, sesame
    seeds, poppy seeds, dried oregano
    leaves

1. Prepare hot roll mix according to package directions.

2. Preheat oven to 375°F. Spray baking sheets with nonstick cooking spray; set aside.

3. Divide dough equally into 16 pieces; roll each piece with hands to form a rope, 7 to 10 inches long. Place on prepared cookie sheets; form into desired shape (hearts, wreaths, pretzels, snails, loops, etc.).

4. Beat together egg white and water in small bowl until foamy. Brush onto dough shapes; sprinkle each shape with 1½ teaspoons of one of the coatings.

5. Bake until golden brown, about 15 minutes. Serve warm or at room temperature. *Makes 8 servings*

Nutrients per Serving: Calories: 214 (23% Calories from Fat), Total Fat: 6 g, Saturated Fat: 1 g, Protein: 8 g, Carbohydrate: 33 g, Cholesterol: 20 mg, Sodium: 315 mg, Fiber: trace, Sugar: 0 g

Dietary Exchanges: 2 Starch/Bread, ½ Lean Meat, 1 Fat

Soft Pretzels

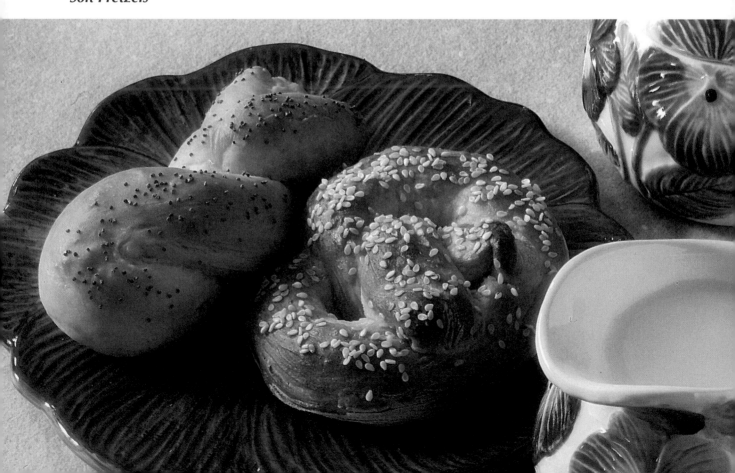

AMAZING APPETIZERS

65 PIZZA BREAD STICKS

1 package (¼ ounce) active dry yeast
¾ cup warm water (105°F to 115°F)
2½ cups all-purpose flour
½ cup (2 ounces) shredded part-skim mozzarella cheese
¼ cup (1 ounce) grated Parmesan cheese
¼ cup chopped red bell pepper
1 green onion with top, sliced
1 medium clove garlic, minced
½ teaspoon dried basil leaves
½ teaspoon dried oregano leaves
¼ teaspoon red pepper flakes (optional)
¼ teaspoon salt
1 tablespoon olive oil

1. Preheat oven to 400°F. Spray 2 large nonstick baking sheets with nonstick cooking spray; set aside.

2. Sprinkle yeast over warm water in small bowl; stir until yeast dissolves. Let stand 5 minutes or until bubbly.

3. Meanwhile, place all remaining ingredients except oil in food processor; process a few seconds to combine. With food processor running, gradually add yeast mixture and oil. Process just until mixture forms a ball. (Add an additional 2 tablespoons flour if dough is too sticky.)

4. Transfer dough to lightly floured surface; knead 1 minute. Let dough rest 5 minutes. Roll out dough with lightly floured rolling pin to form 14×8-inch rectangle; cut dough crosswise into ½-inch-wide strips. Twist dough strips; place on prepared baking sheets.

5. Bake 14 to 16 minutes or until lightly browned.   *Makes 14 servings*

Nutrients per Serving: Calories: 112 (19% Calories from Fat), Total Fat: 2 g, Saturated Fat: 1 g, Protein: 4 g, Carbohydrate: 18 g, Cholesterol: 4 mg, Sodium: 91 mg, Fiber: 1 g, Sugar: trace

Dietary Exchanges: 1 Starch/Bread, ½ Fat

66 SPICED SESAME WONTON CRISPS

20 (3-inch square) wonton wrappers, cut in half
2 teaspoons olive oil
½ teaspoon paprika
½ teaspoon ground cumin or chili powder
¼ teaspoon dry mustard
1 tablespoon sesame seeds

1. Preheat oven to 375°F. Coat 2 large nonstick baking sheets with nonstick cooking spray.

2. Cut each halved wonton wrapper into 2 strips; place in single layer on prepared baking sheets.

3. Combine 1 tablespoon water, oil, paprika, cumin and mustard in small bowl; mix well. Brush oil mixture evenly onto wonton strips; sprinkle evenly with sesame seeds.

4. Bake 6 to 8 minutes or until lightly browned. Remove to wire rack; cool completely. Transfer to serving plate.
Makes 8 servings

Nutrients per Serving: (10 pieces), Calories: 75 (24% Calories from Fat), Total Fat: 2 g, Saturated Fat: trace, Protein: 2 g, Carbohydrate: 12 g, Cholesterol: 3 mg, Sodium: 116 mg, Fiber: trace, Sugar: 0

Dietary Exchanges: 1 Starch/Bread

AMAZING APPETIZERS

67 HERBED POTATO CHIPS

Nonstick olive oil-flavored cooking spray
2 medium-sized red potatoes (about
    ½ pound), unpeeled
1 tablespoon olive oil
2 tablespoons minced fresh dill, thyme or
    rosemary *or* 2 teaspoons dried dill
    weed, thyme or rosemary
¼ teaspoon garlic salt
⅛ teaspoon black pepper
1¼ cups nonfat sour cream

1. Preheat oven to 450°F. Spray large nonstick baking sheets with cooking spray; set aside.

2. Cut potatoes crosswise into very thin slices, about ¹⁄₁₆ inch thick. Pat dry with paper towels. Arrange potato slices in single layer on prepared baking sheets; coat potatoes with cooking spray.

3. Bake 10 minutes; turn slices over. Brush with oil. Combine dill, garlic salt and pepper in small bowl; sprinkle evenly onto potato slices. Continue baking 5 to 10 minutes or until potatoes are golden brown. Cool on baking sheets.

4. Serve with sour cream.

Makes about 60 chips

Nutrients per Serving: (10 chips, about 3 tablespoons sour cream), Calories: 76 (26% Calories from Fat), Total Fat: 2 g, Saturated Fat: trace, Protein: 6 g, Carbohydrate: 9 g, Cholesterol: 0 mg, Sodium: 113 mg, Fiber: trace, Sugar: 0 g

Dietary Exchanges: ½ Starch/Bread, ½ Lean Meat, ½ Fat

68 SOUTHWEST SNACK MIX

4 cups corn cereal squares
2 cups unsalted pretzels
½ cup unsalted pumpkin or squash seeds
1½ teaspoons chili powder
1 teaspoon minced fresh cilantro or
    parsley
½ teaspoon garlic powder
½ teaspoon onion powder
1 egg white
2 tablespoons olive oil
2 tablespoons lime juice

1. Preheat oven to 300°F. Spray large nonstick baking sheet with nonstick cooking spray.

2. Combine cereal, pretzels and pumpkin seeds in large bowl. Combine chili powder, cilantro, garlic powder and onion powder in small bowl.

3. Whisk together egg white, oil and lime juice in separate small bowl. Pour over cereal mixture; toss to coat evenly. Add seasoning mixture; mix lightly to coat evenly. Transfer to prepared baking sheet.

4. Bake 45 minutes, stirring every 15 minutes; cool. Store in airtight container.

Makes 12 servings

VARIATION: Substitute ½ cup unsalted peanuts for pumpkin seeds.

Nutrients per Serving: Calories: 93 (28% Calories from Fat), Total Fat: 3 g, Saturated Fat: trace, Protein: 2 g, Carbohydrate: 15 g, Cholesterol: 0 mg, Sodium: 114 mg, Fiber: 1 g, Sugar: 1 g

Dietary Exchanges: 1 Starch/Bread, ½ Fat

Herbed Potato Chips

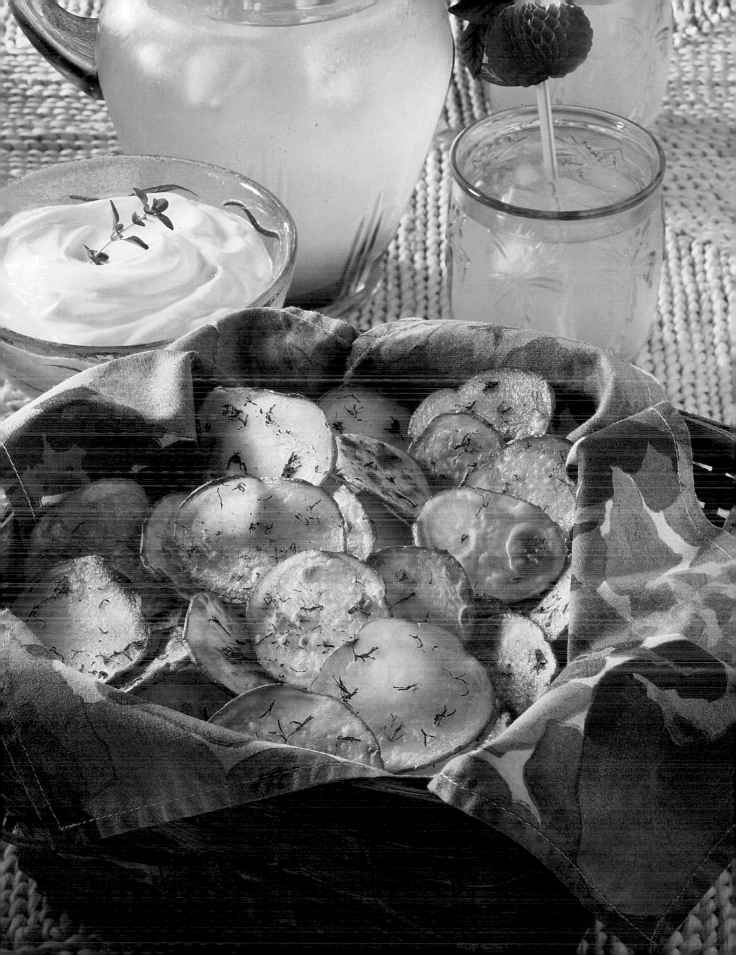

AMAZING APPETIZERS

69 TRAIL MIX TRUFFLES

⅓ **cup dried apples**
¼ **cup dried apricots**
¼ **cup apple butter**
2 **tablespoons golden raisins**
1 **tablespoon reduced-fat peanut butter**
½ **cup low-fat granola**
¼ **cup graham cracker crumbs, divided**
¼ **cup mini chocolate chips**

Blend fruit, apple butter, raisins and peanut butter in food processor until smooth. Stir in granola, 1 tablespoon crumbs, chips and 1 tablespoon water. Place remaining crumbs in bowl. Shape tablespoonfuls mixture into balls; roll in crumbs. Cover; refrigerate until ready to serve.   *Makes 8 servings*

Nutrients per Serving: Calories: 121 (30 % Calories from Fat), Total Fat: 4 g, Saturated Fat: 1 g, Protein: 3 g, Carbohydrate: 20 g, Cholesterol: 0 mg, Sodium: 14 mg, Fiber: 2 g, Sugar: 8 g

Dietary Exchanges: 1 Starch/Bread, ½ Fruit, ½ Fat

70 CINNAMON CARAMEL CORN

8 **cups air-popped popcorn (about** ⅓ **cup kernels)**
2 **tablespoons honey**
4 **teaspoons margarine**
¼ **teaspoon ground cinnamon**

1. Preheat oven to 350°F. Spray jelly-roll pan with nonstick cooking spray. Place popcorn in large bowl.

2. Stir honey, margarine and cinnamon in small saucepan over low heat until margarine is melted and mixture is smooth; immediately pour over popcorn. Toss with

spoon to coat evenly. Pour onto prepared pan; bake 12 to 14 minutes or until coating is golden brown and appears crackled, stirring twice. Let cool on pan 5 minutes. (As popcorn cools, coating becomes crisp. If not crisp enough, or if popcorn softens upon standing, return to oven and heat 5 to 8 minutes more.)   *Makes 4 servings*

Nutrients per Serving: Calories: 117 (29% Calories from Fat), Total Fat: 4 g, Saturated Fat: 1 g, Protein: 2 g, Carbohydrate: 19 g, Cholesterol: 0 mg, Sodium: 45 mg, Fiber: 1 g, Sugar: 9 g

Dietary Exchanges: 1 Starch/Bread, 1 Fat

CAJUN POPCORN: Preheat oven and prepare jelly-roll pan as directed above. Combine 7 teaspoons honey, 4 teaspoons margarine and 1 teaspoon Cajun or Creole seasoning in small saucepan. Proceed with recipe as directed above. Makes 4 servings.

Nutrients per Serving: Calories: 122 (28% Calories from Fat), Total Fat: 4 g, Saturated Fat: 1 g, Protein: 2 g, Carbohydrate: 20 g, Cholesterol: 0 mg, Sodium: 91 mg, Fiber: 1 g, Sugar: 10 g

Dietary Exchanges: 1½ Starch/Bread, ½ Fat

ITALIAN POPCORN: Spray 8 cups of air-popped popcorn with fat-free butter-flavored spray to coat. Sprinkle with 2 tablespoons finely grated Parmesan cheese, ⅛ teaspoon black pepper and ½ teaspoon dried oregano leaves. Gently toss to coat. Makes 4 servings.

Nutrients per Serving: Calories: 65 (14% Calories from Fat), Total Fat: 1 g, Saturated Fat: 1 g, Protein: 3 g, Carbohydrate: 10 g, Cholesterol: 2 mg, Sodium: 58 mg, Fiber: 1 g, Sugar: 0 g

Dietary Exchanges: 1 Starch/Bread

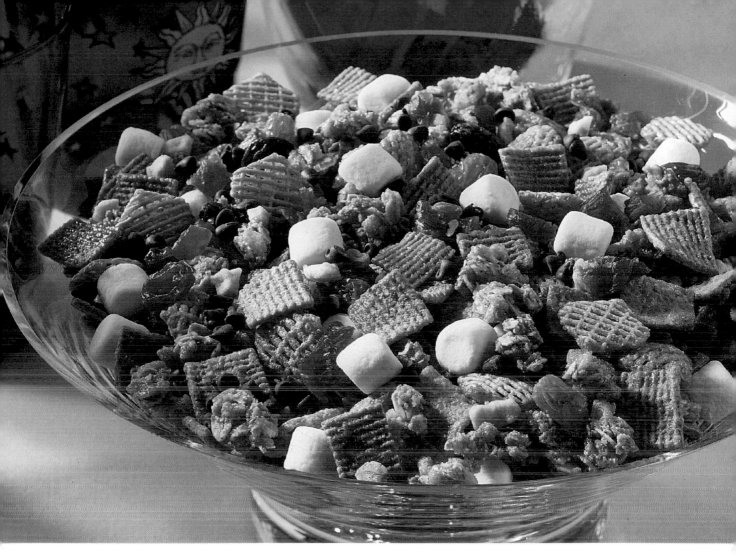

S'More Gorp

71 S'MORE GORP

2 cups honey graham cereal
2 cups low-fat granola cereal
2 cups crispy multi-bran cereal squares
2 tablespoons reduced-calorie margarine
1 tablespoon honey
¼ teaspoon ground cinnamon
¾ cup miniature marshmallows
½ cup dried fruit bits or raisins
¼ cup mini semisweet chocolate chips

1. Preheat oven to 275°F.

2. Combine cereals in nonstick 15×10×1-inch jelly-roll pan. Melt margarine in small saucepan; stir in honey and cinnamon. Pour margarine mixture evenly over cereal mixture; toss until cereals are well coated. Spread mixture evenly onto bottom of pan.

3. Bake 35 to 40 minutes or until crisp, stirring after 20 minutes. Cool completely.

4. Add marshmallows, fruit bits and chocolate chips; toss to mix.

Makes 16 servings

Nutrients per Serving: Calories 137 (17% Calories from Fat), Total Fat: 3 g, Saturated Fat: trace, Protein: 3 g, Carbohydrate: 28 g, Cholesterol: trace, Sodium: 138 mg, Fiber: 1 g, Sugar: 8 g

Dietary Exchanges: 1½ Starch/Bread, ½ Fat

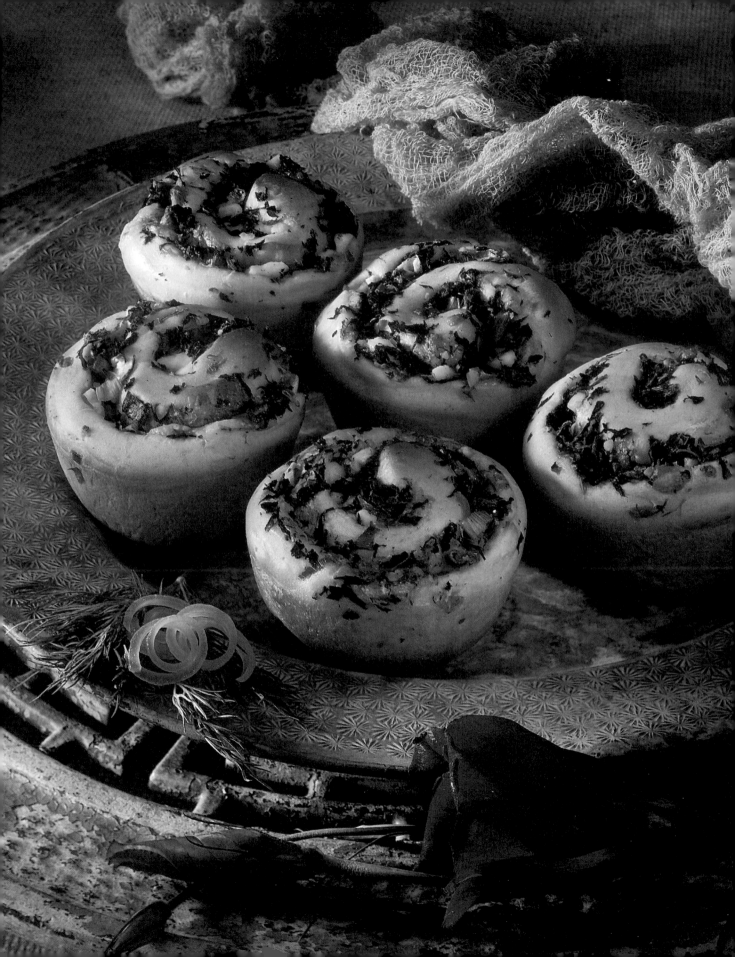

72 GREEK SPINACH–CHEESE ROLLS

1 loaf (1 pound) frozen bread dough
1 package (10 ounces) frozen chopped
   spinach, thawed and squeezed dry
¾ cup (3 ounces) crumbled feta cheese
½ cup (2 ounces) shredded reduced-fat
   Monterey Jack cheese
4 green onions, thinly sliced
1 teaspoon dried dill weed
½ teaspoon garlic powder
½ teaspoon black pepper

1. Thaw bread dough according to package directions. Spray 15 muffin cups with nonstick cooking spray; set aside. Roll out dough on lightly floured surface to 15×9-inch rectangle. (If dough is springy and difficult to roll, cover with plastic wrap and let rest 5 minutes to relax.) Position dough so long edge runs parallel to edge of work surface.

2. Combine spinach, cheeses, green onions, dill weed, garlic powder and pepper in large bowl; mix well.

3. Sprinkle spinach mixture evenly over dough to within 1 inch of long edges. Starting at long edge, roll up snugly, pinching seam closed. Place seam side down; cut roll with serrated knife into 1-inch-wide slices. Place slices cut sides up in prepared muffin cups. Cover with plastic wrap; let stand 30 minutes in warm place until rolls are slightly puffy.

4. Preheat oven to 375°F. Bake 20 to 25 minutes or until golden. Serve warm or at room temperature. Rolls can be stored in refrigerator in airtight container up to 2 days.   *Makes 15 servings (1 roll each)*

Nutrients per Serving: Calories: 111 (24% Calories from Fat), Total Fat: 3 g, Saturated Fat: 2 g, Protein: 5 g, Carbohydrate: 16 g, Cholesterol: 8 mg, Sodium: 267 mg, Fiber: trace, Sugar: trace

Dietary Exchanges: 1 Starch/Bread, ½ Lean Meat, ½ Fat

73 BEAN TORTILLA PINWHEELS

8 corn tortillas (6 inches each)
1 cup GUILTLESS GOURMET® Bean Dip
   (Black or Pinto, mild or spicy)

To soften tortillas, stack 4 tortillas and wrap in damp paper towel. Microwave on HIGH (100% power) 20 seconds. Or, to soften tortillas in oven, preheat oven to 300°F. Wrap tortillas in foil. Bake 10 minutes.

Spread 2 tablespoons bean dip on each tortilla and roll up tightly. Evenly place toothpicks through rolls, using 6 toothpicks per tortilla. Carefully cut between toothpicks to maintain round shape and obtain 6 pinwheels per tortilla. Serve immediately.   *Makes 48 pinwheels*

Nutrients per Serving: (1 bean pinwheel), Calories: 14 (6% of Calories from Fat), Total Fat: trace, Saturated Fat: 0 g, Protein: trace, Carbohydrate: 3 g, Cholesterol: 0 mg, Sodium: 24 mg, Fiber: 0 g

Dietary Exchanges: Free

Greek Spinach-Cheese Rolls

AMAZING APPETIZERS

74 ROASTED EGGPLANT ROLLS

2 medium eggplants (¾ pound each)
2 tablespoons lemon juice
1 teaspoon olive oil
4 tablespoons (2 ounces) fat-free cream cheese
2 tablespoons nonfat sour cream
1 green onion, minced
4 sun-dried tomatoes (packed in oil), drained and minced
1 clove garlic, minced
¼ teaspoon dried oregano leaves
⅛ teaspoon black pepper
16 medium spinach leaves, washed and stemmed
1 cup spaghetti sauce

1. Preheat oven to 450°F. Spray 2 nonstick baking sheets with nonstick cooking spray; set aside. Trim ends from eggplants; cut lengthwise into ¼-inch-thick slices. Discard outside slices that are mostly skin. (You will have about 16 slices.)

2. Combine lemon juice and olive oil in small bowl; brush lightly over both sides of eggplant slices. Arrange slices in single layer on baking sheets. Bake 10 to 12 minutes or until slightly golden brown on bottom. Turn slices over and bake 10 to 12 minutes more or until golden on both sides and tender. (Slices may not brown evenly; turn slices as they brown. Some very dark spots will occur.) Transfer slices to plate; cool.

3. Meanwhile, stir cream cheese in small bowl until smooth. Add sour cream, green onion, tomatoes, garlic, oregano and pepper; stir until blended.

4. Place eggplant slices on work surface; spread about 1 teaspoon cream cheese mixture evenly over each slice. Arrange spinach leaves on top leaving ½-inch border.

Roll up, beginning at narrower end; lay rolls seam sides down on serving platter. (If making ahead, cover and refrigerate up to 2 days. Bring to room temperature before serving.) Serve with warm spaghetti sauce.

Makes 8 servings (2 rolls each)

Nutrients per Serving: Calories: 77 (27% Calories from Fat), Total Fat: 3 g, Saturated Fat: trace, Protein: 3 g, Carbohydrate: 12 g, Cholesterol: 0 mg, Sodium: 213 mg, Fiber: trace, Sugar: trace

Dietary Exchanges: 2 Vegetable, ½ Fat

75 CALIFORNIA ROLLS

1 cup reduced-fat ricotta cheese
2 (11-inch) flour tortillas
1 tomato, thinly sliced
2 cups spinach leaves, washed, stemmed and torn
1 cup chopped onion
½ teaspoon dried oregano leaves
½ teaspoon dried basil leaves
1 cup alfalfa sprouts
4 ounces sliced turkey breast

Spread cheese evenly over tortillas to within ¼ inch of edges. Layer tomato, spinach, onion, oregano, basil, alfalfa sprouts and turkey over ⅔ of each tortilla. Roll up tortillas. Wrap in plastic wrap; refrigerate 1 hour. Cut crosswise into 10 slices.

Makes 4 servings

Nutrients per Serving: Calories: 209 (17 % Calories from Fat), Total Fat: 4 g, Saturated Fat: trace, Protein: 16 g, Carbohydrate: 28 g, Cholesterol: 28 mg, Sodium: 233 mg, Fiber: 2 g, Sugar: 2 g

Dietary Exchanges: 1½ Starch/Bread, 1½ Lean Meat, 1 Vegetable

AMAZING APPETIZERS

76 TURKEY–BROCCOLI ROLL–UPS

2 pounds broccoli
1/3 cup nonfat sour cream
1/4 cup reduced-calorie mayonnaise
2 tablespoons frozen orange juice concentrate, thawed
1 tablespoon Dijon mustard
1 teaspoon dried basil leaves
1 pound smoked turkey, very thinly sliced

1. Trim large leaves and tough ends of lower stalks from broccoli; discard. Wash broccoli. Cut stalks lengthwise, including florets, to form approximately 40 (3-inch) spears.

2. Arrange broccoli spears in single layer in large, shallow microwavable dish. Add 1 tablespoon water. Cover dish tightly with plastic wrap; vent. Microwave at HIGH 6 to 7 minutes or just until broccoli is crisp-tender, rearranging spears after 4 minutes. Carefully remove plastic wrap; drain broccoli. Immediately place broccoli in cold water to prevent additional cooking; drain. Pat dry with paper towels.

3. Combine sour cream, mayonnaise, orange juice concentrate, mustard and basil in small bowl; mix well.

4. Cut turkey slices into 2-inch-wide strips. Spread sour cream mixture evenly onto strips. Place 1 broccoli piece at short end of each strip. Starting at short end, roll up tightly (allow broccoli floret to protrude from one end). Cover and refrigerate until ready to serve. *Makes 20 servings*

Nutrients per Serving: (2 pieces),
Calories: 51 (19% Calories from Fat),
Total Fat: 1 g, Saturated Fat: trace, Protein: 7 g,
Carbohydrate: 4 g, Cholesterol: 10 mg,
Sodium: 259 mg, Fiber: 2 g, Sugar: 2 g

Dietary Exchanges: 1 Lean Meat

77 ROASTED GARLIC & SPINACH SPIRALS

1 whole head garlic
1 can (15 ounces) white beans, rinsed and drained
1 teaspoon dried oregano leaves
1/4 teaspoon black pepper
1/8 teaspoon ground red pepper
3 cups fresh spinach leaves, washed, stemmed and shredded
7 (7-inch) flour tortillas

1. Preheat oven to 400°F. Trim top of garlic just enough to cut tips off center cloves; discard. Moisten head of garlic with water; wrap in foil. Bake 45 minutes or until garlic is soft and has a mellow garlicky aroma; cool. Remove garlic from skin by squeezing between fingers and thumb and place in food processor.

2. Add beans, oregano, black pepper and red pepper to food processor; process until smooth.

3. Place spinach in medium bowl. Add bean mixture; mix well. Spread mixture evenly onto tortillas; roll up. Trim 1/2 inch off ends of rolls; discard. Cut rolls crosswise into 1-inch slices. *Makes 10 servings*

Nutrients per Serving: (4 pieces),
Calories: 139 (13% Calories from Fat),
Total Fat: 2 g, Saturated Fat: trace, Protein: 6 g,
Carbohydrate: 25 g, Cholesterol: 0 mg,
Sodium: 293 mg, Fiber: 1 g, Sugar: trace

Dietary Exchanges: 1½ Starch/Bread,
1 Vegetable

AMAZING APPETIZERS

78 ROCK 'N' ROLLERS

4 (6- to 7-inch) flour tortillas
4 ounces Neufchâtel cheese, softened
⅓ cup peach preserves
1 cup (4 ounces) shredded nonfat Cheddar cheese
½ cup packed washed spinach leaves
3 ounces thinly sliced regular or smoked turkey breast

1. Spread each tortilla evenly with 1 ounce Neufchâtel cheese; cover with thin layer of preserves. Sprinkle with Cheddar cheese.

2. Arrange spinach leaves and turkey over Cheddar cheese. Roll up tortillas; trim ends. Cover and refrigerate until ready to serve.

3. Cut "rollers" crosswise in half or diagonally into 1-inch pieces.

Makes 8 servings

SASSY SALSA ROLLERS: Substitute salsa for peach preserves and shredded iceberg lettuce for spinach leaves.

HAM 'N' APPLE ROLLERS: Omit peach preserves and spinach leaves. Substitute lean ham slices for turkey. Spread tortillas with Neufchâtel cheese as directed; sprinkle with Cheddar cheese. Top each tortilla with about 2 tablespoons finely chopped apple and 2 ham slices; roll up. Continue as directed.

WEDGIES: Prepare Rock 'n' Rollers or any variation as directed, but do not roll up. Top with a second tortilla; cut into wedges.

Nutrients per Serving: Calories: 339 (26% Calories from Fat), Total Fat: 10 g, Saturated Fat: 5 g, Protein: 22 g, Carbohydrate: 40 g, Cholesterol: 48 mg, Sodium: 505 mg, Fiber: 1 g, Sugar: 16 g

Dietary Exchanges: 2½ Starch/Bread, 2 Lean Meat, 1 Fat

79 CINNAMON–RAISIN ROLL–UPS

4 ounces Neufchâtel cheese, softened
½ cup shredded carrot
¼ cup golden or regular raisins
1 tablespoon honey
¼ teaspoon ground cinnamon
4 (7- to 8-inch) whole wheat or flour tortillas
8 thin apple wedges (optional)

1. Combine Neufchâtel cheese, carrot, raisins, honey and cinnamon in small bowl; mix well.

2. Spread tortillas evenly with Neufchâtel mixture, leaving ½-inch border around edge of each tortilla. Place 2 apple wedges down center of each tortilla; roll up. Wrap in plastic wrap. Refrigerate until ready to serve. *Makes 4 servings*

Nutrients per Serving: Calories: 240 (32% Calories from Fat), Total Fat: 9 g, Saturated Fat: 4 g, Protein: 7 g, Carbohydrate: 34 mg, Cholesterol: 25 mg, Sodium: 127 mg, Fiber: 1 g, Sugar: 12 g

Dietary Exchanges: 1½ Starch/Bread, ½ Lean Meat, ½ Fruit, ½ Vegetable, 1½ Fat

Rock 'n' Rollers

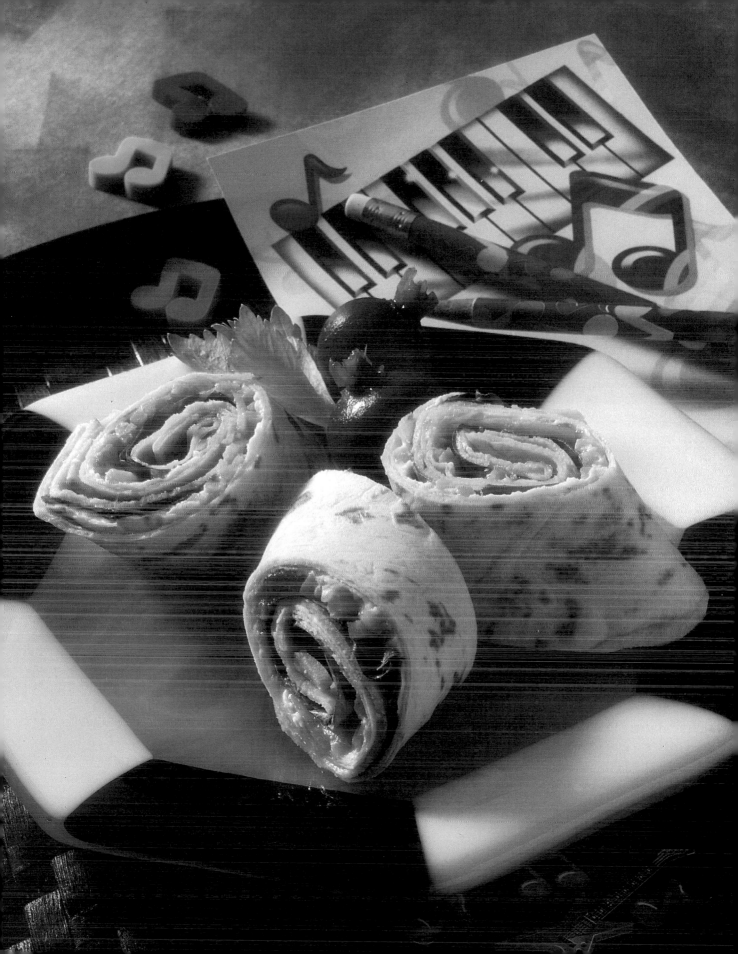

AMAZING APPETIZERS

80 JICAMA & SHRIMP COCKTAIL WITH ROASTED RED PEPPER SAUCE

2 large red bell peppers
6 ounces (about 24 medium-large) shrimp, peeled and deveined
1 medium clove garlic
1½ cups fresh cilantro sprigs
2 tablespoons lime juice
2 tablespoons orange juice
½ teaspoon hot pepper sauce
1 small jicama (about ¾ pound), peeled and cut into strips
1 plum tomato, halved, seeded and thinly sliced

1. Place bell peppers on broiler pan. Broil, 4 to 6 inches from heat, about 6 minutes, turning every 2 to 3 minutes or until all sides are charred. Transfer peppers to paper bag; close bag tightly. Let stand 10 minutes or until peppers are cool enough to handle and skins are loosened. Peel peppers; cut in half. Remove cores, seeds and membranes; discard.

2. Add shrimp to large saucepan of boiling water. Reduce heat to medium-low; simmer, uncovered, 2 to 3 minutes or until shrimp turn pink. Drain shrimp; rinse under cold running water. Cover; refrigerate until ready to use.

3. Place peppers and garlic in food processor; process until peppers are

Jicama & Shrimp Cocktail with Roasted Red Pepper Sauce

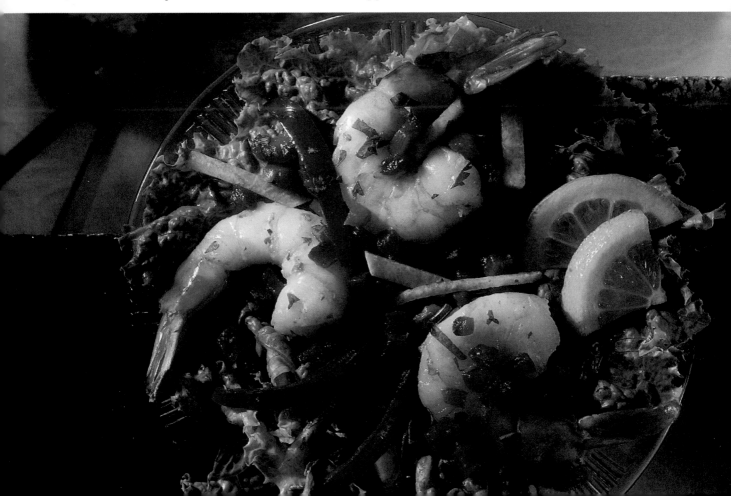

AMAZING APPETIZERS

coarsely chopped. Add cilantro, lime juice, orange juice and pepper sauce; process until cilantro is finely chopped but mixture is not puréed.

4. Combine jicama, shrimp and tomato in large bowl. Add bell pepper mixture; toss to coat evenly. Serve over lettuce.

Makes 8 servings

Nutrients per Serving: Calories: 69 (7% Calories from Fat), Total Fat: 1 g, Saturated Fat: trace, Protein: 6 g, Carbohydrate: 10 g, Cholesterol: 42 mg, Sodium: 120 mg, Fiber: 1 g, Sugar: 1 g

Dietary Exchanges: ½ Lean Meat, 2 Vegetable

81 CRAB CANAPÉS

⅔ cup fat-free cream cheese, softened
2 teaspoons lemon juice
1 teaspoon hot pepper sauce
1 package (8 ounces) imitation crabmeat or lobster, flaked
⅓ cup chopped red bell pepper
2 green onions with tops, sliced
64 cucumber slices (about 2½ medium cucumbers cut ⅜ inch thick) or melba toast rounds

1. Combine cream cheese, lemon juice and pepper sauce in medium bowl; mix well. Stir in crabmeat, bell pepper and green onions; cover. Chill until ready to serve.

2. When ready to serve, spoon 1½ teaspoons crab mixture onto each cucumber slice.

Makes 16 servings

Nutrients per Serving: (4 pieces), Calories: 31 (8% Calories from Fat), Total Fat: trace, Saturated Fat: trace, Protein: 4 g, Carbohydrate: 4 g, Cholesterol: 5 mg, Sodium: 178 mg, Fiber: trace, Sugar: trace

Dietary Exchanges: ½ Lean Meat

82 SMOKED SALMON APPETIZERS

¼ cup Neufchâtel or fat-free cream cheese, softened
1 tablespoon chopped fresh dill *or* 1 teaspoon dried dill weed
⅛ teaspoon ground red pepper
4 ounces thinly sliced smoked salmon or lox
24 melba toast rounds or other low-fat crackers

1. Combine Neufchâtel cheese, dill and pepper in small bowl; stir to blend. Spread evenly over each slice of salmon. Starting with short side, roll up salmon slices jelly-roll fashion. Place on plate; cover with plastic wrap. Chill at least 1 hour or up to 4 hours before serving.

2. Using a sharp knife, cut salmon rolls crosswise into ¾-inch pieces. Place pieces, cut side down, on serving plate. Garnish each piece with dill sprig, if desired. Serve cold or at room temperature with melba rounds.

Makes 8 servings

Nutrients per Serving: (3 appetizers per serving), Calories: 80 (21% Calories from Fat), Total Fat: 2 g, Saturated Fat: 1 g, Protein: 6 g, Carbohydrate: 10 g, Cholesterol: 6 mg, Sodium: 241 mg, Fiber: 1 g, Sugar: 0 g

Dietary Exchanges: ½ Starch/Bread, ½ Lean Meat

AMAZING APPETIZERS

83 SOUTHERN CRAB CAKES WITH RÉMOULADE DIPPING SAUCE

10 ounces fresh lump crabmeat
1½ cups fresh white bread crumbs, divided
¼ cup chopped green onions
½ cup nonfat or reduced-fat mayonnaise, divided
2 tablespoons coarse grain or spicy brown mustard, divided
¾ teaspoon hot pepper sauce, divided
1 egg white, lightly beaten
2 teaspoons olive oil, divided
Lemon wedges

1. Preheat oven to 200°F. Combine crabmeat, ¾ cup bread crumbs and green onions in medium bowl. Add ¼ cup mayonnaise, 1 tablespoon mustard, ½ teaspoon pepper sauce and egg white; mix well. Using ¼ cup mixture per cake, shape eight ½-inch-thick cakes. Roll crab cakes lightly in remaining ¾ cup bread crumbs.

2. Heat large nonstick skillet over medium heat until hot; add 1 teaspoon oil. Add 4 crab cakes; cook 4 to 5 minutes per side or until golden brown. Transfer to serving platter; keep warm in oven. Repeat with remaining 1 teaspoon oil and crab cakes.

3. To prepare dipping sauce, combine remaining ¼ cup mayonnaise, 1 tablespoon mustard and ¼ teaspoon pepper sauce in small bowl; mix well.

4. Serve warm crab cakes with lemon wedges and dipping sauce.

Makes 8 servings

Nutrients per Serving: Calories: 81 (25% Calories from Fat), Total Fat: 2 g, Saturated Fat: trace, Protein: 7 g, Carbohydrate: 8 g, Cholesterol: 30 mg, Sodium: 376 mg, Fiber: trace, Sugar: trace

Dietary Exchanges: ½ Starch/Bread, 1 Lean Meat

84 PINEAPPLE GINGER SHRIMP COCKTAIL

9 fresh pineapple spears (about 1 package), divided
¼ cup all-fruit apricot preserves
1 tablespoon finely chopped onion
½ teaspoon grated fresh ginger
⅛ teaspoon black pepper
8 ounces cooked medium shrimp (about 30)
1 red or green bell pepper, cut into 12 strips

1. Chop 3 pineapple spears into bite-sized pieces; combine with preserves, onion, ginger and black pepper in medium bowl.

2. Evenly arrange shrimp, bell pepper strips and remaining pineapple spears on 6 small plates lined with lettuce leaves, if desired. Add one spoonful of pineapple mixture to each plate. *Makes 6 servings*

Nutrients per Serving: Calories: 108 (6% Calories from Fat), Total Fat: 1 g, Saturated Fat: trace, Protein: 7 g, Carbohydrate: 20 g, Cholesterol: 58 mg, Sodium: 69 mg, Fiber: 2 g, Sugar 7 g

Dietary Exchanges: 1 Lean Meat, ½ Fruit, 1 Vegetable

Southern Crab Cakes with Rémoulade Dipping Sauce

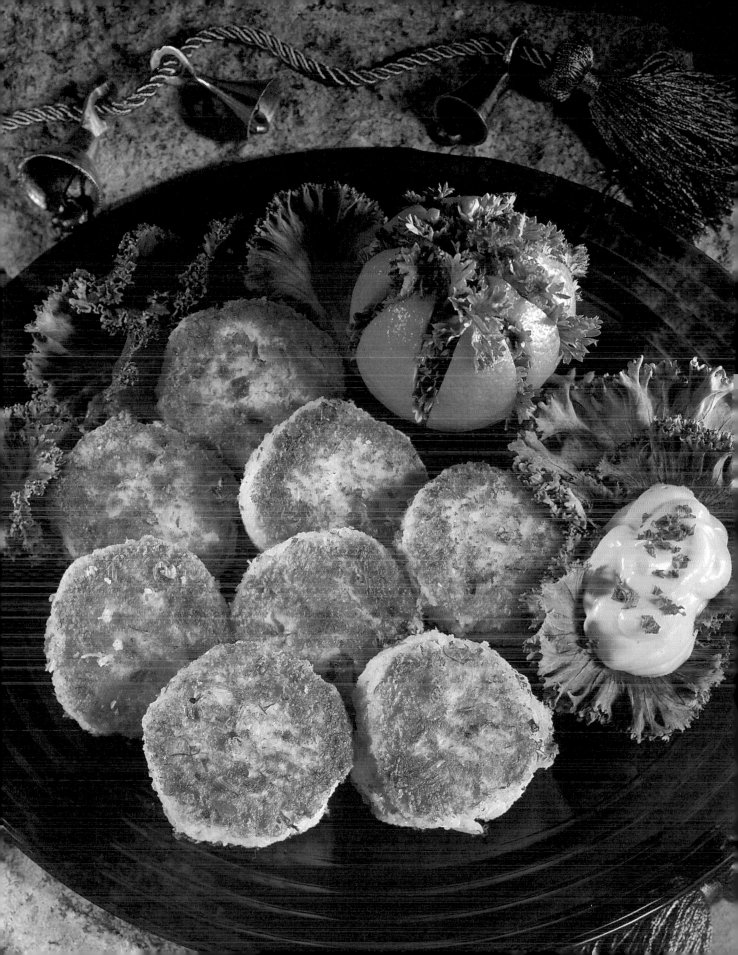

85 TUSCAN WHITE BEAN CROSTINI

2 cans (15 ounces each) Great Northern
   or cannellini beans, rinsed and
   drained
½ large red bell pepper, finely chopped *or*
   ⅓ cup finely chopped roasted red bell
   pepper
⅓ cup finely chopped onion
⅓ cup red wine vinegar
3 tablespoons chopped parsley
1 tablespoon olive oil
2 cloves garlic, minced
½ teaspoon dried oregano leaves
¼ teaspoon black pepper
18 French bread slices, about ¼ inch thick

1. Combine beans, bell pepper and onion in large bowl.

2. Whisk together vinegar, parsley, oil, garlic, oregano and black pepper in small bowl. Pour over bean mixture; toss to coat. Cover; refrigerate 2 hours or overnight.

3. Arrange bread slices in single layer on large nonstick baking sheet or broiler pan. Broil, 6 to 8 inches from heat, 30 to 45 seconds or until bread slices are lightly toasted. Remove; cool completely.

4. Top each toasted bread slice with about 3 tablespoons of bean mixture.

Makes 6 servings

Nutrients per Serving: Calories: 317 (12% Calories from Fat), Total Fat: 4 g, Saturated Fat: 1 g, Protein: 15 g, Carbohydrate: 57 g, Cholesterol: 0 mg, Sodium: 800 mg, Fiber: 1 g, Sugar: trace

Dietary Exchanges: 2 Starch/Bread, 1 Vegetable, ½ Fat

86 MEDITERRANEAN PITA PIZZAS

1 cup rinsed and drained canned
   cannellini beans
2 teaspoons lemon juice
2 medium cloves garlic, minced
2 (8-inch) rounds pita bread
1 teaspoon olive oil
½ cup thinly sliced radicchio or escarole
   lettuce (optional)
½ cup chopped seeded tomato
½ cup finely chopped red onion
¼ cup (1 ounce) crumbled feta cheese
2 tablespoons thinly sliced pitted black
   olives

1. Preheat oven to 450°F.

2. Place beans in small bowl; mash lightly with fork. Stir in lemon juice and garlic.

3. Arrange pitas on baking sheet; brush tops with oil. Bake 6 minutes.

4. Spread bean mixture evenly onto pita rounds to within ½ inch of edges. Arrange remaining ingredients evenly on pitas. Bake 5 minutes or until topping is thoroughly heated and crust is crisp. Cut into quarters. Serve hot. *Makes 8 servings*

Nutrients per Serving: Calories: 98 (29% Calories from Fat), Total Fat: 3 g, Saturated Fat: 1 g, Protein: 4 g, Carbohydrate: 14 g, Cholesterol: 7 mg, Sodium: 282 mg, Fiber: 2 g, Sugar: 1 g

Dietary Exchanges: 1 Starch/Bread, ½ Fat

Mediterranean Pita Pizzas

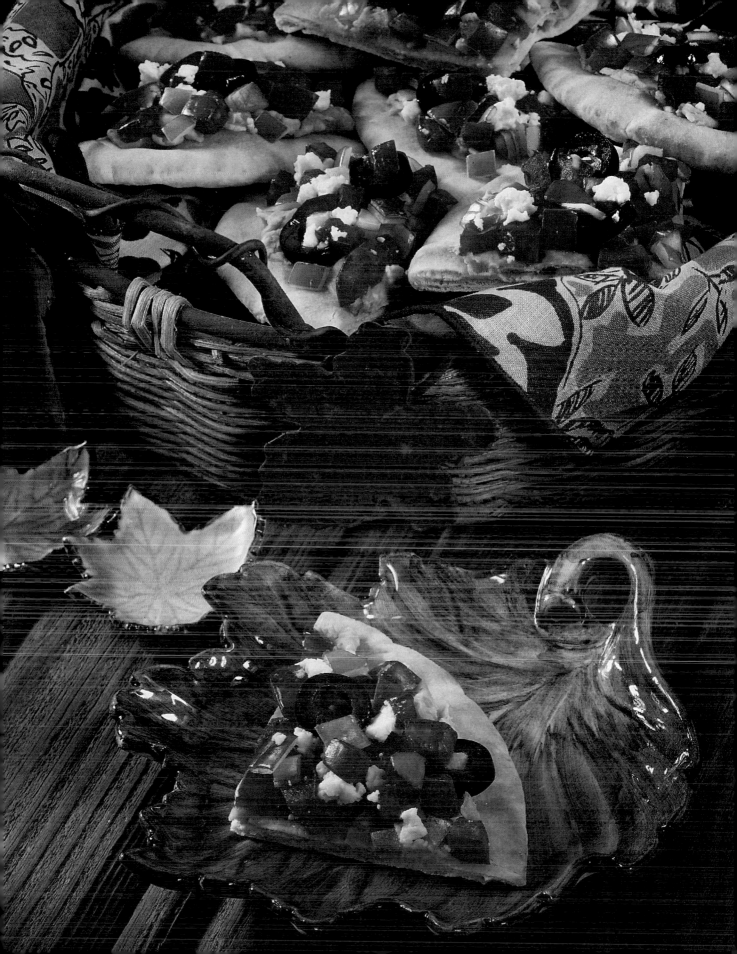

87 HERBED BLUE CHEESE SPREAD WITH GARLIC TOASTS

1⅓ cups 1% low-fat cottage cheese
1¼ cups (5 ounces) crumbled blue, feta or
    goat cheese
1 large clove garlic
2 teaspoons lemon juice
2 green onions with tops, sliced
¼ cup chopped fresh basil or oregano *or*
    1 teaspoon dried basil or oregano
    leaves
2 tablespoons toasted slivered almonds
2 teaspoons lemon juice
    Garlic Toasts (recipe follows)

1. Combine cottage cheese, blue cheese, garlic and lemon juice in food processor; process until smooth. Add green onions, basil and almonds; pulse until well blended but still chunky.

2. Spoon cheese spread into small serving bowl; cover. Refrigerate until ready to serve.

3. When ready to serve, prepare Garlic Toasts. Spread 1 tablespoon cheese spread onto each toast slice.

Makes 16 servings

GARLIC TOASTS
32 French bread slices, ½ inch thick
    Nonstick cooking spray
¼ teaspoon garlic powder
⅛ teaspoon salt

1. Place bread slices on nonstick baking sheet. Lightly coat both sides of bread slices with cooking spray. Combine garlic powder and salt in small bowl; sprinkle evenly onto bread slices. Broil, 6 to 8 inches from heat, 30 to 45 seconds on each side or until bread slices are lightly toasted on both sides.

Makes 32 pieces

Nutrients per Serving: (2 pieces),
Calories: 189 (23% Calories from Fat),
Total Fat: 5 g, Saturated Fat: 2 g, Protein: 9 g,
Carbohydrate: 27 g, Cholesterol: 7 mg,
Sodium: 521 mg, Fiber: trace, Sugar: 1 g

Dietary Exchanges: 2 Starch/Bread, 1 Fat

88 TOASTED PESTO ROUNDS

¼ cup thinly sliced fresh basil or chopped
    fresh dill
¼ cup (1 ounce) grated Parmesan cheese
1 medium clove garlic, minced
3 tablespoons reduced-calorie mayonnaise
12 French bread slices, about ¼ inch thick
4 teaspoons drained chopped tomato
1 green onion with top, sliced
    Black pepper

1. Preheat broiler.

2. Combine basil, cheese, garlic and mayonnaise in small bowl; mix well.

3. Arrange bread slices in single layer on large nonstick baking sheet or broiler pan. Broil, 6 to 8 inches from heat, 30 to 45 seconds or until bread slices are lightly toasted.

4. Turn bread slices over; spread evenly with basil mixture. Broil 1 minute or until lightly browned. Top evenly with tomato and green onion. Season to taste with pepper. Transfer to serving plate. *Makes 12 servings*

Nutrients per Serving: Calories: 90
(25% Calories from Fat), Total Fat: 2 g,
Saturated Fat: 1 g, Protein: 3 g,
Carbohydrate: 14 g, Cholesterol: 3 mg,
Sodium: 195 mg, Fiber: trace, Sugar: trace

Dietary Exchanges: 1 Starch/Bread, ½ Fat

AMAZING APPETIZERS

89 BRUSCHETTA

Nonstick cooking spray
1 cup thinly sliced onion
½ cup chopped seeded tomato
2 tablespoons capers
¼ teaspoon black pepper
3 cloves garlic, finely chopped
1 teaspoon olive oil
4 slices French bread
½ cup (2 ounces) shredded reduced-fat
    Monterey Jack cheese

1. Spray large skillet with cooking spray; heat over medium heat until hot. Add onion; cook and stir 5 minutes. Stir in tomato, capers and pepper; cook 3 minutes.

2. Preheat broiler. Combine garlic and oil in small bowl; brush slices with mixture. Top with onion mixture; sprinkle with cheese. Place slices on baking sheet. Broil 3 minutes or until cheese melts.　　*Makes 4 servings*

Nutrients per Serving: Calories: 90 (20 % Calories from Fat),Total Fat: 2 g, Saturated Fat: trace, Protein: 3 g, Carbohydrate: 17 g, Cholesterol: 0 mg, Sodium: 104 mg, Fiber: trace, Sugar: 1 g

Dietary Exchanges: 1 Starch/Bread

Bruschetta

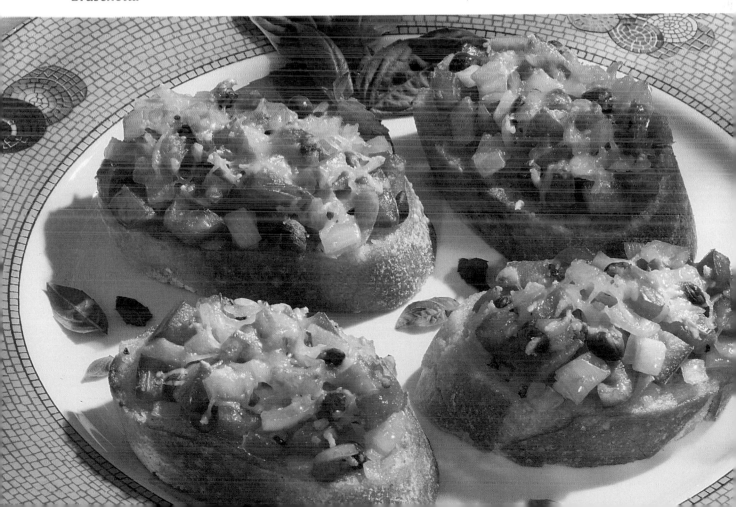

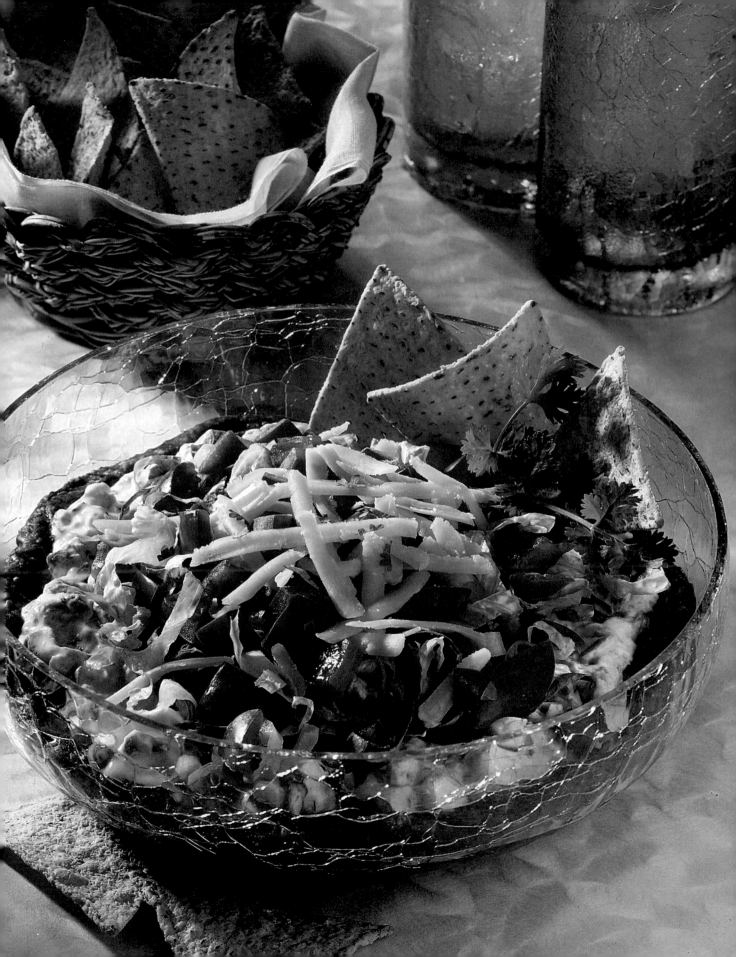

AMAZING APPETIZERS

90 FIVE–LAYERED MEXICAN DIP

½ cup low fat sour cream
½ cup GUILTLESS GOURMET® Salsa (medium)
1 jar (12.5 ounces) GUILTLESS GOURMET® Bean Dip (Black or Pinto, mild or spicy)
2 cups shredded lettuce
½ cup chopped tomato
¼ cup (1 ounce) shredded sharp Cheddar cheese
Chopped fresh cilantro and cilantro sprigs (optional)
1 large bag (7 ounces) GUILTLESS GOURMET® Baked Tortilla Chips (yellow, white or blue corn)

Mix together sour cream and salsa in small bowl. Spread bean dip in shallow glass bowl. Top with sour cream-salsa mixture, spreading to cover bean dip.* Just before serving, top with lettuce, tomato and cheese. Garnish with cilantro, if desired. Serve with tortilla chips.   *Makes 8 servings*

Dip may be prepared to this point; cover and refrigerate up to 24 hours.

Nutrients per Serving: (⅔ cup dip and 20 chips), Calories: 199 (18% Calories from Fat), Total Fat: 4 g, Saturated Fat: 1 g, Protein: 7 g, Carbohydrate: 31 g, Cholesterol: 8 mg, Sodium: 425 mg, Fiber: 3 g

Dietary Exchanges: 2 Starch/Bread, ½ Lean Meat, ½ Vegetable

91 TACO CHICKEN NACHOS

2 small boneless skinless chicken breasts (about 8 ounces)
1 tablespoon plus 1½ teaspoons taco seasoning mix
1 teaspoon olive oil
¾ cup nonfat sour cream
1 can (4 ounces) diced green chilies, drained
¼ cup minced red onion
1 bag (8 ounces) baked fat-free tortilla chips
1 cup (4 ounces) shredded reduced-fat Cheddar or Monterey Jack cheese
½ cup chopped tomato
¼ cup pitted black olive slices (optional)
2 tablespoons chopped fresh cilantro

1. Bring 2 cups water to a boil in small saucepan. Add chicken. Reduce heat to low; cover. Simmer 10 minutes or until chicken is no longer pink in center. Remove from saucepan; cool. Chop chicken.

2. Combine taco seasoning mix and oil in small bowl; mix until smooth paste forms. Stir in sour cream. Add chicken, green chilies and onion; mix lightly.

3. Preheat broiler. Arrange tortilla chips on large platter; cover chips with chicken mixture and cheese. Broil, 4 inches from heat, 2 to 3 minutes or until chicken mixture is hot and cheese is melted. Sprinkle with tomatoes, olives, if desired, and cilantro.
          Makes 12 servings

Nutrients per Serving: Calories: 148 (20% Calories from Fat), Total Fat: 3 g, Saturated Fat: 1 g, Protein: 12 g, Carbohydrate: 18 g, Cholesterol: 20 mg, Sodium: 431 mg, Fiber: 1 g, Sugar: trace

Dietary Exchanges: 1 Starch/Bread, 1½ Lean Meat

Five-Layered Mexican Dip

AMAZING APPETIZERS

92 SOUTH–OF–THE–BORDER NACHOS

4 ounces low-fat tortilla chips
  Nonstick cooking spray
¾ cup chopped onion
2 jalapeño peppers,* seeded and chopped
3 cloves garlic, finely chopped
2 teaspoons chili powder
½ teaspoon ground cumin
1 boneless skinless chicken breast (about 6 ounces), cooked and chopped
1 can (14½ ounces) Mexican-style diced tomatoes, drained
1 cup (4 ounces) shredded reduced-fat Monterey Jack cheese
2 tablespoons chopped black olives

Jalapeño peppers can sting and irritate the skin. Wear rubber gloves when handling peppers and do not touch eyes. Wash hands after handling.

1. Preheat oven to 350°F. Place chips in 13×9-inch baking pan.

2. Spray large nonstick skillet with cooking spray; heat over medium heat until hot. Add onion, peppers, garlic, chili powder and cumin; cook 5 minutes or until vegetables are tender, stirring occasionally. Stir in chicken and tomatoes.

3. Spoon tomato mixture, cheese and olives over chips. Bake 5 minutes or until cheese melts. Serve immediately.

Makes 4 servings

Nutrients per Serving: Calories: 226, (26 % Calories from Fat), Total Fat: 7 g, Saturated Fat: 2 g, Protein: 22 g, Carbohydrate: 21 g, Cholesterol: 34 mg, Sodium: 273 mg, Fiber: 2 g, Sugar: 2 g

Dietary Exchanges: 1 Starch/Bread, 2 Lean Meat, 1 Vegetable, ½ Fat

93 BLACK BEAN QUESADILLAS

  Nonstick cooking spray
4 (8-inch) flour tortillas
¾ cup (3 ounces) shredded reduced-fat Monterey Jack or Cheddar cheese
½ cup rinsed and drained canned black beans
2 green onions with tops, sliced
¼ cup minced fresh cilantro
½ teaspoon ground cumin
½ cup salsa
2 tablespoons plus 2 teaspoons nonfat sour cream

1. Preheat oven to 450°F. Spray large nonstick baking sheet with cooking spray. Place 2 tortillas on prepared baking sheet; sprinkle each with half the cheese.

2. Combine beans, green onions, cilantro and cumin in small bowl; mix lightly. Spoon bean mixture evenly over cheese; top with remaining tortillas. Coat tops with cooking spray.

3. Bake 10 to 12 minutes or until cheese is melted and tortillas are lightly browned. Cut into quarters; top each wedge with 1 tablespoon salsa and 1 teaspoon sour cream. Transfer to serving plate.

Makes 8 servings

Nutrients per Serving: Calories: 105 (30% Calories from Fat), Total Fat: 4 g, Saturated Fat: 1 g, Protein: 7 g, Carbohydrate: 13 g, Cholesterol: 8 mg, Sodium: 259 mg, Fiber: 1 g, Sugar: trace

Dietary Exchanges: 1 Starch/Bread, ½ Lean Meat

Black Bean Quesadillas

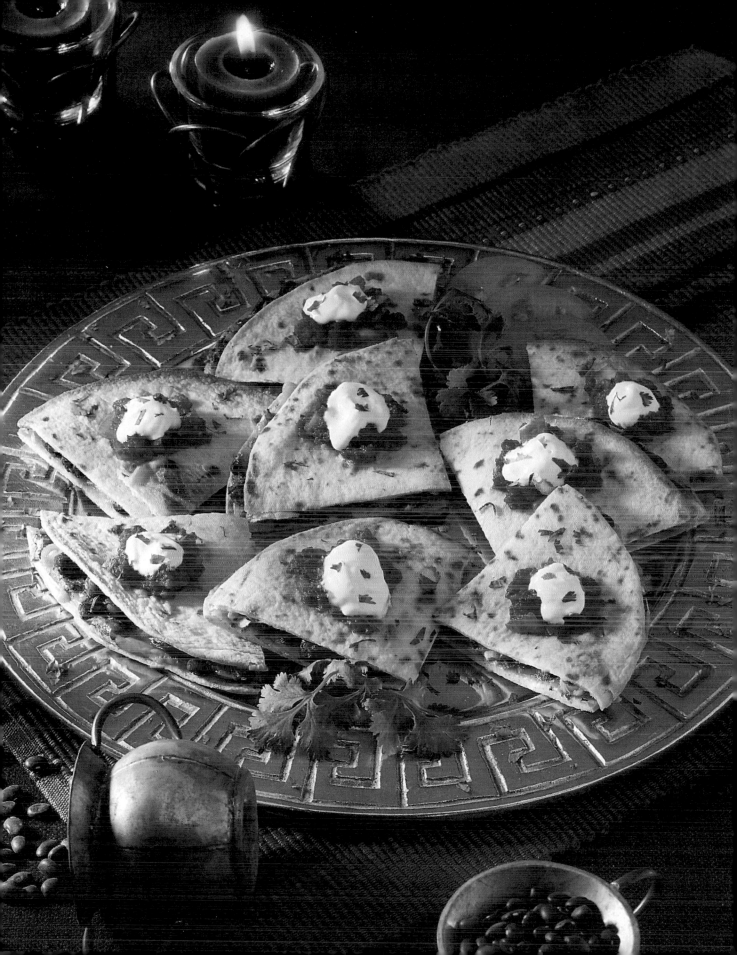

94 TOASTED RAVIOLI WITH SALSA

1 package (9 ounces) refrigerated cheese
  ravioli
  Nonstick olive oil-flavored cooking spray
¾ cup plain dry bread crumbs
2 tablespoons grated Parmesan cheese
1 teaspoon dried basil leaves
1 teaspoon dried oregano leaves
¼ teaspoon black pepper
2 egg whites
  Fresh Tomato-Basil Salsa (recipe follows)

1. Cook ravioli according to package directions, omitting salt. Rinse under cold running water until cool; drain.

2. Preheat oven to 375°F. Spray large nonstick baking sheet with cooking spray.

3. Combine bread crumbs, cheese, basil, oregano and pepper in medium bowl.

4. Beat egg whites lightly in shallow dish. Add ravioli; toss lightly to coat. Transfer ravioli, a few at a time, to crumb mixture; toss to coat evenly. Arrange on prepared baking sheet. Repeat with remaining ravioli. Spray tops of ravioli with cooking spray.

5. Bake 12 to 14 minutes or until crisp. Meanwhile, prepare Fresh Tomato-Basil Salsa; serve with ravioli.

Makes 8 servings

FRESH TOMATO–BASIL SALSA

1 pound fresh tomatoes, peeled and
  seeded
½ cup loosely packed fresh basil leaves
¼ small onion (about 2×1-inch piece)
1 teaspoon red wine vinegar
¼ teaspoon salt

1. Combine ingredients in food processor; process until finely chopped but not smooth.

Makes about 1 cup

Nutrients per Serving: Calories: 167 (29% Calories from Fat), Total Fat: 5 g, Saturated Fat: 3 g, Protein: 8 g, Carbohydrate: 22 g, Cholesterol: 29 mg, Sodium: 337 mg, Fiber: 1 g, Sugar: 1 g

Dietary Exchanges: 1 Starch/Bread, 1 Lean Meat, 1 Vegetable, ½ Fat

95 REUBEN BITES

24 party rye bread slices
½ cup prepared fat-free Thousand Island
  dressing
6 ounces turkey pastrami, very thinly
  sliced
1 cup (4 ounces) shredded reduced-fat
  Swiss cheese
1 cup alfalfa sprouts

1. Preheat oven to 400°F.

2. Arrange bread slices on nonstick baking sheet. Bake 5 minutes or until lightly toasted.

3. Spread 1 teaspoon dressing onto each bread slice; top with pastrami, folding slices to fit bread slices. Sprinkle evenly with cheese.

4. Bake 5 minutes or until hot. Top evenly with sprouts. Transfer to serving plate.

Makes 12 servings

Nutrients per Serving: (2 pieces), Calories: 142 (21% Calories from Fat), Total Fat: 3 g, Saturated Fat: 1 g, Protein: 9 g, Carbohydrate: 19 g, Cholesterol: 15 mg, Sodium: 516 mg, Fiber: trace, Sugar: 0 g

Dietary Exchanges: 1 Starch/Bread, 1 Lean Meat

Toasted Ravioli with Salsa

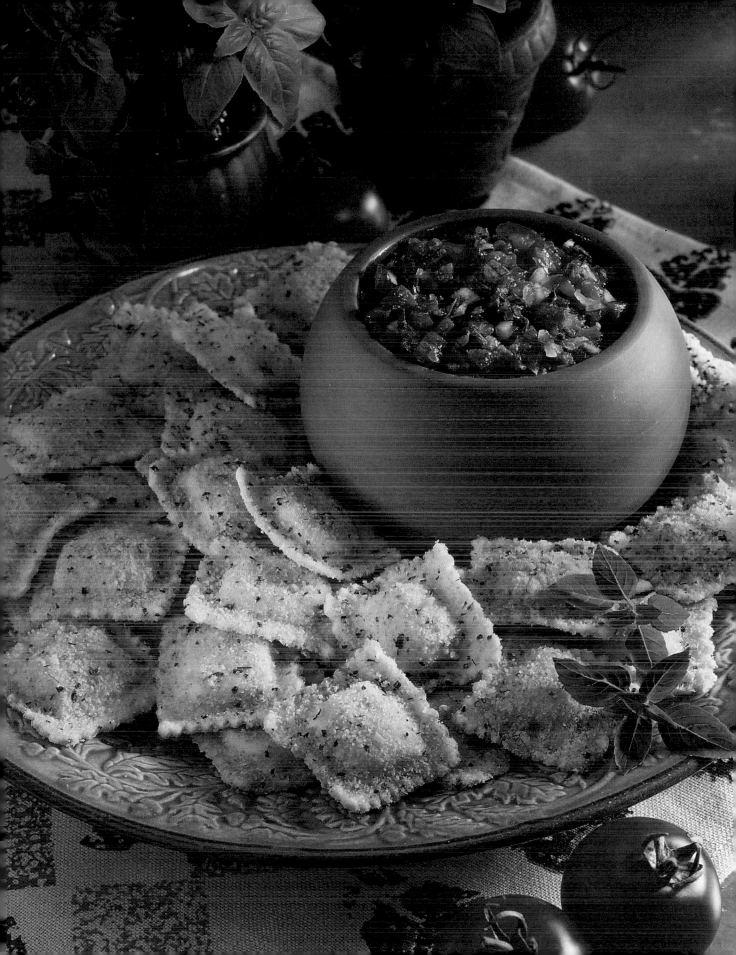

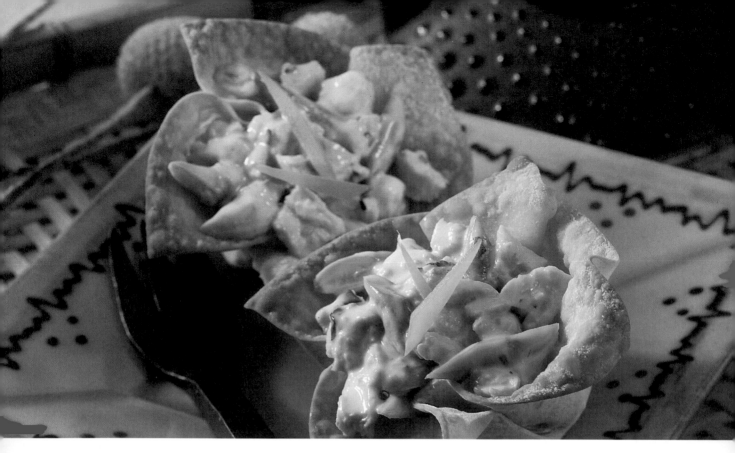

Sesame Chicken Salad Wonton Cups

96 SESAME CHICKEN SALAD WONTON CUPS

    Nonstick cooking spray
 20 (3-inch) wonton wrappers
  1 tablespoon sesame seeds
  2 small boneless skinless chicken breasts
       (about 8 ounces)
  1 cup fresh green beans, cut diagonally
       into ½-inch pieces
 ¼ cup reduced-calorie mayonnaise
  1 tablespoon chopped fresh cilantro
       (optional)
  2 teaspoons honey
  1 teaspoon reduced-sodium soy sauce
 ⅛ teaspoon ground red pepper

1. Preheat oven to 350°F. Spray miniature muffin pan with nonstick cooking spray. Press 1 wonton wrapper into each muffin cup; spray with nonstick cooking spray. Bake 8 to 10 minutes or until golden brown. Cool in pan on wire rack before filling.

2. Place sesame seeds in shallow baking pan. Bake 5 minutes or until lightly toasted, stirring occasionally. Set aside to cool.

3. Meanwhile, bring 2 cups water to a boil in medium saucepan. Add chicken; reduce heat to low. Simmer, covered, 10 minutes or until chicken is no longer pink in center, adding green beans after 7 minutes. Drain.

4. Finely chop chicken; place in medium bowl. Add green beans and remaining ingredients; mix lightly. Spoon lightly rounded tablespoonful of chicken mixture into each wonton cup.

Makes 10 servings

Nutrients per Serving: (2 filled wonton cups), Calories: 103 (25% Calories from Fat), Total Fat: 3 g, Saturated Fat: 1 g, Protein: 7 g, Carbohydrate: 12 g, Cholesterol: 18 mg, Sodium: 128 mg, Fiber: trace, Sugar: 1 g

Dietary Exchanges: 1 Starch/Bread, ½ Lean Meat

97 TURKEY MEATBALLS IN CRANBERRY– BARBECUE SAUCE

1 can (16 ounces) jellied cranberry sauce
½ cup barbecue sauce
1 egg white
1 pound ground turkey
1 green onion with top, sliced
2 teaspoons grated orange peel
1 teaspoon reduced-sodium soy sauce
¼ teaspoon black pepper
⅛ teaspoon ground red pepper (optional)
    Nonstick cooking spray

1. Combine cranberry sauce and barbecue sauce in slow cooker. Set on highest temperature; cover. Cook 20 to 30 minutes or until cranberry sauce is melted and mixture is hot, stirring every 10 minutes.

2. Meanwhile, place egg white in medium bowl; beat lightly. Add turkey, green onion, orange peel, soy sauce, black pepper and red pepper, if desired; mix with hands until well blended. Shape into 24 balls.

3. Spray large nonstick skillet with cooking spray. Add meatballs to skillet; cook over medium heat 8 to 10 minutes or until meatballs are no longer pink in center, carefully turning occasionally to brown evenly. Add to heated sauce in slow cooker; stir gently to coat evenly with sauce.

4. Reduce heat setting to medium or low. Cook up to 3 hours. When ready to serve, transfer meatballs to serving plate.
Makes 12 servings

Nutrients per Serving: (2 meatballs with 2 tablespoons sauce), Calories: 137 (27% Calories from Fat), Total Fat: 4 g, Saturated Fat: 1 g, Protein: 7 g, Carbohydrate: 18 g, Cholesterol: 19 mg, Sodium: 206 mg, Fiber: 1 g, Sugar: 0 g

Dietary Exchanges: 1 Lean Meat, ½ Fat, 1 Fruit

98 SPINACH–CHEDDAR SQUARES

1½ cups EGG BEATERS® Healthy Real Egg Substitute
¾ cup skim milk
1 tablespoon dried onion flakes
1 tablespoon grated Parmesan cheese
¼ teaspoon garlic powder
⅛ teaspoon ground black pepper
¼ cup plain dry bread crumbs
¾ cup shredded fat-free Cheddar cheese, divided
1 (10-ounce) package frozen chopped spinach, thawed and well drained
¼ cup diced pimientos

In medium bowl, combine Egg Beaters, milk, onion flakes, Parmesan cheese, garlic powder and pepper; set aside.

Sprinkle bread crumbs evenly into bottom of lightly greased 8×8×2-inch baking dish. Top with ½ cup Cheddar cheese and spinach. Pour egg mixture evenly over spinach; top with remaining Cheddar cheese and pimientos.

Bake at 350°F for 35 to 40 minutes or until knife inserted in center comes out clean. Let stand 10 minutes before serving.
Makes 16 appetizer servings

Prep Time: 15 minutes
Cook Time: 40 minutes

Nutrients per Serving: Calories: 39, Total Fat: 0 g, Saturated Fat: 0 g, Cholesterol: 1 mg, Sodium: 134 mg, Fiber: 0 g

Dietary Exchanges: 1 Lean Meat

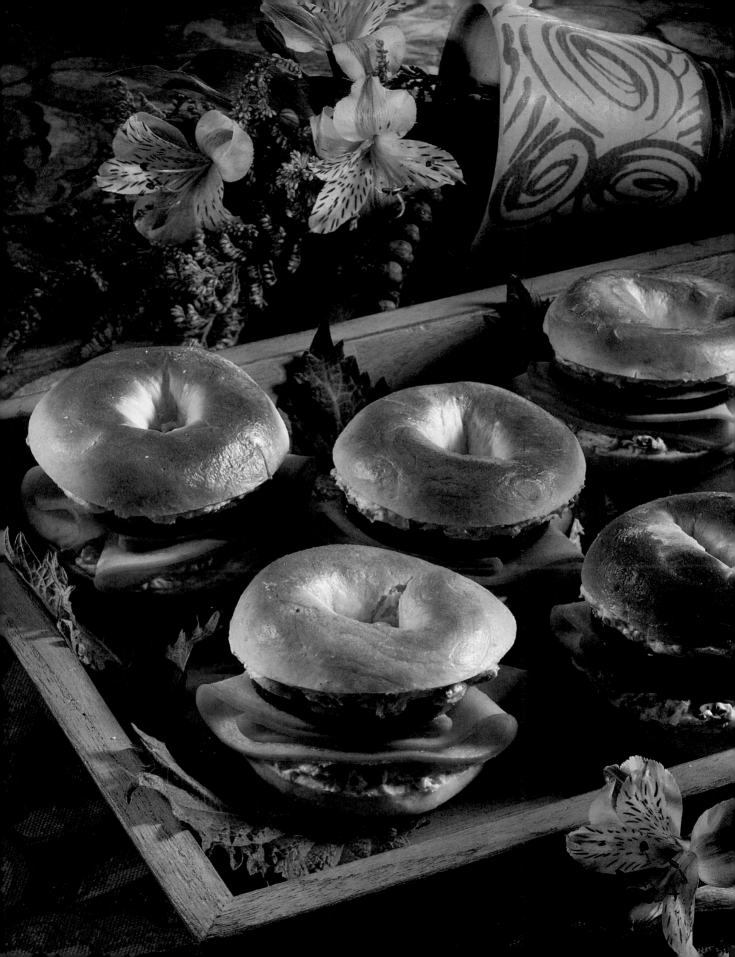

99 SMOKED CHICKEN BAGEL SNACKS

⅓ cup fat-free cream cheese, softened
2 teaspoons spicy brown mustard
¼ cup chopped roasted red peppers
1 green onion with top, sliced
5 mini-bagels, split
3 ounces smoked chicken or turkey, cut into 10 very thin slices
¼ medium cucumber, cut into 10 thin slices

1. Combine cream cheese and mustard in small bowl; mix well. Stir in peppers and green onion.

2. Spread cream cheese mixture evenly onto cut sides of bagels. Cover bottom halves of bagels with chicken, folding chicken to fit onto bagels; top with cucumber slices and tops of bagels.   *Makes 5 servings*

Nutrients per Serving: Calories: 139 (7% Calories from Fat), Total Fat: 1 g, Saturated Fat: trace, Protein: 10 g, Carbohydrate: 21 g, Cholesterol: 12 mg, Sodium: 502 mg, Fiber: trace, Sugar: 0 g

Dietary Exchanges: 1 Starch/Bread, 1 Lean Meat

100 CRANBERRY–ALMOND PEAR WEDGES

3 firm ripe pears
¼ cup triple sec*
2 tablespoons orange juice
½ cup prepared cranberry fruit relish
¼ cup finely chopped walnuts
¼ cup (1 ounce) crumbled blue cheese

Omit liqueur, if desired. Increase orange juice to ¼ cup. Add 2 tablespoons honey and 2 tablespoons balsamic vinegar to marinade.

1. Cut each pear lengthwise into quarters. Using a melon ball scoop, grapefruit spoon or sharp knife, remove cores.

2. Place pears in resealable plastic food storage bag. Pour liqueur and orange juice over pears; seal bag. Turn bag over several times to coat pears evenly. Refrigerate at least 1 hour, turning bag occasionally.

3. Drain pears; discard marinade. Place pears on serving platter. Spoon cranberry relish evenly into cavities in pears; sprinkle with walnuts and cheese.

Makes 12 servings

Nutrients per Serving: Calories 77 (27% Calories from Fat), Total Fat: 3 g, Saturated Fat: 1 g, Protein: 1 g, Carbohydrate: 13 g, Cholesterol: 2 mg, Sodium: 43 mg, Fiber: 1 g, Sugar: 5 g

Dietary Exchanges: ½ Fat, 1 Fruit

Smoked Chicken Bagel Snacks

AMAZING APPETIZERS

101 COCKTAIL STUFFED MUSHROOMS

30 to 40 medium-size mushrooms
1 (14-ounce) package HEALTHY CHOICE®
    Low Fat Polska Kielbasa
    Vegetable cooking spray
¾ cup minced onion
½ cup minced fresh parsley
2 teaspoons minced garlic
½ teaspoon ground fennel
½ teaspoon salt (optional)
¼ teaspoon black pepper
⅛ teaspoon crushed red pepper
1 can HEALTHY CHOICE® RECIPE
    CREATIONS™ Cream of Roasted
    Garlic Condensed Soup
⅓ cup fat free shredded Parmesan cheese

Wash mushrooms well. Remove stems and mince; set caps aside. In food processor, process Kielbasa until ground. In large nonstick skillet sprayed with vegetable cooking spray, sauté minced mushroom stems, Kielbasa, onion, parsley, garlic, fennel, salt, black pepper and red pepper. Cook until onion is tender.

Remove skillet from heat; add soup to meat mixture and blend well. Fill mushroom caps, dividing meat mixture evenly among caps. Sprinkle with Parmesan cheese. Bake at 400°F 20 to 22 minutes.

Makes 20 servings

Nutrients per Serving: Calories: 45
(16% Calories from Fat), Fat: 1 g, Protein: 4 g,
Sodium: 310 mg

Dietary Exchanges: ½ Lean Meat, 1 Vegetable

102 CARIBBEAN CHUTNEY KABOBS

20 (4-inch) bamboo skewers
½ medium pineapple
1 medium red bell pepper, cut into 1-inch
    pieces
¾ pound boneless skinless chicken breasts,
    cut into 1-inch pieces
½ cup bottled mango chutney
2 tablespoons orange juice or pineapple
    juice
1 teaspoon vanilla
¼ teaspoon ground nutmeg

1. To prevent burning, soak skewers in water at least 20 minutes before assembling kabobs.

2. Peel and core pineapple. Cut pineapple into 1-inch chunks. Alternately thread bell pepper, pineapple and chicken onto skewers. Place in shallow baking dish.

3. Combine chutney, orange juice, vanilla and nutmeg in small bowl; mix well. Pour over kabobs; cover. Refrigerate up to 4 hours.

4. Preheat broiler. Spray broiler pan with nonstick cooking spray; place kabobs on prepared broiler pan. Broil, 6 to 8 inches from heat, 4 to 5 minutes on each side or until chicken is no longer pink in center. Transfer to serving plates.

Makes 10 servings

Nutrients per Serving: Calories: 108
(10% Calories from Fat), Total Fat: 1 g,
Saturated Fat: trace, Protein: 8 g,
Carbohydrate: 16 g, Cholesterol: 21 mg,
Sodium: 22 mg, Fiber: 2 g, Sugar 14 g

Dietary Exchanges: 1 Lean Meat, 1 Fruit

AMAZING APPETIZERS

103 APRICOT–CHICKEN POT STICKERS

2 cups plus 1 tablespoon water, divided
2 small boneless skinless chicken breasts
    (about 8 ounces)
2 cups chopped finely shredded cabbage
½ cup all-fruit apricot preserves
2 green onions with tops, finely chopped
2 teaspoons soy sauce
½ teaspoon grated fresh ginger
⅛ teaspoon black pepper
30 (3-inch) wonton wrappers
    Prepared sweet & sour sauce (optional)

1. Bring 2 cups water to boil in medium saucepan. Add chicken. Reduce heat to low; simmer, covered, 10 minutes or until chicken is no longer pink in center. Remove from saucepan; drain.

2. Add cabbage and remaining 1 tablespoon water to saucepan. Cook over high heat 1 to 2 minutes or until water evaporates, stirring occasionally. Remove from heat; cool slightly.

3. Finely chop chicken. Add to saucepan along with preserves, green onions, soy sauce, ginger and pepper; mix well.

4. To assemble pot stickers, remove 3 wonton wrappers at a time from package. Spoon slightly rounded tablespoonful of chicken mixture onto center of each wrapper; brush edges with water. Bring 4 corners together; press to seal. Repeat with remaining wrappers and filling.

5. Spray steamer with nonstick cooking spray. Assemble steamer so that water is ½ inch below steamer basket. Fill steamer basket with pot stickers, leaving enough space between them to prevent sticking. Cover; steam 5 minutes. Transfer pot stickers to serving plate. Serve with prepared sweet & sour sauce, if desired.

Makes 10 servings (3 pot stickers each)

Nutrients per Serving: Calories: 145 (6% Calories from Fat), Total Fat: 1 g, Saturated Fat: trace, Protein: 8 g, Carbohydrate: 26 g, Cholesterol: 17 mg, Sodium: 223 mg, Fiber: 1 g, Sugar: 10 g

Dietary Exchanges: 1½ Starch/Bread, ½ Lean Meat

104 CHEESY POTATO SKINS

2 tablespoons grated Parmesan cheese
3 cloves garlic, finely chopped
2 teaspoons dried rosemary
½ teaspoon salt
¼ teaspoon black pepper
4 baked potatoes
2 egg whites, slightly beaten
½ cup (2 ounces) shredded part-skim
    mozzarella cheese

Preheat oven to 400°F. Combine Parmesan cheese and seasonings. Cut potatoes lengthwise in half. Remove pulp, leaving ¼-inch-thick shells. Cut lengthwise into wedges. Place on baking sheet. Brush with egg whites; sprinkle with cheese mixture. Bake 20 minutes. Sprinkle with mozzarella cheese; bake until melted. Serve with salsa, if desired.
Makes 8 servings

Nutrients per Serving: Calories: 90 (17% Calories from Fat), Total Fat: 2 g, Saturated Fat: 1 g, Protein: 5 g, Carbohydrate: 14 g, Cholesterol: 5 mg, Sodium: 215 mg, Fiber: 2 g, Sugar: trace

Dietary Exchanges: 1 Starch/Bread, ½ Lean Meat

Sensational Soups

105 SPICY PUMPKIN SOUP WITH GREEN CHILI SWIRL

1 can (4 ounces) diced green chilies, drained
¼ cup reduced-fat sour cream
¼ cup fresh cilantro leaves
1 can (15 ounces) solid-pack pumpkin
1 can (about 14 ounces) fat-free reduced-sodium chicken broth
½ cup water
1 teaspoon ground cumin
½ teaspoon chili powder
¼ teaspoon garlic powder
⅛ teaspoon ground red pepper (optional)

1. Combine green chilies, sour cream and cilantro in food processor or blender; process until smooth.*

2. Combine pumpkin, chicken broth, water, cumin, chili powder, garlic powder and pepper, if desired, in medium saucepan; stir in ¼ cup green chili mixture. Bring to a boil; reduce heat to medium. Simmer, uncovered, 5 minutes, stirring occasionally.

3. Pour into serving bowls. Top each serving with small dollops of remaining green chili mixture and additional sour cream, if desired. Run tip of spoon through dollops to swirl. *Makes 4 servings*

Omit food processor step by adding green chilies directly to soup. Finely chop cilantro and combine with sour cream. Dollop with sour cream mixture as directed.

Nutrients per Serving: Calories: 72 (17% Calories from Fat), Total Fat: 1 g, Saturated Fat: trace, Protein: 4 g, Carbohydrate: 12 g, Cholesterol: 5 mg, Sodium: 276 mg, Fiber: 4 g, Sugar: 0 g

Dietary Exchanges: 1 Starch/Bread

Spicy Pumpkin Soup with Green Chili Swirl

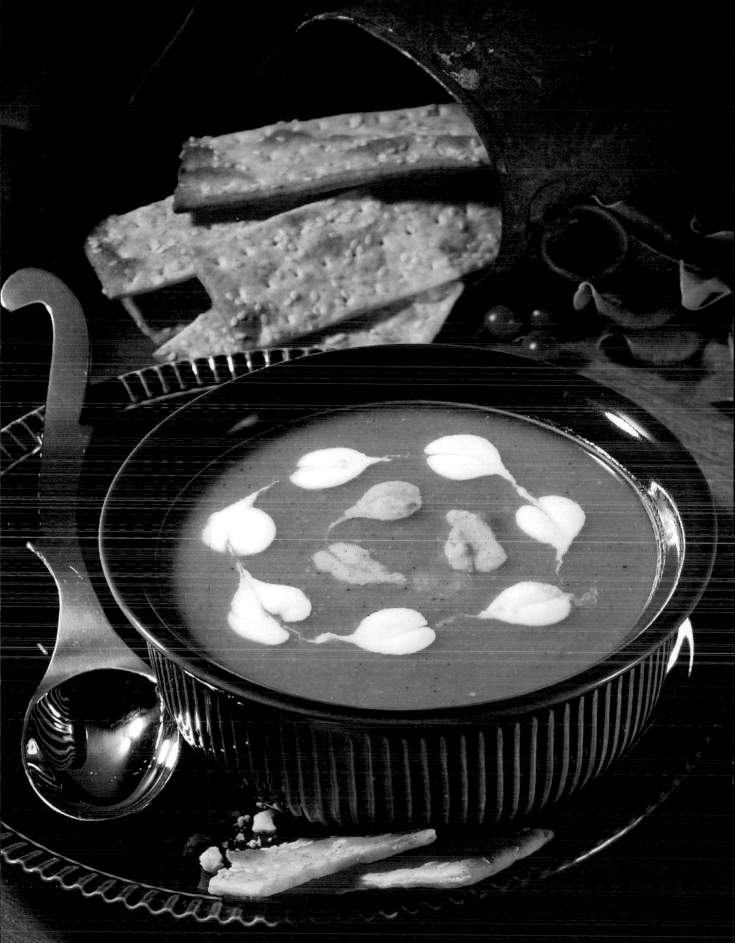

SENSATIONAL SOUPS

106 SPICY LENTIL AND PASTA SOUP

  2 medium onions, thinly sliced
½ cup chopped carrot
½ cup chopped celery
½ cup peeled and chopped turnip
  1 small jalapeño pepper,* finely chopped
  2 cans (about 14 ounces each) vegetable broth
  1 can (14½ ounces) no-salt-added stewed tomatoes
  2 cups water
  8 ounces dried lentils, sorted, rinsed and drained
  2 teaspoons chili powder
½ teaspoon dried oregano
  3 ounces uncooked whole wheat spaghetti, broken
¼ cup minced fresh cilantro

*Jalapeño peppers can sting and irritate the skin; wear rubber gloves when handling peppers and do not touch eyes. Wash hands after handling.

1. Spray large nonstick saucepan with nonstick cooking spray; heat over medium heat until hot. Add onions, carrot, celery, turnip and jalapeño; cook and stir 10 minutes or until vegetables are crisp-tender.

2. Add vegetable broth, tomatoes, water, lentils, chili powder and oregano; bring to a boil. Reduce heat; simmer, covered, 20 to 30 minutes or until lentils are tender.

3. Add pasta; cook 10 minutes or until tender.

4. Ladle soup into bowls; sprinkle with cilantro.   *Makes 6 servings*

Nutrients per Serving: Calories: 261 (7% Calories from Fat), Total Fat: 2 g, Saturated Fat: trace, Protein: 15 g, Carbohydrate: 49 g, Cholesterol: 1 mg, Sodium: 771 mg, Fiber: 5 g, Sugar: 2 g

Dietary Exchanges: 2½ Starch/Bread, ½ Lean Meat, 2 Vegetable

107 WILD RICE SOUP

½ cup dried lentils, sorted, rinsed and drained
  3 cups water
  1 package (6 ounces) long grain and wild rice blend
  1 can (about 14 ounces) vegetable broth
  1 package (10 ounces) frozen mixed vegetables
  1 cup skim milk
½ cup (2 ounces) reduced-fat processed American cheese, cut into pieces

1. Combine lentils and water in small saucepan; bring to a boil. Reduce heat to low; simmer, covered, 5 minutes. Let stand, covered, 1 hour. Drain and rinse lentils.

2. Cook rice according to package directions in medium saucepan. Add lentils and remaining ingredients. Bring to a boil; reduce heat to low. Simmer, uncovered, 20 minutes.   *Makes 6 servings*

Nutrients per Serving: Calories: 199 (25% Calories from Fat), Total Fat: 6 g, Saturated Fat: 1 g, Protein: 12 g, Carbohydrate: 26 g, Cholesterol: 6 mg, Sodium: 697 mg, Fiber: 2 g, Sugar: 3 g

Dietary Exchanges: 1½ Starch/Bread, 1 Lean Meat, 1 Vegetable, ½ Fat

Wild Rice Soup

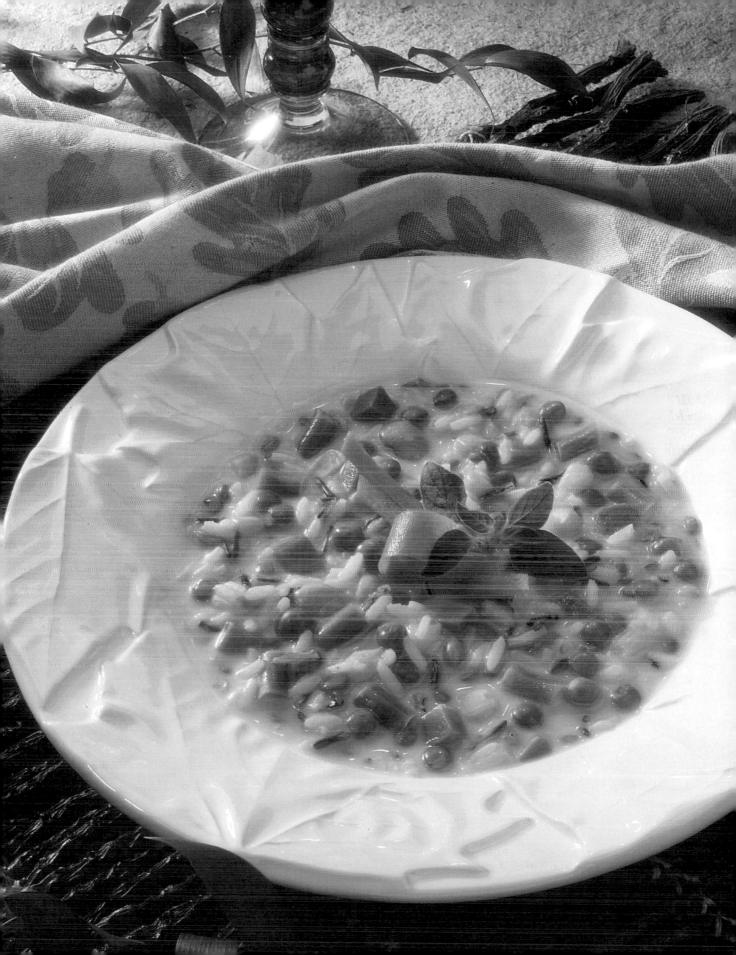

SENSATIONAL SOUPS

108 MOROCCAN LENTIL & VEGETABLE SOUP

1 tablespoon olive oil
1 cup chopped onion
4 medium cloves garlic, minced
½ cup dry lentils, sorted, rinsed and drained
1½ teaspoons ground coriander
1½ teaspoons ground cumin
½ teaspoon black pepper
½ teaspoon ground cinnamon
3¾ cups fat-free reduced-sodium chicken broth
½ cup chopped celery
½ cup chopped sun-dried tomatoes (not packed in oil)
1 medium yellow summer squash, chopped
½ cup chopped green bell pepper
½ cup chopped parsley
1 cup chopped plum tomatoes
¼ cup chopped cilantro or basil

1. Heat oil in medium saucepan over medium heat. Add onion and garlic; cook 4 to 5 minutes or until onion is tender, stirring occasionally. Stir in lentils, coriander, cumin, black pepper and cinnamon; cook 2 minutes. Add chicken broth, celery and sun-dried tomatoes; bring to a boil over high heat. Reduce heat to low; simmer, covered, 25 minutes.

2. Stir in squash, bell pepper and parsley. Continue cooking, covered, 10 minutes or until lentils are tender.

3. Top with plum tomatoes and cilantro just before serving. *Makes 6 servings*

Nutrients per Serving: Calories: 131 (20% Calories from Fat), Total Fat: 3 g, Saturated Fat: trace, Protein: 8 g, Carbohydrate: 20 g, Cholesterol: 0 mg, Sodium: 264 mg, Fiber: 2 g, Sugar: 2 g

Dietary Exchanges: 1 Starch/Bread, 1 Vegetable, ½ Fat

109 TUSCANY BEAN & PASTA SOUP

Vegetable cooking spray
½ cup chopped onion
2 cloves garlic, minced
1 can HEALTHY CHOICE® RECIPE CREATIONS™ Cream of Mushroom with Cracked Pepper & Herbs Condensed Soup
2½ cups nonfat milk
1 (15-ounce) can cannellini beans, drained and rinsed
1 cup cooked small macaroni (shells or elbow)
2 teaspoons chopped fresh parsley
½ teaspoon chili powder
½ teaspoon salt (optional)
Crumbled cooked bacon for garnish (optional)

In medium saucepan sprayed with vegetable cooking spray, sauté onion and garlic until tender. Add soup, milk, beans, macaroni, parsley, chili powder and salt; mix well. Simmer 10 minutes, stirring occasionally. Garnish with bacon, if desired.

Makes 6 servings

Nutrients per Serving: Calories: 150 (5% Calories from Fat), Fat: 1 g, Protein: 8 g, Sodium: 410 mg

Dietary Exchanges: 2 Starch/Bread

Moroccan Lentil & Vegetable Soup

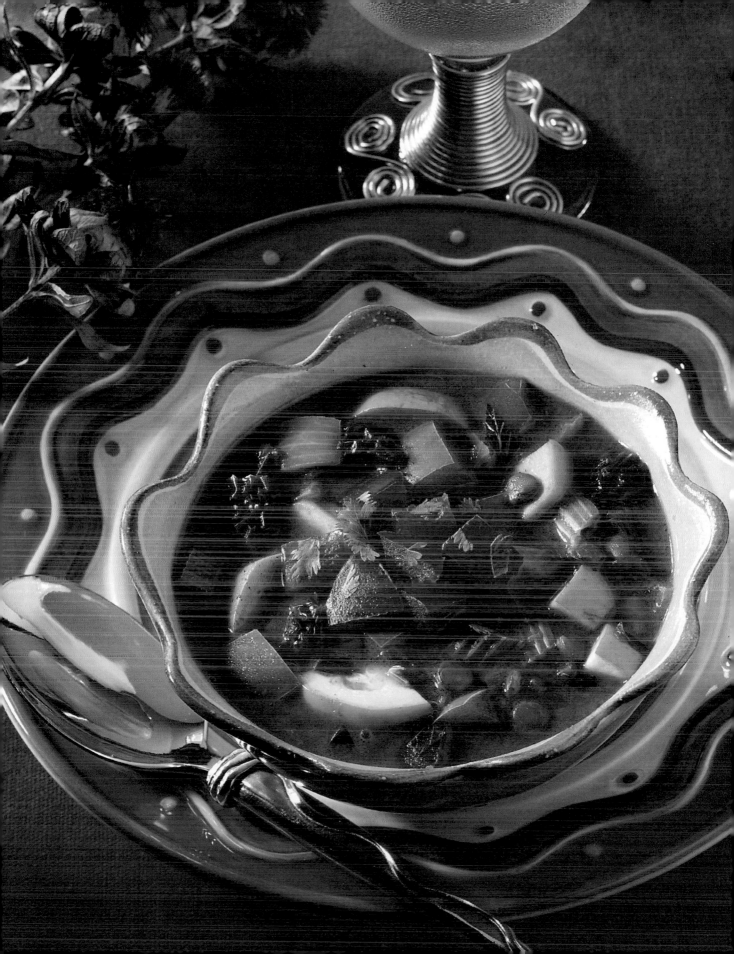

110 GAZPACHO

2 cups HUNT'S® Low Sodium Tomato Juice
1 (14½-ounce) can fat free, low sodium beef broth
1 can HEALTHY CHOICE® RECIPE CREATIONS™ Tomato with Garden Herbs Condensed Soup
1½ cups *each* peeled and diced cucumbers and diced green bell peppers
1¼ cups *each* shredded carrots and diced celery
½ cup sliced green onions
¼ cup chopped fresh parsley
2 cloves garlic, minced
1 tablespoon lime juice
2 teaspoons low sodium Worcestershire sauce
½ teaspoon salt (optional)
Fat free sour cream
Chopped cilantro

In large bowl, combine tomato juice, beef broth, soup, cucumbers, peppers, carrots, celery, green onions, parsley, garlic, lime juice, Worcestershire sauce and salt. Chill at least 2 hours to blend flavors. Top with desired amount of sour cream and cilantro.

Makes 4 to 6 servings

Nutrients per Serving: Calories: 80 (6% Calories from Fat), Fat: 1 g, Protein: 4 g, Sodium: 210 mg

Dietary Exchanges: 2 Starch/Bread

Gazpacho

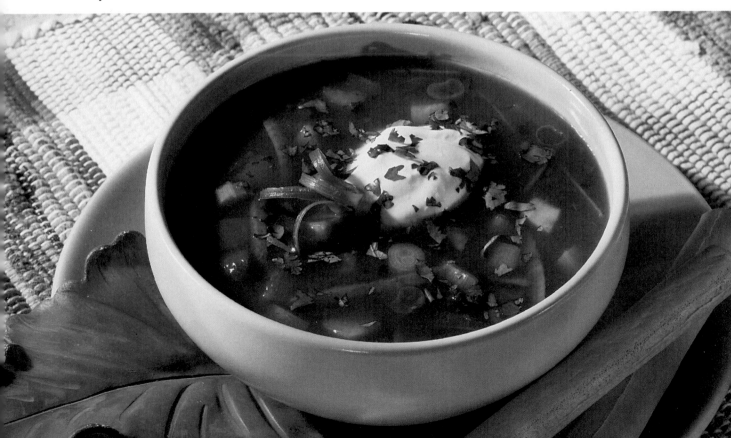

SENSATIONAL SOUPS

111 CREAM OF BROCCOLI AND CHEESE SOUP

Nonstick cooking spray
1 cup chopped onion
3 cloves garlic, minced
3 tablespoons all-purpose flour
4 cans (about 14 ounces each) fat-free reduced-sodium chicken broth
1½ pounds fresh broccoli, chopped
1½ pounds potatoes, peeled and cubed
½ cup skim milk, divided
1 cup (4 ounces) shredded reduced-fat Cheddar cheese
½ teaspoon salt
¼ teaspoon white pepper

1. Spray 4-quart Dutch oven or large saucepan with cooking spray; heat over medium heat until hot. Add onion and garlic; cook until tender. Add flour; stir over low heat 1 to 2 minutes.

2. Add chicken broth; bring to a boil. Add broccoli and potatoes; reduce heat and simmer, covered, about 15 minutes or until vegetables are tender. Remove 1½ cups broccoli mixture with slotted spoon; reserve.

3. Process remaining broccoli mixture in batches in food processor or blender until smooth; return to Dutch oven. Stir in reserved broccoli mixture and milk; cook over medium heat until heated through. Remove from heat; stir in cheese until melted. Stir in salt and pepper.

Makes 8 servings

Nutrients per Serving: Calories: 168 (16% Calories from Fat), Total Fat: 3 g, Saturated Fat: 1 g, Protein: 10 g, Carbohydrate: 26 g, Cholesterol: 8 mg, Sodium: 413 mg, Fiber: 0 g, Sugar: 1 g

Dietary Exchanges: 1 Starch/Bread, ½ Lean Meat, 2 Vegetable, ½ Fat

112 TOMATO PASTINA SOUP

2 teaspoons olive oil
⅔ cup coarsely chopped green bell pepper
½ cup coarsely chopped onion
½ cup coarsely chopped cucumber
3 cloves garlic, minced
1½ pounds fresh tomatoes, coarsely chopped
1 can (14½ ounces) whole tomatoes, undrained
2 tablespoons balsamic vinegar
2 teaspoons ground cumin
1 teaspoon coriander seeds
½ teaspoon black pepper
¼ teaspoon salt
1 ounce uncooked pastina
1 cup water

1. Heat oil in large saucepan over medium heat until hot. Add green pepper, onion, cucumber and garlic; cook and stir until pepper and onion are tender. Add fresh and canned tomatoes, vinegar, cumin, coriander, pepper and salt; bring to a boil over high heat. Reduce heat to low; simmer, covered, 15 minutes. Remove from heat; cool.

2. Place tomato mixture in food processor or blender; process in small batches until smooth. Return to saucepan; bring to a boil over high heat. Add pasta; cook 4 to 6 minutes or until pasta is tender. Stir in water; transfer to serving bowls.

Makes 6 servings

Nutrients per Serving: Calories: 93 (21% Calories from Fat), Total Fat: 2 g, Saturated Fat: trace, Protein: 3 g, Carbohydrate: 17 g, Cholesterol: 0 mg, Sodium: 214 mg, Fiber: 3 g, Sugar: 6 g

Dietary Exchanges: ½ Starch/Bread, 2 Vegetable, ½ Fat

SENSATIONAL SOUPS

113 GREEN CHILI SOUP WITH SPICY BAKED WONTONS

½ teaspoon chili powder
⅛ teaspoon garlic powder
⅛ teaspoon onion powder
1 teaspoon water
1 teaspoon vegetable oil
12 (3-inch) wonton wrappers
1 tablespoon reduced-calorie margarine
1 leek (white part only) thinly sliced
1 cup chopped celery
2 cloves garlic, minced
½ can (7 ounces) fat-free reduced-sodium chicken broth
1 cup water
2 cans (4 ounces each) diced green chilies, drained
2 cups skim milk
3 tablespoons all-purpose flour
½ teaspoon ground cumin

1. Preheat oven to 375°F. Combine chili powder, garlic powder and onion powder in small bowl; stir in water and oil.

2. Cut wonton wrappers in half diagonally; place on large ungreased baking sheet. Brush wontons with chili powder mixture; bake 5 to 6 minutes or until crisp. Cool completely on wire rack.

3. Heat margarine in medium saucepan. Add leek, celery and garlic; cook 4 minutes or until softened, stirring occasionally. Stir in chicken broth, water and chilies; bring to a boil.

4. Whisk together milk, flour and cumin until smooth. Add milk mixture to saucepan and cook until thickened, stirring constantly, about 4 minutes.

5. Ladle into soup bowls; serve with wontons. Garnish with fresh cilantro, if desired.   *Makes 4 servings*

Nutrients per Serving: Calories: 150 (24% Calories from Fat), Total Fat: 4 g, Saturated Fat: 1 g, Cholesterol: 5 mg, Sodium: 605 mg, Carbohydrate: 32 g, Fiber: 2 g, Protein: 5 g, Sugar: 6 g

Dietary Exchanges: 1½ Starch/Bread, ½ Milk, 1 Vegetable, ½ Fat

114 BUTTONS & BOWS

1 teaspoon olive oil
⅓ cup minced onion
⅓ cup sliced carrot
3 cups sliced fresh mushrooms
1 teaspoon ground sage
¼ teaspoon ground thyme
¼ teaspoon black pepper
¼ cup dry red wine
2 cans (about 14 ounces each) fat-free reduced-sodium beef broth
¼ cup tomato paste
2 ounces uncooked small bow tie pasta

Heat oil in large saucepan over medium heat until hot. Add onion and carrot; cook 2 minutes. Add mushrooms, sage, thyme and pepper; cook and stir 5 minutes or until mushrooms are soft. Add wine; cook 2 minutes or until wine is reduced by half. Add beef broth; bring to a boil over medium-high heat. Add tomato paste and pasta; cover. Cook, stirring occasionally, 10 to 12 minutes or until pasta is tender. Serve immediately.   *Makes 4 servings*

Nutrients per Serving: Calories: 160 (14% Calories from Fat), Total Fat: 3 g, Saturated Fat: trace, Protein: 7 g, Carbohydrate: 26 g, Cholesterol: 0 mg, Sodium: 204 mg, Fiber: 2 g, Sugar: 2 g

Dietary Exchanges: 1 Starch/Bread, 2 Vegetable, ½ Fat

Green Chili Soup with Spicy Baked Wontons

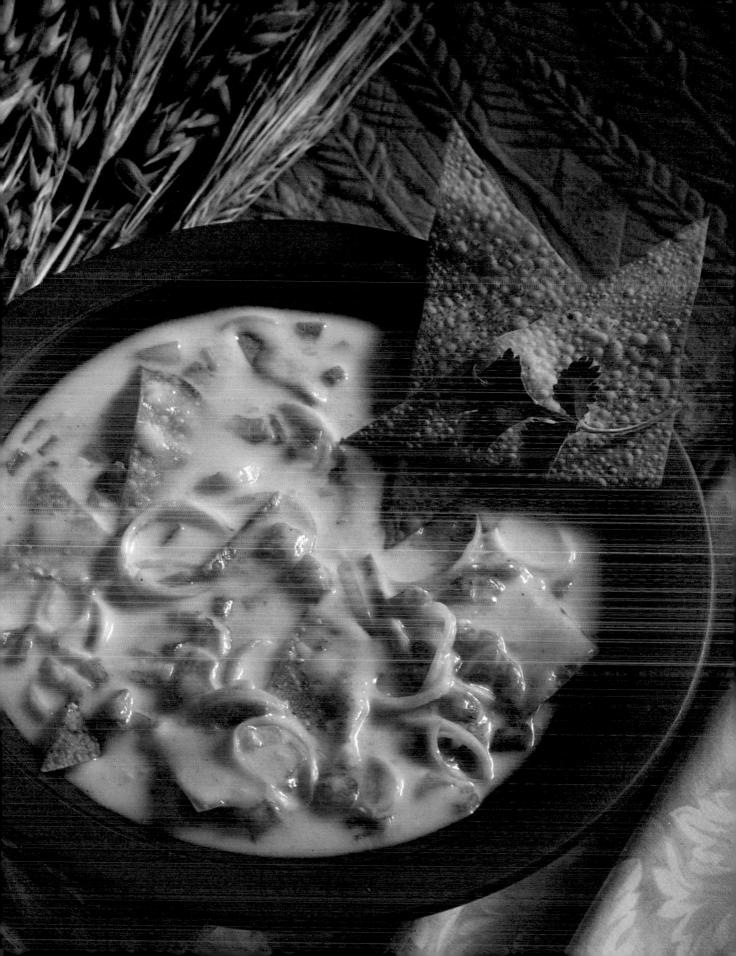

SENSATIONAL SOUPS

115 INDIAN CARROT SOUP

    Nonstick cooking spray
1 small onion, chopped
1 tablespoon minced fresh ginger
1 teaspoon olive oil
1½ teaspoons curry powder
  ½ teaspoon ground cumin
2 cans (about 14 ounces each) fat-free reduced-sodium chicken broth, divided
1 pound peeled baby carrots
1 tablespoon sugar
  ¼ teaspoon ground cinnamon
    Pinch ground red pepper
2 teaspoons lime juice
3 tablespoons chopped cilantro
  ¼ cup plain nonfat yogurt

1. Spray large saucepan with cooking spray; heat over medium heat until hot. Add onion and ginger; reduce heat to low. Cook, covered, 3 to 4 minutes or until onion is transparent, stirring occasionally. Add olive oil; cook and stir, 3 to 4 minutes or until onion is golden. Add curry powder and cumin; cook and stir 30 seconds. Add 1 can chicken broth and carrots; bring to a boil. Reduce heat to low; simmer, covered, 15 minutes or until carrots are tender.

2. Ladle carrot mixture into food processor; process until smooth. Return to saucepan; stir in remaining 1 can chicken broth, sugar, cinnamon and red pepper; bring to a boil over medium heat. Remove from heat; stir in lime juice. Sprinkle with cilantro. Top with yogurt. *Makes 4 servings*

Nutrients per Serving: Calories: 99 (20% Calories from Fat), Total Fat: 2 g, Saturated Fat: trace, Protein: 3 g, Carbohydrate: 17 g, Cholesterol: trace, Sodium: 77 mg, Fiber: 1 g, Sugar: 4 g

Dietary Exchanges: ½ Starch/Bread, 3 Vegetable, 1 Fat

116 JAPANESE NOODLE SOUP

1 package (8½ ounces) Japanese udon noodles
1 teaspoon vegetable oil
1 medium red bell pepper, cut into thin strips
1 medium carrot, diagonally sliced
2 green onions, thinly sliced
2 cans (about 14 ounces each) fat-free reduced-sodium beef broth
1 cup water
1 teaspoon reduced-sodium soy sauce
½ teaspoon grated fresh ginger
½ teaspoon black pepper
2 cups thinly sliced fresh shiitake mushrooms, stems removed
4 ounces daikon (Japanese radish), peeled and cut into thin strips
4 ounces firm tofu, drained and cut into ½-inch cubes

1. Cook noodles according to package directions, omitting salt; drain. Rinse; set aside.

2. Heat oil in large nonstick saucepan until hot. Add red bell pepper, carrot and green onions; cook until slightly softened, about 3 minutes. Stir in beef broth, water, soy sauce, ginger and black pepper; bring to a boil. Add mushrooms, daikon and tofu; reduce heat and simmer 5 minutes.

3. Place noodles in soup tureen; ladle soup over noodles. *Makes 6 servings*

Nutrients per Serving: Calories: 144 (16% Calories from Fat), Total Fat: 3 g, Saturated Fat: trace, Protein: 9 g, Carbohydrate: 24 g, Cholesterol: 0 mg, Sodium: 107 mg, Fiber: 3 g, Sugar: 2 g

Dietary Exchanges: 1½ Starch/Bread, ½ Vegetable, ½ Fat

Indian Carrot Soup

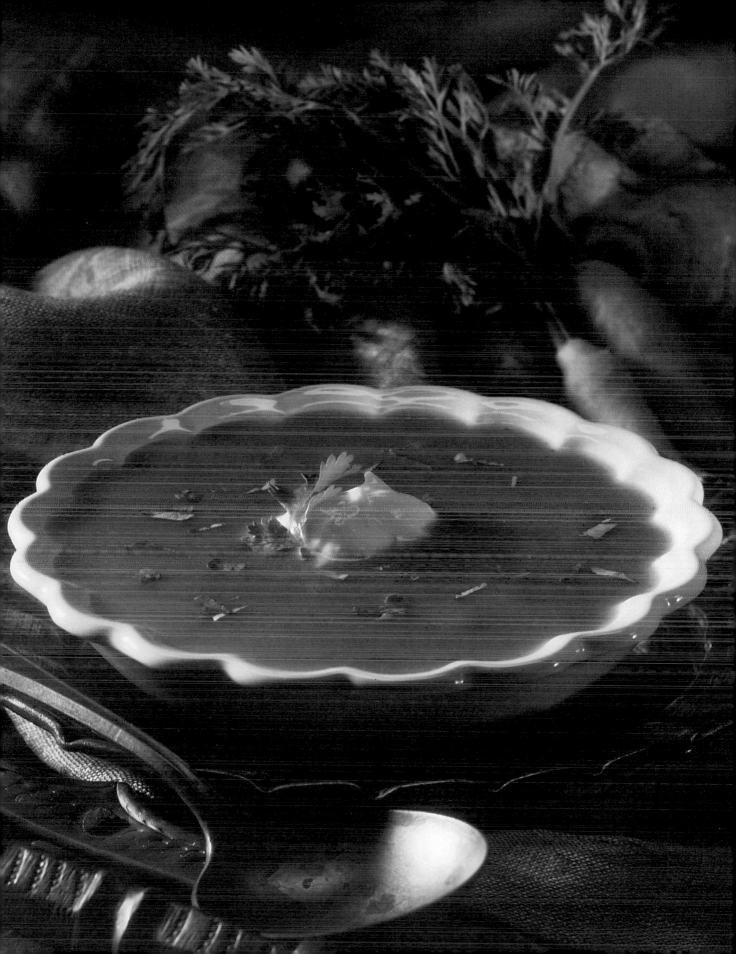

SENSATIONAL SOUPS

117 VEGETABLE–CHICKEN NOODLE SOUP

1 cup chopped celery
½ cup thinly sliced leek (white part only)
½ cup chopped carrot
½ cup chopped turnip
6 cups fat-free reduced-sodium chicken broth, divided
1 tablespoon minced fresh parsley
1 teaspoon balsamic vinegar
1½ teaspoons fresh thyme *or* ½ teaspoon dried thyme leaves
1 teaspoon fresh rosemary *or* ¼ teaspoon dried rosemary
¼ teaspoon black pepper
2 ounces uncooked yolk-free wide noodles
1 cup diced cooked chicken

1. Place celery, leek, carrot, turnip and ⅓ cup chicken broth in large saucepan. Cover; cook over medium heat until vegetables are tender, stirring occasionally.

2. Stir in remaining chicken broth, parsley, vinegar, thyme, rosemary and pepper. Bring to a boil; add noodles. Cook until noodles are tender; stir in chicken. Reduce heat to medium. Simmer until heated through.

Makes 6 servings

Nutrients per Serving: Calories: 98 (14% Calories from Fat), Total Fat: 2 g, Saturated Fat: trace, Protein: 10 g, Carbohydrate: 12 g, Cholesterol: 18 mg, Sodium: 73 mg, Fiber: 1 g, Sugar: 1 g

Dietary Exchanges: ½ Starch/Bread, 1 Lean Meat, ½ Vegetable

118 CHICKEN CURRY SOUP

6 ounces boneless skinless chicken breast, cut into ½-inch pieces
3½ teaspoons curry powder, divided
1 teaspoon olive oil
¾ cup chopped apple
½ cup sliced carrot
⅓ cup sliced celery
¼ teaspoon ground cloves
2 cans (about 14 ounces each) fat-free reduced-sodium chicken broth
½ cup orange juice
4 ounces uncooked radiatore pasta
Plain nonfat yogurt (optional)

1. Coat chicken with 3 teaspoons curry powder. Heat oil in large saucepan over medium heat until hot. Add chicken; cook and stir 3 minutes or until no longer pink in center. Remove from pan; set aside.

2. Add apple, carrot, celery, remaining ½ teaspoon curry powder and cloves to same pan; cook, stirring occasionally, 5 minutes. Add chicken broth and juice; bring to a boil over high heat. Reduce heat to medium-low. Add pasta; cover. Cook, stirring occasionally, 8 to 10 minutes or until pasta is tender. Add chicken; remove from heat. Ladle into bowls; top each serving with a dollop of plain nonfat yogurt, if desired.

Makes 4 servings

Nutrients per Serving: Calories: 153 (15% Calories from Fat), Total Fat: 3 g, Saturated Fat: trace, Protein: 11 g, Carbohydrate: 22 g, Cholesterol: 17 mg, Sodium: 64 mg, Fiber: 1 g, Sugar: 5 g

Dietary Exchanges: 1 Starch/Bread, 1 Lean Meat, ½ Fruit

Vegetable-Chicken Noodle Soup

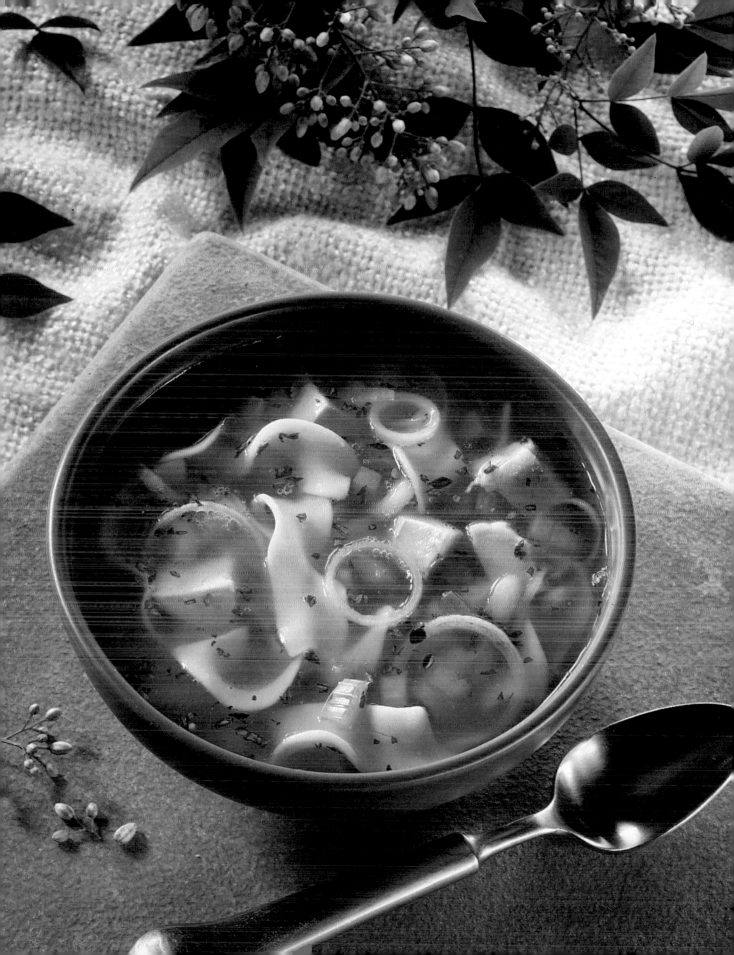

SENSATIONAL SOUPS

119 CREAM OF CHICKEN SOUP

1 cup uncooked white rice
3 cans (10¾ ounces each) fat-free
 reduced-sodium chicken broth
1 skinless bone-in chicken breast half
 (about 6 ounces)
1 rib celery, coarsely chopped
1 carrot, thinly sliced
¼ cup coarsely chopped onion
3 sprigs fresh parsley
1¼ cups evaporated skim milk
¼ teaspoon dried thyme leaves
⅛ teaspoon white pepper
⅛ teaspoon ground nutmeg
2 tablespoons finely chopped fresh parsley
1 green onion, finely chopped

1. Cook rice according to package
directions, omitting salt.

2. Meanwhile, combine chicken broth and
chicken in large saucepan; bring to a boil
over high heat. Reduce heat to medium-low;
simmer 10 minutes, skimming off any foam
that rises to surface. Add celery, carrot,
onion and parsley sprigs; simmer 10 minutes
or until chicken is no longer pink in center
and vegetables are tender, skimming off any
foam that rises to surface.

3. Remove chicken breast from saucepan;
let stand 10 minutes or until cool enough to
handle. Remove chicken from bone; cut into
1-inch pieces.

4. Add rice, chicken pieces, milk, thyme,
pepper and nutmeg to saucepan; cook over
medium-high heat 8 minutes or until soup
thickens, stirring constantly.

5. Top servings with chopped parsley and
green onion.   *Makes 4 servings*

Nutrients per Serving: Calories: 326
(11% Calories from Fat), Total Fat: 4 g,
Saturated Fat: 1 g, Protein: 21 g,
Carbohydrate: 50 g, Cholesterol: 28 mg,
Sodium: 173 mg, Fiber: 1 g, Sugar: 2 g

Dietary Exchanges: 2½ Starch/Bread,
1½ Lean Meat, ½ Milk, 1 Vegetable

120 CHICKEN AND DUMPLINGS STEW

2 cans (about 14 ounces) fat-free
 reduced-sodium chicken broth
1 pound boneless skinless chicken breast
 halves, cut into bite-sized pieces
1 cup diagonally sliced carrots
¾ cup diagonally sliced celery
1 onion, halved and cut into small wedges
3 small new potatoes, unpeeled, cut into
 cubes
½ teaspoon dried rosemary
¼ teaspoon pepper
1 can (14½ ounces) diced tomatoes,
 drained *or* 1½ cups diced fresh
 tomatoes
3 tablespoons all-purpose flour blended
 with ⅓ cup water

DUMPLINGS
¾ cup all-purpose flour
1 teaspoon baking powder
¼ teaspoon onion powder
¼ teaspoon salt
1 to 2 tablespoons finely chopped parsley
¼ cup cholesterol-free egg substitute
¼ cup 1% low-fat milk
1 tablespoon vegetable oil

SENSATIONAL SOUPS

1. Bring chicken broth to a boil in Dutch oven; add chicken. Cover; simmer 3 minutes. Add carrots, celery, onion, potatoes, rosemary and pepper. Cover; simmer 10 minutes. Reduce heat; stir in tomatoes and dissolved flour. Cook and stir until stew thickens.

2. Combine ¾ cup flour, baking powder, onion powder and salt in medium bowl; blend in parsley. Combine egg substitute, milk and oil in small bowl; stir into flour mixture. *Do not overmix.*

3. Return stew to a boil. Drop 8 tablespoons of dumpling batter into broth; cover tightly. Reduce heat; simmer 18 to 20 minutes. *Do not lift lid.* Dumplings are done when wooden pick inserted comes out clean.

Makes 4 servings

Nutrients per Serving: (2 dumplings and stew), Calories: 422 (15% Calories from Fat), Total Fat: 7 g, Saturated Fat: 1 g, Protein: 37 g, Carbohydrate: 51 g, Cholesterol: 70 mg, Sodium: 968 mg, Fiber: 3 g, Sugar: 7

Dietary Exchanges: 2½ Starch/Bread, 3½ Lean Meat, 2 Vegetable

Chicken and Dumplings Stew

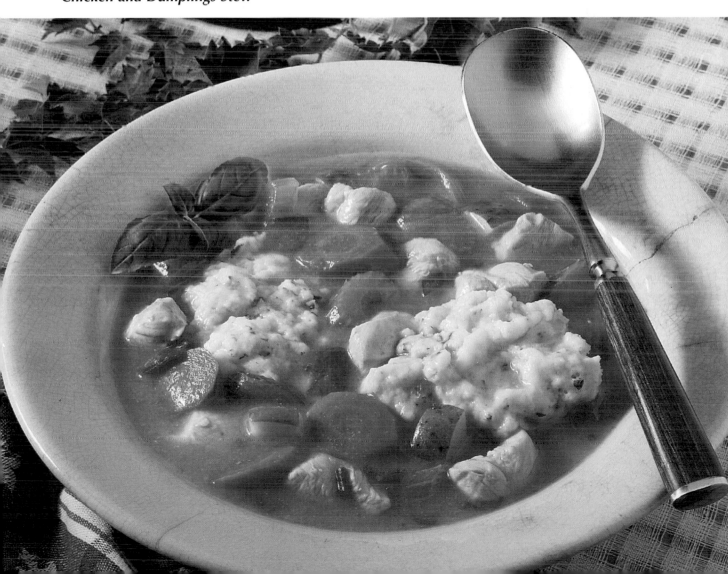

121 SOUTHWEST CORN AND TURKEY SOUP

3 dried ancho chilies *or* 6 dried New
    Mexico chilies
2 small zucchini
1 medium onion, thinly sliced
3 cloves garlic, minced
1 teaspoon ground cumin
3 cans (about 14 ounces each) fat-free
    reduced-sodium chicken broth
1½ to 2 cups (8 to 12 ounces) shredded
    cooked dark turkey meat
1 can (15 ounces) chick-peas or black
    beans, rinsed and drained
1 package (10 ounces) frozen corn
¼ cup cornmeal
1 teaspoon dried oregano leaves
⅓ cup chopped cilantro

1. Cut stems from chilies; shake out seeds.
Place chilies in medium bowl; cover with
boiling water. Let stand 20 to 40 minutes or
until soft; drain. Cut open lengthwise; lay flat
on work surface. Scrape chili pulp from skin
with small knife; set aside.

2. Cut zucchini in half lengthwise; slice
crosswise into ½-inch-wide pieces. Set aside.

3. Spray large saucepan with cooking spray;
heat over medium heat. Add onion; cook,
covered, 3 to 4 minutes or until golden
brown, stirring several times. Add garlic and
cumin; cook and stir about 30 seconds. Add
reserved chili pulp and remaining
ingredients; bring to a boil. Reduce heat;
simmer 15 minutes. *Makes 6 servings*

Nutrients per Serving: Calories: 243
(19% Calories from Fat), Total Fat: 5 g,
Saturated Fat: 1 g, Protein: 19 g,
Carbohydrate: 32 g, Cholesterol: 32 mg,
Sodium: 408 mg, Fiber: 7 g, Sugar 2 g

Dietary Exchanges: 2 Bread/Starch,
2 Lean Meat

122 VEGETABLE BEEF NOODLE SOUP

8 ounces beef stew meat, cut into ½-inch
    pieces
¾ cup unpeeled cubed potato (1 medium)
½ cup sliced carrots
1 tablespoon balsamic vinegar
¾ teaspoon dried thyme leaves
¼ teaspoon black pepper
2½ cups fat-free reduced-sodium beef broth
1 cup water
¼ cup prepared chili sauce or ketchup
2 ounces uncooked thin egg noodles
¾ cup jarred or canned pearl onions,
    rinsed and drained
¼ cup frozen peas

1. Heat large saucepan over high heat until
hot; add beef. Cook 3 minutes or until
browned on all sides, stirring occasionally.
Remove from pan.

2. Cook potato, carrots, vinegar, thyme and
pepper 3 minutes in same saucepan over
medium heat. Add beef broth, water and
chili sauce; bring to a boil over medium-high
heat. Add beef; reduce heat to medium-low.
Simmer, covered, 30 minutes or until meat is
almost fork tender.

3. Bring beef mixture to a boil over medium-
high heat. Add noodles; cook, covered, 7 to
10 minutes or until noodles are tender,
stirring occasionally. Add onions and peas;
heat 1 minute. *Makes 6 servings*

Nutrients per Serving: Calories: 182
(14% Calories from Fat), Total Fat: 3 g,
Saturated Fat: 1 g, Protein: 15 g,
Carbohydrate: 24 g, Cholesterol: 28 mg,
Sodium: 258 mg, Fiber: 1 g, Sugar: 3 g

Dietary Exchanges: 1 Starch/Bread,
1½ Lean Meat, 1 Vegetable

Southwest Corn and Turkey Soup

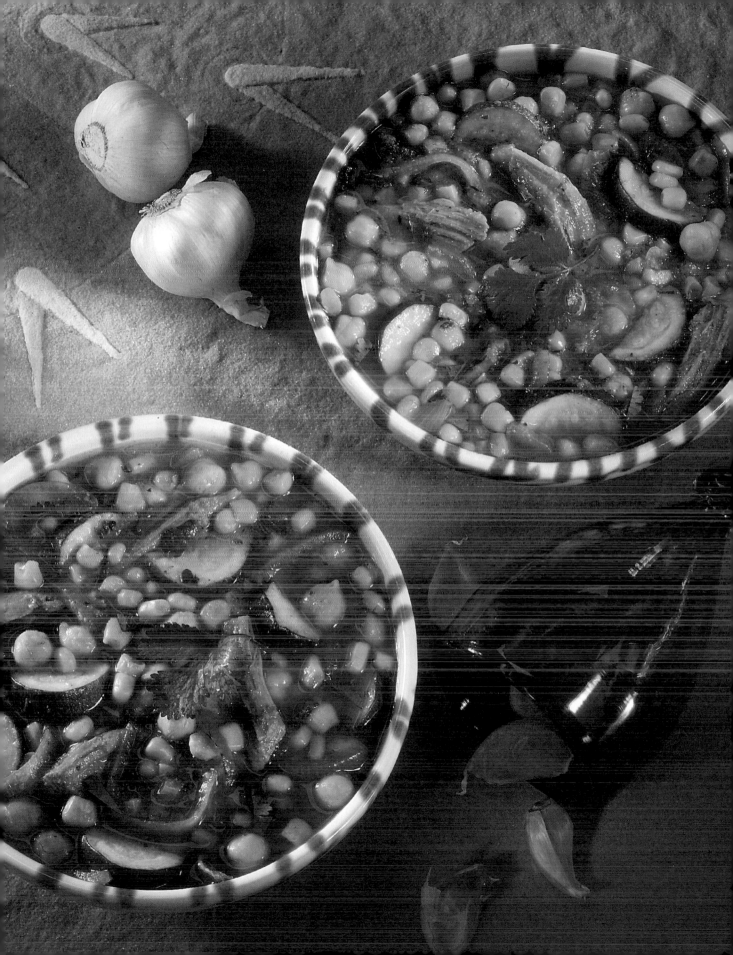

SENSATIONAL SOUPS

123 VIETNAMESE BEEF SOUP

¾ **pound boneless lean beef, such as sirloin or round steak**

3 cups water

1 can (about 14 ounces) beef broth

1 can (10½ ounces) condensed consommé

2 tablespoons reduced-sodium soy sauce

2 tablespoons minced fresh ginger

1 cinnamon stick (3 inches long)

4 ounces uncooked rice noodles, ⅛ inch wide

½ **cup thinly sliced or julienned carrots**

2 cups fresh mung bean sprouts

1 small red onion, halved and thinly sliced

½ **cup chopped cilantro**

½ **cup chopped fresh basil leaves**

1 to 3 teaspoons Chinese chili sauce or paste

1. Place beef in freezer 45 minutes or until firm. Meanwhile, combine water, beef broth, consommé, soy sauce, ginger and cinnamon stick in large saucepan; bring to a boil over high heat. Reduce heat to low; simmer, covered, 20 to 30 minutes. Remove cinnamon stick; discard. Meanwhile, place rice noodles in large bowl and cover with warm water; let stand until pliable, about 20 minutes.

2. Slice beef across grain into very thin strips. Drain noodles. Place noodles and carrots in simmering broth; cook 2 to 3 minutes or until noodles are tender. Add beef and bean sprouts; cook 1 minute or until beef is no longer pink.

3. Remove from heat; stir in red onion, cilantro, basil and chili sauce. To serve, lift noodles from soup with fork and place in bowls. Ladle remaining ingredients and broth over noodles. *Makes 6 servings*

Nutrients per Serving: Calories: 180 (15% Calories from Fat), Total Fat: 3 g, Saturated Fat: 1 g, Protein: 16 g, Carbohydrate: 23 g, Cholesterol: 32 mg, Sodium: 800 mg, Fiber: 1 g, Sugar: 3 g

Dietary Exchanges: 1 Starch/Bread, 1½ Lean Meat, 1 Vegetable

124 KANSAS CITY STEAK SOUP

Nonstick cooking spray

½ **pound ground sirloin**

1 cup chopped onion

3 cups frozen mixed vegetables

1 cup sliced celery

1 can (14½ ounces) stewed tomatoes, undrained

1 beef bouillon cube

½ **to 1 teaspoon black pepper**

2 cups water

½ **cup all-purpose flour**

1 can (10½ ounces) fat-free reduced-sodium beef broth

Spray Dutch oven with cooking spray; heat over medium-high heat until hot. Add beef and onion; cook and stir 5 minutes. Add mixed vegetables, celery, tomatoes, bouillon cube, pepper and water; bring to a boil. Whisk together flour and beef broth until smooth; add to beef mixture, stirring constantly. Return mixture to a boil. Reduce heat to low; simmer, covered, 15 minutes, stirring frequently. *Makes 6 servings*

Nutrients per Serving: Calories: 198 (23% Calories from Fat), Total Fat: 5 g, Saturated Fat: 2 g, Protein: 13 g, Carbohydrate: 27 g, Cholesterol: 23 mg, Sodium: 598 mg, Fiber: 5 g, Sugar: 7 g

Dietary Exchanges: ½ Starch/Bread, 1 Lean Meat, 3½ Vegetable, ½ Fat

Vietnamese Beef Soup

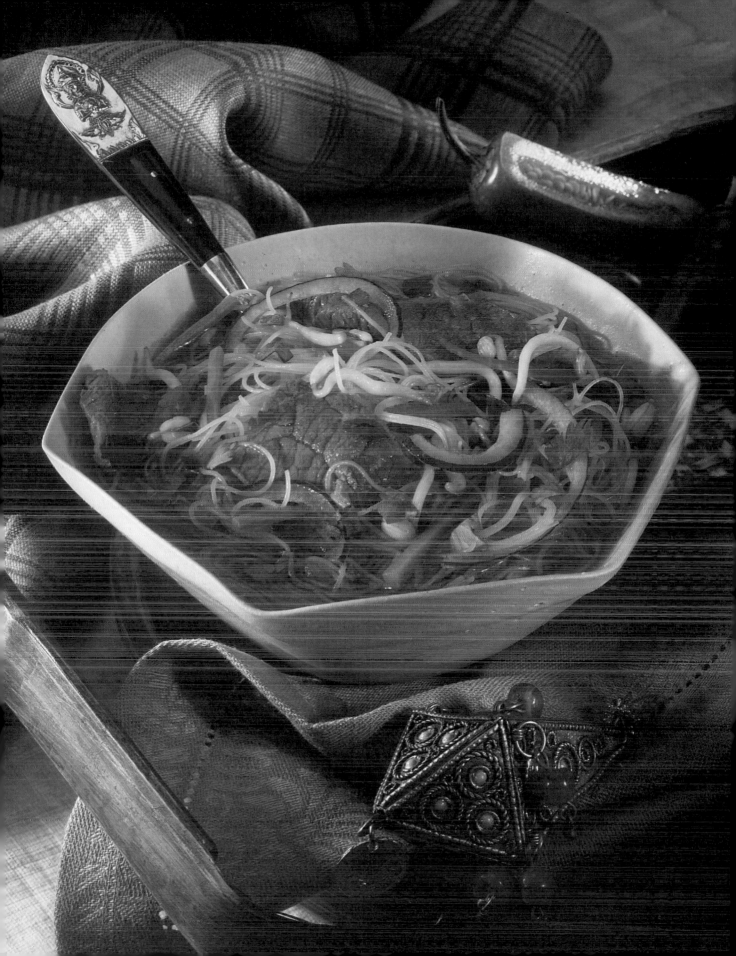

SENSATIONAL SOUPS

125 GINGER WONTON SOUP

4 ounces lean ground pork
½ cup reduced-fat ricotta cheese
½ tablespoon minced fresh cilantro
½ teaspoon black pepper
⅛ teaspoon Chinese five-spice powder
20 (3-inch) wonton wrappers
1 teaspoon vegetable oil
⅓ cup chopped red bell pepper
1 teaspoon grated fresh ginger
2 cans (about 14 ounces each) fat-free reduced-sodium chicken broth
2 teaspoons reduced-sodium soy sauce
4 ounces fresh snow peas
1 can (8¾ ounces) baby corn, rinsed and drained
2 green onions, thinly sliced

1. Cook pork in small nonstick skillet over medium-high heat 4 minutes or until no longer pink. Cool slightly; stir in ricotta cheese, cilantro, black pepper and five-spice powder.

2. Place 1 teaspoon filling in center of each wonton wrapper. Fold top corner of wonton over filling. Lightly brush remaining corners with water. Fold left and right corners over filling. Tightly roll filled end toward remaining corner in jelly-roll fashion. Moisten edges with water to seal. Cover and set aside.

3. Heat oil in large saucepan. Add bell pepper and ginger; cook 1 minute. Add chicken broth and soy sauce; bring to a boil. Add snow peas, baby corn and wontons. Reduce heat to medium-low and simmer 4 to 5 minutes or until wontons are tender. Sprinkle with green onions.

Makes 4 servings

Nutrients per Serving: Calories: 259 (17% Calories from Fat), Total Fat: 5 g, Saturated Fat: 1 g, Protein: 16 g, Carbohydrate: 39 g, Cholesterol: 53 mg, Sodium: 261 mg, Fiber: 3 g, Sugar: 2 g

Dietary Exchanges: 2½ Starch/Bread, 1 Lean Meat, ½ Vegetable, ½ Fat

126 ASIAN RAMEN NOODLE SOUP

2 cans (about 14 ounces each) fat-free reduced-sodium chicken broth
4 ounces boneless pork loin, sliced into thin strips
¾ cup thinly sliced mushrooms
½ cup firm tofu, diced (optional)
3 tablespoons white vinegar
3 tablespoons sherry
1 tablespoon reduced-sodium soy sauce
½ teaspoon ground red pepper
2 ounces uncooked low-fat ramen noodles
1 egg, beaten
¼ cup finely chopped green onion tops

1. Bring chicken broth to a boil in large saucepan; add pork, mushrooms and tofu, if desired. Reduce heat; simmer, covered, 5 minutes.

2. Stir in vinegar, sherry, soy sauce and pepper; return to a boil. Stir in noodles; cook, stirring occasionally, 5 to 7 minutes or until noodles are tender. Slowly stir in beaten egg and onions.

Makes 4 servings

Nutrients per Serving: Calories: 148 (24% Calories from Fat), Total Fat: 4 g, Saturated Fat: 1 g, Protein: 10 g, Carbohydrate: 15 g, Cholesterol: 66 mg, Sodium: 269 mg, Fiber: 1 g, Sugar: 2 g

Dietary Exchanges: ½ Starch/Bread, 1½ Lean Meat, 1 Vegetable

Ginger Wonton Soup

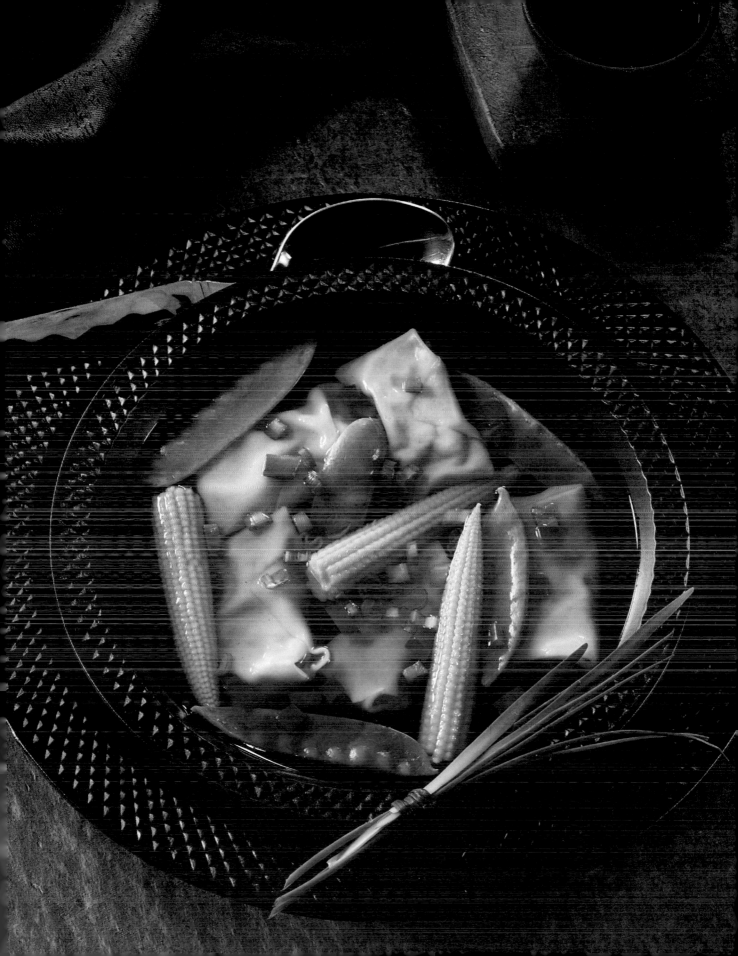

SENSATIONAL SOUPS

127 SHANTUNG TWIN MUSHROOM SOUP

1 package (1 ounce) dried black Chinese
 mushrooms
2 teaspoons vegetable oil
1 large onion, coarsely chopped
2 cloves garlic, minced
2 cups sliced fresh button mushrooms
2 cans (about 14 ounces each) fat-free
 reduced-sodium chicken broth
2 ounces cooked ham, cut into thin slivers
½ cup thinly sliced green onions
1 tablespoon reduced-sodium soy sauce
1 tablespoon dry sherry
1 tablespoon cornstarch
6 whole wheat dinner rolls

1. Place dried mushrooms in small bowl;
cover with warm water. Soak 20 minutes to
soften. Drain; squeeze out excess water.
Discard stems; slice caps.

2. Heat oil in large saucepan over medium
heat until hot. Add chopped onion and garlic;
cook 1 minute. Add both types of mushrooms;
cook 4 minutes, stirring occasionally.

3. Add chicken broth; bring to a boil over
high heat. Reduce heat to medium; simmer,
covered, 15 minutes.

4. Stir in ham and green onions; heat
through. Blend soy sauce and sherry into
cornstarch in small bowl until smooth; stir
into soup. Cook 2 minutes or until soup is
thickened, stirring occasionally. Serve with
whole wheat dinner rolls.

Makes 6 servings

Nutrients per Serving: (including 1 dinner
roll), Calories: 154 (25% Calories from Fat),
Total Fat: 4 g, Saturated Fat: trace, Protein: 7 g,
Carbohydrate: 22 g, Cholesterol: 5 mg,
Sodium: 363 mg, Fiber: 3 g, Sugar: 2 g

Dietary Exchanges: 1½ Starch/Bread,
1 Vegetable, ½ Fat

128 MEDITERRANEAN FISH SOUP

4 ounces uncooked pastina or other small
 pasta
 Nonstick cooking spray
¾ cup chopped onion
2 cloves garlic, minced
1 teaspoon fennel seeds
1 can (14½ ounces) no-salt-added stewed
 tomatoes
1 can (about 14 ounces) fat-free
 reduced-sodium chicken broth
1 tablespoon minced fresh parsley
½ teaspoon black pepper
¼ teaspoon ground turmeric
8 ounces firm, white-fleshed fish, cut into
 1-inch pieces
3 ounces small shrimp, peeled and
 deveined

1. Cook pasta according to package
directions, omitting salt. Drain; set aside.

2. Spray large nonstick saucepan with
cooking spray; heat over medium heat until
hot. Add onion, garlic and fennel seeds; cook
and stir 3 minutes or until onion is soft.

3. Stir in tomatoes, chicken broth, parsley,
black pepper and turmeric; bring to a boil.
Reduce heat; simmer 10 minutes. Add fish;
cook 1 minute. Add shrimp; cook until
shrimp just begins to turn opaque.

4. Divide pasta among bowls; ladle soup
over pasta. *Makes 4 servings*

Nutrients per Serving: Calories: 209
(10% Calories from Fat), Total Fat: 2 g,
Saturated Fat: trace, Protein: 19 g,
Carbohydrate: 28 g, Cholesterol: 59 mg,
Sodium: 111 mg, Fiber: 3 g, Sugar: 4 g

Dietary Exchanges: 1½ Starch/Bread,
1½ Lean Meat, 1½ Vegetable

Mediterranean Fish Soup

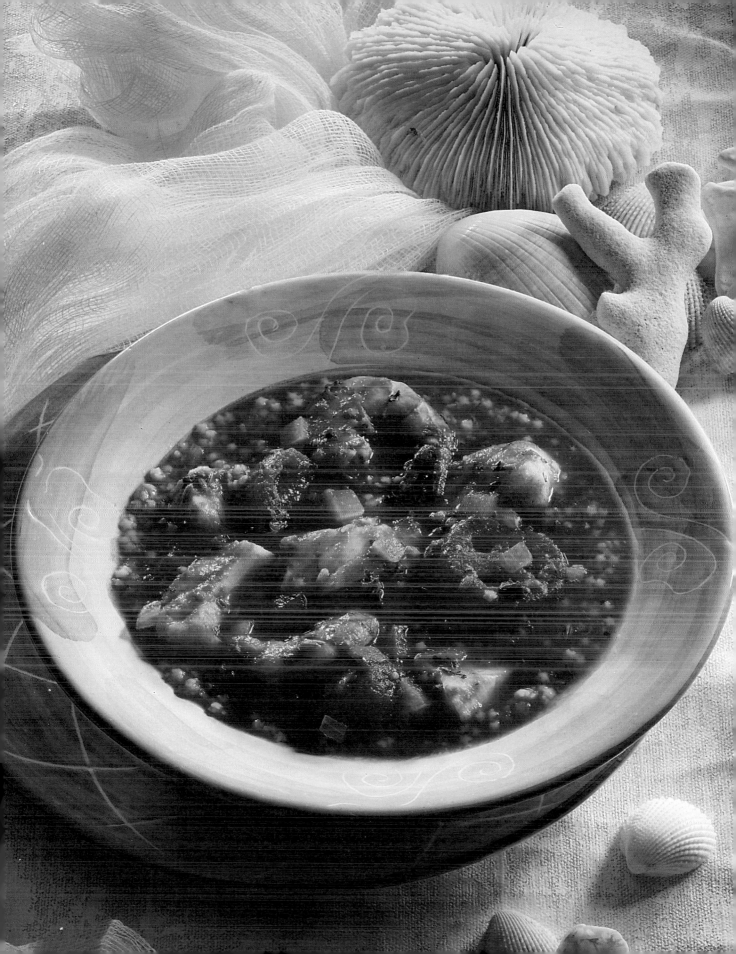

129 VEGETABLE–BEAN CHOWDER

Nonstick cooking spray
½ cup chopped onion
½ cup chopped celery
2 cups water
½ teaspoon salt
2 cups cubed and peeled potatoes
1 cup carrot slices
1 can (15 ounces) cream-style corn
1 can (15 ounces) cannellini beans, rinsed
    and drained
¼ teaspoon dried tarragon leaves
¼ teaspoon black pepper
2 cups 1% low-fat milk
2 tablespoons cornstarch

1. Spray 4-quart Dutch oven or large saucepan with cooking spray; heat over medium heat until hot. Add onion and celery; cook and stir 3 minutes or until crisp-tender.

2. Add water and salt; bring to a boil over high heat. Add potatoes and carrot; reduce heat to medium-low. Simmer, covered, 10 minutes or until potatoes and carrot are tender. Stir in corn, beans, tarragon and pepper; simmer, covered, 10 minutes or until heated through.

3. Stir milk into cornstarch in medium bowl until smooth. Stir into vegetable mixture. Simmer, uncovered, until thickened.

Makes 5 servings

Nutrients per Serving: Calories: 273 (6% Calories from Fat), Total Fat: 2 g, Saturated Fat: 1 g, Protein: 13 g, Carbohydrate: 60 g, Cholesterol: 4 mg, Sodium: 696 mg, Fiber: 8 g, Sugar: 7 g

Dietary Exchanges: 2½ Starch/Bread, ½ Milk, 1 Vegetable, ½ Fat

130 BLACK BEAN BISQUE WITH CRAB

3 cups low sodium chicken broth, defatted
1 jar (12.5 ounces) GUILTLESS
    GOURMET® Black Bean Dip
    (mild or spicy)
1 can (6 ounces) crabmeat, drained
2 tablespoons brandy (optional)
8 tablespoons low fat sour cream
    Chopped fresh chives (optional)

MICROWAVE DIRECTIONS: Combine broth and bean dip in 2-quart glass measure or microwave-safe casserole. Cover with vented plastic wrap or lid; microwave on HIGH (100% power) 6 minutes or until soup starts to bubble.

Stir in crabmeat and brandy, if desired; microwave on MEDIUM (50% power) 2 minutes or to desired serving temperature. To serve, ladle bisque into 8 individual ramekins or soup bowls, dividing evenly. Swirl 1 tablespoon sour cream into each serving. Garnish with chives, if desired.

Makes 8 servings

STOVE TOP DIRECTIONS: Combine broth and bean dip in 2-quart saucepan; bring to a boil over medium heat. Stir in crabmeat and brandy, if desired; cook 2 minutes or to desired serving temperature. Serve as directed.

Nutrients per Serving: Calories: 90 (14% Calories from Fat), Total Fat: 1 g, Saturated Fat: 0 g, Protein: 9 g, Carbohydrate: 9 g, Cholesterol: 22 mg, Sodium: 260 mg, Fiber: 1 g

Dietary Exchanges: ½ Starch/Bread, 1 Lean Meat

Vegetable-Bean Chowder

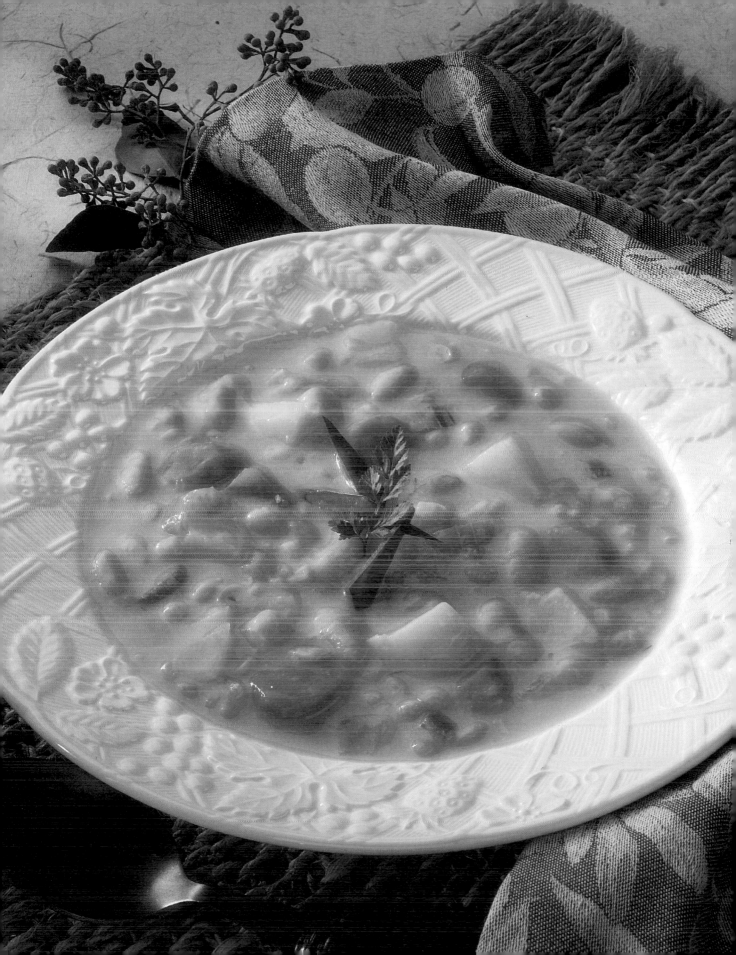

SENSATIONAL SOUPS

131 NEW ENGLAND CLAM CHOWDER

1 can (5 ounces) whole baby clams, undrained
1 baking potato, peeled and coarsely chopped
¼ cup finely chopped onion
⅔ cup evaporated skim milk
¼ teaspoon white pepper
¼ teaspoon dried thyme leaves
1 tablespoon reduced-calorie margarine

1. Drain clams; reserve juice. Add enough water to reserved juice to measure ⅔ cup. Combine clam juice mixture, potato and onion in medium saucepan; bring to a boil over high heat. Reduce heat; simmer 8 minutes or until potato is tender.

2. Add milk, pepper and thyme to saucepan. Increase heat to medium-high; cook and stir 2 minutes. Add margarine; cook 5 minutes or until chowder thickens, stirring occasionally.

3. Add clams; cook and stir 5 minutes or until clams are firm.   *Makes 2 servings*

Nutrients per Serving: Calories: 191 (18% Calories from Fat), Total Fat: 4 g, Saturated Fat: 1 g, Protein: 14 g, Carbohydrate: 27 g, Cholesterol: 47 mg, Sodium: 205 mg, Fiber: 1 g, Sugar: 2 g

Dietary Exchanges: 1 Starch/Bread, 1 Lean Meat, 1 Milk

132 DOUBLE CORN & CHEDDAR CHOWDER

1 tablespoon margarine
1 cup chopped onion
2 tablespoons all-purpose flour
2½ cups fat-free reduced-sodium chicken broth
1 can (16 ounces) cream-style corn
1 cup frozen corn
½ cup finely diced red bell pepper
½ teaspoon hot pepper sauce
¾ cup (3 ounces) shredded sharp Cheddar cheese
Freshly ground black pepper (optional)

1. Melt margarine in large saucepan over medium heat. Add onion; cook and stir 5 minutes. Sprinkle onion with flour; cook and stir 1 minute.

2. Add chicken broth; bring to a boil, stirring frequently. Add cream-style corn, frozen corn, bell pepper and pepper sauce; bring to a simmer. Cover; simmer 15 minutes.

3. Remove from heat; gradually stir in cheese until melted. Ladle into soup bowls; sprinkle with black pepper, if desired.
     Makes 6 servings

DOUBLE CORN, CHEDDAR & RICE CHOWDER: Add 1 cup cooked white or brown rice with corn.

Nutrients per Serving: Calories: 180 (28% Calories from Fat), Total Fat: 6 g, Saturated Fat: 2 g, Protein: 7 g, Carbohydrate: 28 g, Cholesterol: 10 mg, Sodium: 498 mg, Fiber: 2 g, Sugar: 1 g

Dietary Exchanges: 1½ Starch/Bread, ½ Lean Meat, 1 Fat

New England Clam Chowder

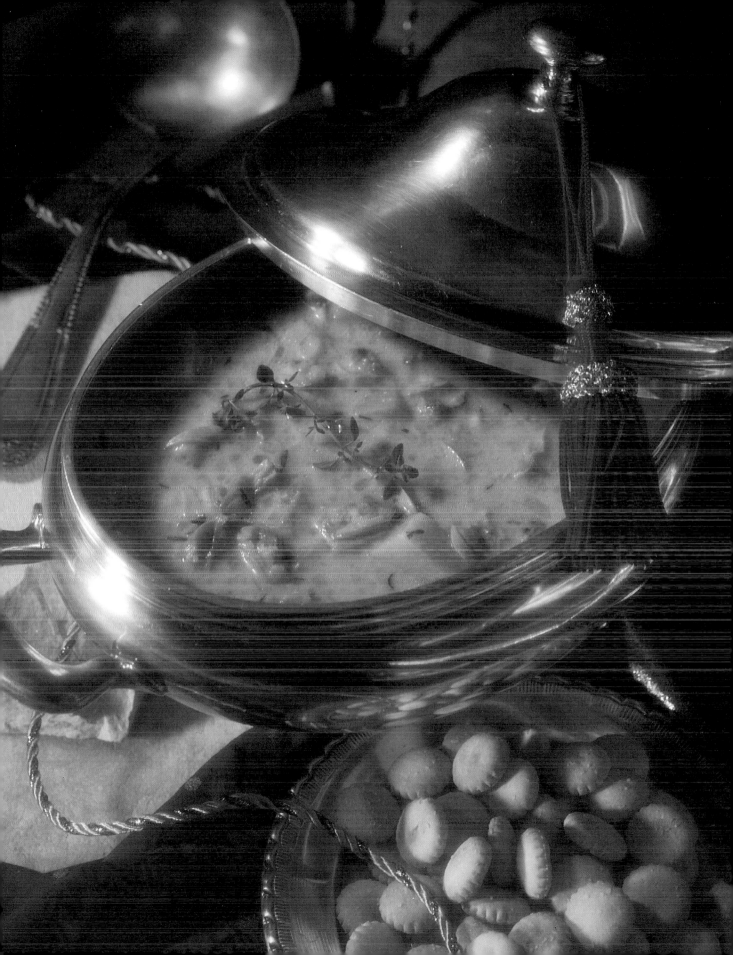

SENSATIONAL SOUPS

133 TURKEY CHILI WITH BLACK BEANS

1 pound ground turkey breast
1 can (about 14 ounces) fat-free
    reduced-sodium chicken broth
1 large onion, finely chopped
1 green bell pepper, diced
2 teaspoons chili powder
½ teaspoon ground allspice
¼ teaspoon ground cinnamon
¼ teaspoon paprika
1 can (15 ounces) black beans,
    rinsed and drained
1 can (14 ounces) crushed tomatoes in
    tomato puree, undrained
2 teaspoons cider vinegar

1. Heat large nonstick skillet over high heat. Add turkey, chicken broth, onion and bell pepper; cook and stir, breaking up turkey until turkey is no longer pink.

2. Add chili powder, allspice, cinnamon and paprika. Reduce heat to medium-low; simmer 10 minutes. Add black beans, tomatoes and vinegar; bring to a boil.

3. Reduce heat to low; simmer 20 to 25 minutes or until thickened to desired consistency.   *Makes 4 servings*

Nutrients per Serving: Calories: 272 (7% Calories from Fat), Total Fat: 2 g, Saturated Fat: 0 g, Protein: 40 g, Carbohydrate: 31 g, Cholesterol: 75 mg, Sodium: 873 mg, Fiber: 10 g, Sugar: 5 g

Dietary Exchanges: 1 Starch/Bread, 4 Lean Meat, 2 Vegetable

134 MEDITERRANEAN CHILI

1 can HEALTHY CHOICE® RECIPE
    CREATIONS™ Tomato with Garden
    Herbs Condensed Soup
¼ cup water
1 cup fat free refried beans
    Vegetable cooking spray
10 ounces extra-lean ground beef
1 small eggplant, diced
½ cup *each* diced onion and diced green
    bell pepper
2 cloves garlic, minced
½ teaspoon chili powder
½ teaspoon salt (optional)

In medium bowl, combine soup, water and beans; mix well. Set aside. In large saucepan sprayed with vegetable cooking spray, cook beef until no longer pink; drain and set aside.

In same saucepan, sauté eggplant, onion, pepper, garlic, chili powder and salt over medium-high heat until vegetables are tender. Add soup mixture and beef; mix well. Simmer until hot and bubbly.

Makes 4 servings

Nutrients per Serving: Calories: 220 (29% Calories from Fat), Fat: 6 g, Protein: 6 g, Sodium: 470 mg

Dietary Exchanges: 1½ Starch/Bread, 2 Lean Meat, 2 Vegetable, 1 Fat

Turkey Chili with Black Beans

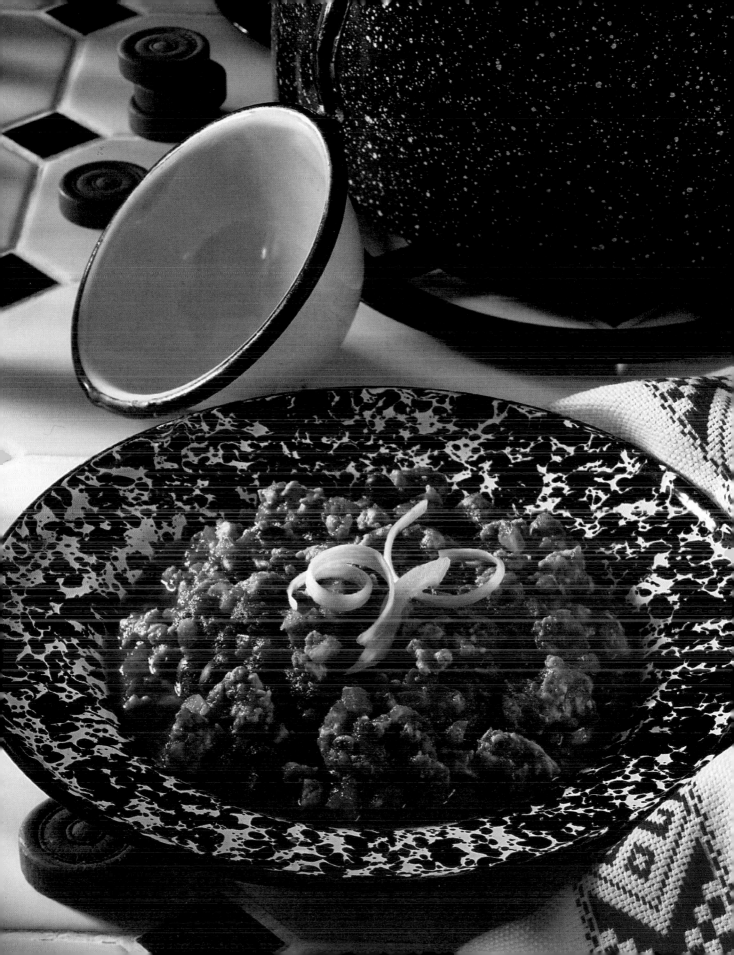

SENSATIONAL SOUPS

135 TEXAS–STYLE CHILI

Nonstick cooking spray
1 pound lean boneless beef chuck, cut into 1/2-inch pieces
2 cups chopped onions
5 cloves garlic, minced
2 tablespoons chili powder
1 tablespoon ground cumin
1 teaspoon ground coriander
1 teaspoon dried oregano leaves
2 1/2 cups fat-free reduced-sodium beef broth
1 cup prepared salsa or picante sauce
2 cans (16 ounces each) pinto or red beans (or one of each), rinsed and drained
1/2 cup chopped fresh cilantro
1/2 cup nonfat sour cream
1 cup chopped ripe tomatoes

1. Spray Dutch oven or large saucepan with nonstick cooking spray; heat over medium-high heat until hot. Add beef, onions and garlic; cook and stir until beef is no longer pink, about 5 minutes. Sprinkle mixture with chili powder, cumin, coriander and oregano; mix well. Add beef broth and salsa; bring to a boil. Cover; simmer 45 minutes.

2. Stir in beans; continue to simmer uncovered 30 minutes or until beef is tender and chili has thickened, stirring occasionally.

3. Stir in cilantro. Ladle into bowls; top with sour cream and tomatoes. Garnish with pickled jalapeño peppers, if desired.

Makes 8 servings

Nutrients per Serving: Calories: 268 (21% Calories from Fat), Total Fat: 7 g, Saturated Fat: 2 g, Protein: 25 g, Carbohydrate: 31 g, Cholesterol: 37 mg, Sodium: 725 mg, Fiber: 2 g, Sugar: 2 g

Dietary Exchanges: 1 1/2 Starch/Bread, 2 1/2 Lean Meat, 1 Vegetable

136 VEGETARIAN CHILI

1 tablespoon vegetable oil
2 cloves garlic, finely chopped
1 1/2 cups thinly sliced mushrooms
2/3 cup chopped red onion
2/3 cup chopped red bell pepper
2 teaspoons chili powder
1/4 teaspoon ground cumin
1/8 teaspoon ground red pepper
1/8 teaspoon dried oregano leaves
1 can (28 ounces) peeled whole tomatoes
2/3 cup frozen baby lima beans
1/2 cup canned Great Northern beans, rinsed and drained
3 tablespoons nonfat sour cream
3 tablespoons shredded reduced-fat Cheddar cheese

1. Heat oil in large nonstick saucepan over medium-high heat until hot. Add garlic; cook and stir 3 minutes. Add mushrooms, onion and bell pepper; cook 5 minutes, stirring occasionally. Add chili powder, cumin, red pepper and oregano; cook and stir 1 minute. Add tomatoes and beans; reduce heat to medium-low. Simmer 15 minutes, stirring occasionally.

2. Top servings with sour cream and cheese.

Makes 4 servings

Nutrients per Serving: Calories: 189 (24% Calories from Fat), Total Fat: 5 g, Saturated Fat: 1 g, Protein: 10 g, Carbohydrate: 29 g, Cholesterol: 3 mg, Sodium: 428 mg, Fiber: 7 g, Sugar: 7 g

Dietary Exchanges: 1 Starch/Bread, 3 Vegetable, 1 Fat

Texas-Style Chili

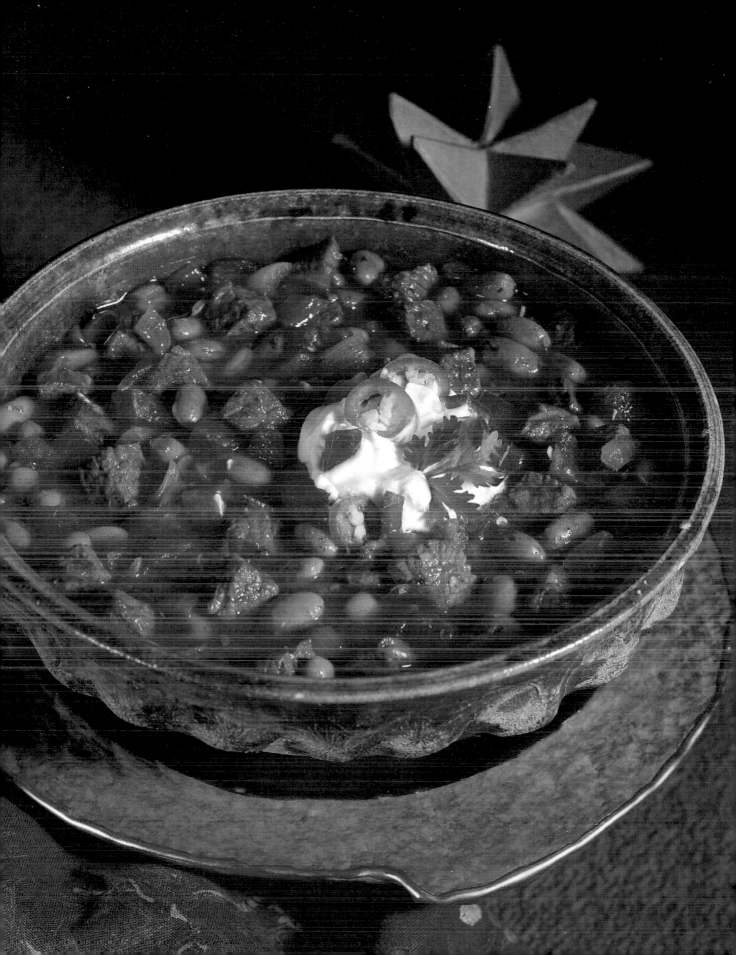

Satisfying Salads & Sandwiches

137 FAJITA SALAD

1 beef sirloin steak (6 ounces)
¼ cup lime juice
2 tablespoons chopped fresh cilantro
1 clove garlic, minced
1 teaspoon chili powder
2 red bell peppers
1 medium onion
1 teaspoon olive oil
1 cup rinsed and drained canned chick-peas
4 cups mixed salad greens
1 tomato, cut into wedges
1 cup salsa

1. Cut beef into strips, about $2 \times 1 \times \frac{1}{4}$-inch. Place in resealable plastic food storage bag. Combine lime juice, cilantro, garlic and chili powder in small bowl. Pour over beef; seal bag. Let stand for 10 minutes, turning once.

2. Cut peppers into strips. Cut onion into slices. Heat olive oil in large nonstick skillet over medium-high heat until hot. Add peppers and onion; cook and stir for 6 minutes or until vegetables are crisp-tender. Remove from skillet; set aside. Add beef and marinade to skillet; cook and stir 3 minutes or until meat is cooked through. Remove from heat. Add peppers, onion and chick-peas to skillet; toss to coat with pan juices. Cool slightly.

3. Divide lettuce evenly among serving plates; top with beef mixture and tomato wedges. Serve with salsa; garnish with sour cream and sprigs of cilantro, if desired.

Makes 4 servings

Nutrients per Serving: Calories: 160 (23% Calories from Fat), Total Fat: 5 g, Saturated Fat: 1 g, Protein: 17 g, Carbohydrate: 20 g, Cholesterol: 30 mg, Sodium: 667 mg, Fiber: 6 g, Sugar: 4 g

Dietary Exchanges: ½ Starch/Bread, 1½ Lean Meat, 2 Vegetable

Fajita Salad

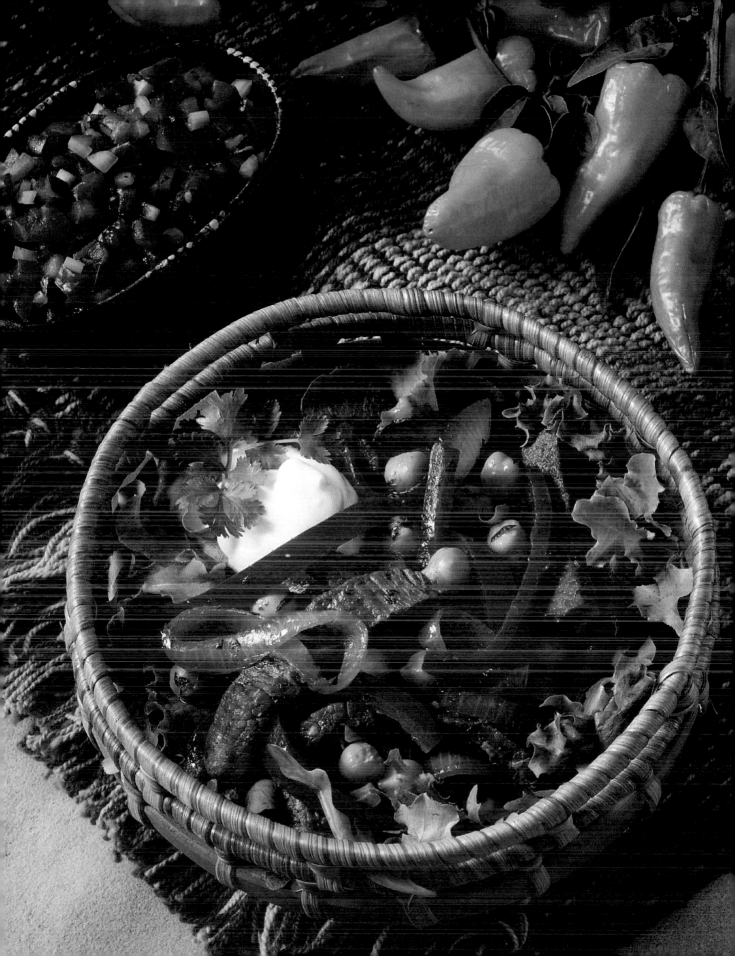

SATISFYING SALADS & SANDWICHES

138 CHICKEN CAESAR SALAD

4 small boneless skinless chicken breast halves
6 ounces uncooked gnocchi or other dried pasta
1 package (9 ounces) frozen artichoke hearts, thawed
1½ cups cherry tomatoes, quartered
¼ cup plus 2 tablespoons plain nonfat yogurt
2 tablespoons reduced-calorie mayonnaise
2 tablespoons grated Romano cheese
1 tablespoon sherry or red wine vinegar
1 clove garlic, minced
½ teaspoon anchovy paste
½ teaspoon Dijon mustard
½ teaspoon white pepper
1 small head romaine lettuce, washed and torn into bite-size pieces
1 cup toasted bread cubes

1. Grill or broil chicken breasts until no longer pink in center; set aside.

2. Cook pasta according to package directions, omitting salt; drain. Rinse under cold running water until cool; drain. Combine pasta, artichoke hearts and tomatoes in large bowl; set aside.

3. Combine yogurt, mayonnaise, Romano cheese, sherry, garlic, anchovy paste, mustard and white pepper in small bowl; whisk until smooth. Pour over pasta mixture; toss to coat evenly.

4. Arrange lettuce on platter or individual plates. Spoon pasta mixture over lettuce. Thinly slice chicken breasts; place on top of pasta. Sprinkle with bread cubes.

Makes 4 servings

Nutrients per Serving: Calories: 379 (19% Calories from Fat), Total Fat: 8 g, Saturated Fat: 2 g, Protein: 32 g, Carbohydrate: 45 g, Cholesterol: 56 mg, Sodium: 294 mg, Fiber: 7 g, Sugar: 5 g

Dietary Exchanges: 2 Starch/Bread, 3 Lean Meat, 3 Vegetable

139 SUNBURST CHICKEN SALAD

1 tablespoon fat-free mayonnaise
1 tablespoon nonfat sour cream
2 teaspoons frozen orange juice concentrate, thawed
¼ teaspoon grated orange peel
1 boneless skinless chicken breast, cooked and chopped
1 large kiwi, thinly sliced
⅓ cup mandarin oranges
¼ cup finely chopped celery
4 lettuce leaves, washed
2 tablespoons coarsely chopped cashews

Combine mayonnaise, sour cream, concentrate and peel in small bowl. Add chicken, kiwi, oranges and celery; toss to coat. Cover; refrigerate 2 hours. Serve on lettuce leaves. Top with cashews.

Makes 2 servings

Nutrients per Serving: Calories: 195 (29% Calories from Fat), Total Fat: 6 g, Saturated Fat: 1 g, Protein: 18 g, Carbohydrate: 18 g, Cholesterol: 39 mg, Sodium: 431 mg, Fiber: 2 g, Sugar: 8 g

Dietary Exchanges: 2 Lean Meat, 1 Fruit, ½ Fat

Sunburst Chicken Salad

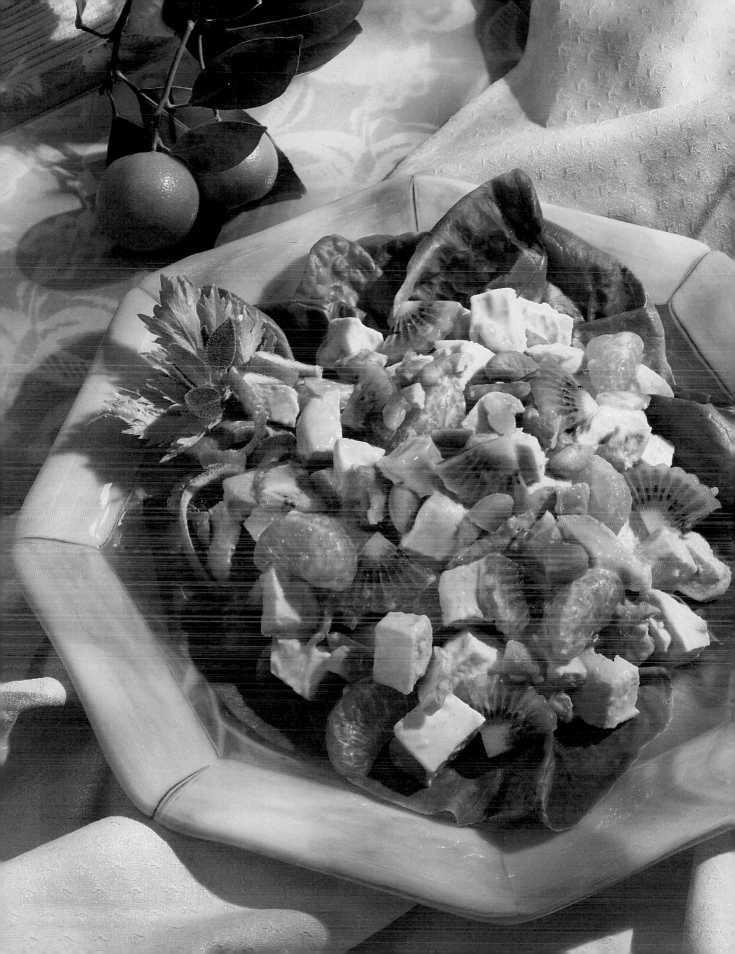

SATISFYING SALADS & SANDWICHES

140 CHICKEN AND SPINACH SALAD

12 ounces chicken tenders
   Nonstick cooking spray
4 cups shredded spinach leaves
2 cups washed and torn romaine lettuce
   leaves
8 thin slices red onion
2 tablespoons (1 ounce) crumbled blue
   cheese
1 large grapefruit, peeled and sectioned
½ cup frozen citrus blend concentrate,
   thawed
¼ cup prepared fat-free Italian salad
   dressing

1. Cut chicken tenders into 2×½-inch strips. Spray large nonstick skillet with cooking spray; heat over medium heat until hot. Add chicken tenders; cook and stir 5 minutes or until no longer pink in center. Remove from skillet.

2. Divide spinach, lettuce, onion, cheese, grapefruit and chicken among 4 salad plates. Combine concentrate and Italian dressing in small bowl; drizzle over salads. Garnish with assorted greens, if desired.

Makes 4 servings

Nutrients per Serving: Calories: 218 (15% Calories from Fat), Total Fat: 4 g, Saturated Fat: 1 g, Protein: 23 g, Carbohydrate: 23 g, Cholesterol: 55 mg, Sodium: 361 mg, Fiber: 3 g, Sugar: 5 g

Dietary Exchanges: 2 Lean Meat, 1½ Fruit, 1 Vegetable

Chicken and Spinach Salad

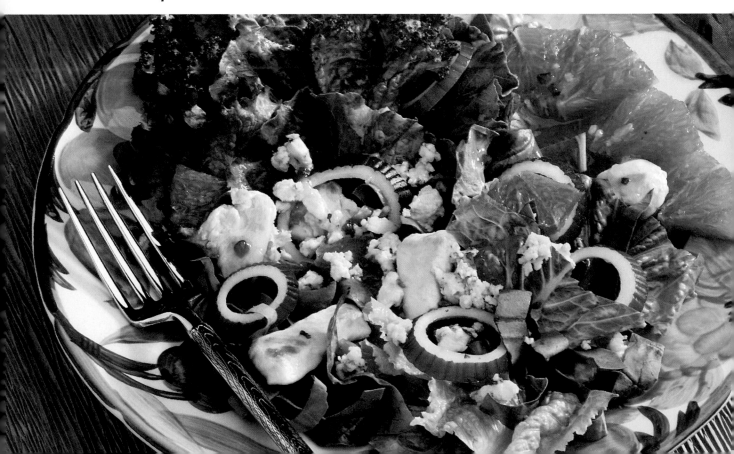

141 CHICKEN AND FRUIT SALAD

½ cup plain nonfat yogurt
½ to 1 teaspoon lemon-pepper seasoning
½ teaspoon dry mustard
¼ teaspoon garlic salt
¼ teaspoon poppy seed
1¼ teaspoons EQUAL® MEASURE™ or
    4 packets EQUAL® sweetener or
    3 tablespoons EQUAL® SPOONFUL™
1 to 2 tablespoons orange juice
4 cups torn spinach leaves
8 ounces thinly sliced cooked chicken breast
2 cups sliced strawberries
1 cup halved seedless green grapes
1½ cups thinly sliced yellow summer squash
2 medium oranges, peeled and sectioned
½ cup toasted pecan pieces (optional)

• Combine yogurt, lemon-pepper seasoning, mustard, garlic salt, poppy seed and Equal® in small bowl. Add enough orange juice to reach drizzling consistency; set aside.

• Line platter with spinach. Arrange chicken, strawberries, grapes, squash and orange sections over spinach. Drizzle salad with dressing. Sprinkle with pecans, if desired.
Makes 4 servings

Nutrients per Serving: Calories: 202, Fat: 5 g, Protein: 21 g, Carbohydrate: 20 g, Cholesterol: 51 mg, Sodium: 380 mg

Dietary Exchanges: 2½ Lean Meat, ½ Vegetable, 1 Fruit

142 ZESTY TACO SALAD

2 tablespoons vegetable oil
1 clove garlic, finely chopped
¾ pound ground turkey
1¾ teaspoons chili powder
¼ teaspoon ground cumin
3 cups washed and torn lettuce leaves
1 can (14½ ounces) Mexican-style diced tomatoes, drained
1 cup rinsed and drained canned chick-peas or pinto beans
⅔ cup chopped peeled cucumber
⅓ cup frozen corn, thawed
¼ cup chopped red onion
1 to 2 jalapeño peppers,* seeded and finely chopped (optional)
1 tablespoon red wine vinegar
12 fat-free baked tortilla chips

*Jalapeño peppers can sting and irritate the skin. Wear rubber gloves when handling peppers and do not touch eyes. Wash hands after handling.

1. Combine oil and garlic in small bowl; let stand 1 hour at room temperature.

2. Combine turkey, chili powder and cumin in large nonstick skillet. Cook over medium heat 5 minutes or until turkey is no longer pink, stirring to separate turkey.

3. Combine turkey, lettuce, tomatoes, beans, cucumber, corn, onion and jalapeño in large bowl. Remove garlic from oil; discard garlic. Combine oil and vinegar in small bowl. Drizzle over salad; toss to coat. Serve on tortilla chips.
Makes 4 servings

Nutrients per Serving: Calories: 285 (33% Calories from Fat), Total Fat: 11 g, Saturated Fat: 1 g, Protein: 21 g, Carbohydrate: 28 g, Cholesterol: 33 mg, Sodium: 484 mg, Fiber: 5 g, Sugar: 4 g

Dietary Exchanges: 1½ Starch/Bread, 2 Lean Meat, 1 Vegetable, 1 Fat

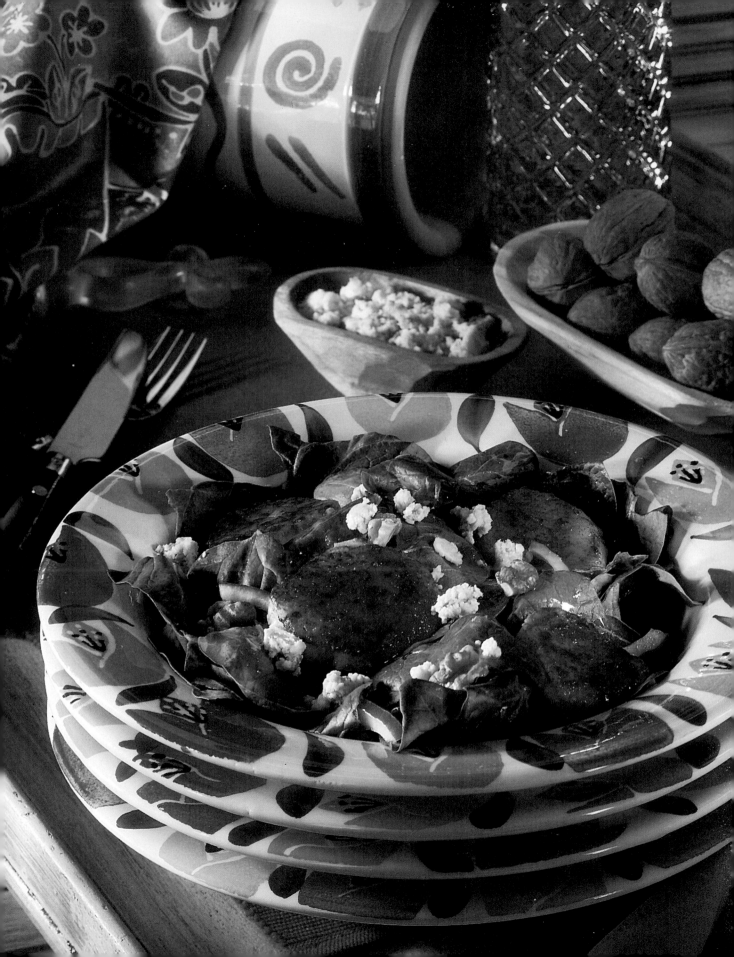

SATISFYING SALADS & SANDWICHES

143 SCALLOP AND SPINACH SALAD

1 package (10 ounces) spinach leaves, washed, stemmed and torn
3 thin slices red onion, halved and separated
12 ounces sea scallops
   Ground red pepper
   Paprika
   Nonstick cooking spray
½ cup prepared fat-free Italian salad dressing
¼ cup crumbled blue cheese
2 tablespoons toasted walnuts

1. Pat spinach dry; place in large bowl with red onion. Cover; set aside.

2. Rinse scallops. Cut in half horizontally (to make 2 thin rounds); pat dry. Sprinkle top side lightly with red pepper and paprika. Spray large nonstick skillet with cooking spray; heat over high heat until very hot. Add half of scallops, seasoned side down, in single layer, placing ½ inch or more apart. Sprinkle with red pepper and paprika. Cook 2 minutes or until browned on bottom. Turn scallops; cook 1 to 2 minutes or until opaque in center. Transfer to plate; cover to keep warm. Wipe skillet clean; repeat procedure with remaining scallops.

3. Place dressing in small saucepan; bring to a boil over high heat. Pour dressing over spinach and onion; toss to coat. Divide among 4 plates. Place scallops on top of spinach; sprinkle with blue cheese and walnuts. *Makes 4 servings*

Nutrients per Serving: Calories: 169 (29% Calories from Fat), Total Fat: 6 g, Saturated Fat: 2 g, Protein: 24 g, Carbohydrate: 6 g, Cholesterol: 50 mg, Sodium: 660 mg, Fiber: 2 g, Sugar: trace

Dietary Exchanges: 3 Lean Meat, 1 Vegetable

144 STILTON SALAD DRESSING

½ cup buttermilk
¼ cup silken firm tofu
2 ounces Stilton cheese
1 teaspoon lemon juice
1 clove garlic, peeled
¼ teaspoon salt
⅛ teaspoon black pepper
2 tablespoons 1% low-fat cottage cheese
   Romaine lettuce hearts, torn into bite-sized pieces (optional)
   Toasted chopped walnuts (optional)

1. Place buttermilk, tofu, Stilton cheese, lemon juice, garlic, salt and black pepper in blender or food processor; process until smooth. Pour mixture into small bowl; fold in cottage cheese. Store in airtight container and refrigerate 3 hours or overnight before serving. Serve with romaine lettuce and toasted walnuts, if desired.

Makes 6 servings

Nutrients per Serving: Calories: 51 (55% Calories from Fat), Total Fat: 3 g, Saturated Fat: 2 g, Protein: 4 g, Carbohydrate: 2 g, Cholesterol: 8 mg, Sodium: 265 mg, Fiber: trace, Sugar: 1 g

Dietary Exchanges: ½ Lean Meat, ½ Fat

Scallop and Spinach Salad

SATISFYING SALADS & SANDWICHES

145 ITALIAN CROUTON SALAD

6 ounces French or Italian bread
¼ cup plain nonfat yogurt
¼ cup red wine vinegar
4 teaspoons olive oil
1 tablespoon water
3 cloves garlic, minced
6 medium (about 12 ounces) plum
   tomatoes
½ medium red onion, thinly sliced
3 tablespoons slivered fresh basil leaves
2 tablespoons finely chopped parsley
12 leaves red leaf lettuce *or* 4 cups
   prepared Italian salad mix
2 tablespoons grated Parmesan cheese

1. Preheat broiler. Cut bread into ¾-inch cubes. Place in single layer on jelly-roll pan. Broil, 4 inches from heat, 3 minutes or until bread is golden, stirring every 30 seconds to 1 minute. Remove from pan; place in large bowl.

2. Whisk together yogurt, vinegar, oil, water and garlic in small bowl until blended; set aside. Core tomatoes; cut into ¼-inch-wide slices. Add to bread along with onion, basil and parsley; stir until blended. Pour yogurt mixture over crouton mixture; toss to coat. Cover; refrigerate 30 minutes or up to 1 day. (Croutons will be more tender the following day.)

3. To serve, place lettuce on plates. Spoon crouton mixture over lettuce. Sprinkle with Parmesan cheese.   *Makes 6 servings*

Nutrients per Serving: Calories: 160 (28% Calories from Fat), Total Fat: 5 g, Saturated Fat: 1 g, Protein: 6 g, Carbohydrate: 25 g, Cholesterol: 2 mg, Sodium: 234 mg, Fiber: 2 g, Sugar: 5 g

Dietary Exchanges: 1 Starch/Bread, 1½ Vegetable, 1 Fat

146 SPINACH SALAD WITH HOT APPLE DRESSING

6 strips turkey bacon
¾ cup apple cider
2 tablespoons brown sugar
4 teaspoons rice wine vinegar
¼ teaspoon black pepper
6 cups washed, stemmed and torn spinach
   leaves
2 cups sliced mushrooms
1 medium tomato, cut into wedges
½ cup thinly sliced red onion

1. Heat medium nonstick skillet over medium heat until hot; add bacon and cook 2 to 3 minutes per side or until crisp. Remove from pan. Coarsely chop 3 pieces; set aside. Finely chop remaining 3 pieces; return to skillet. Add apple cider, sugar, vinegar and pepper. Heat just to a simmer; remove from heat.

2. Combine spinach, mushrooms, tomato and onion in large bowl. Add dressing; toss to coat. Top with reserved bacon.
Makes 6 servings

Nutrients per Serving: Calories: 95 (28% Calories from Fat), Total Fat: 3 g, Saturated Fat: 1 g, Protein: 5 g, Carbohydrate: 14 g, Cholesterol: 9 mg, Sodium: 256 mg, Fiber: 2 g, Sugar: 1 g

Dietary Exchanges: ½ Fruit, 1½ Vegetable, ½ Fat

Italian Crouton Salad

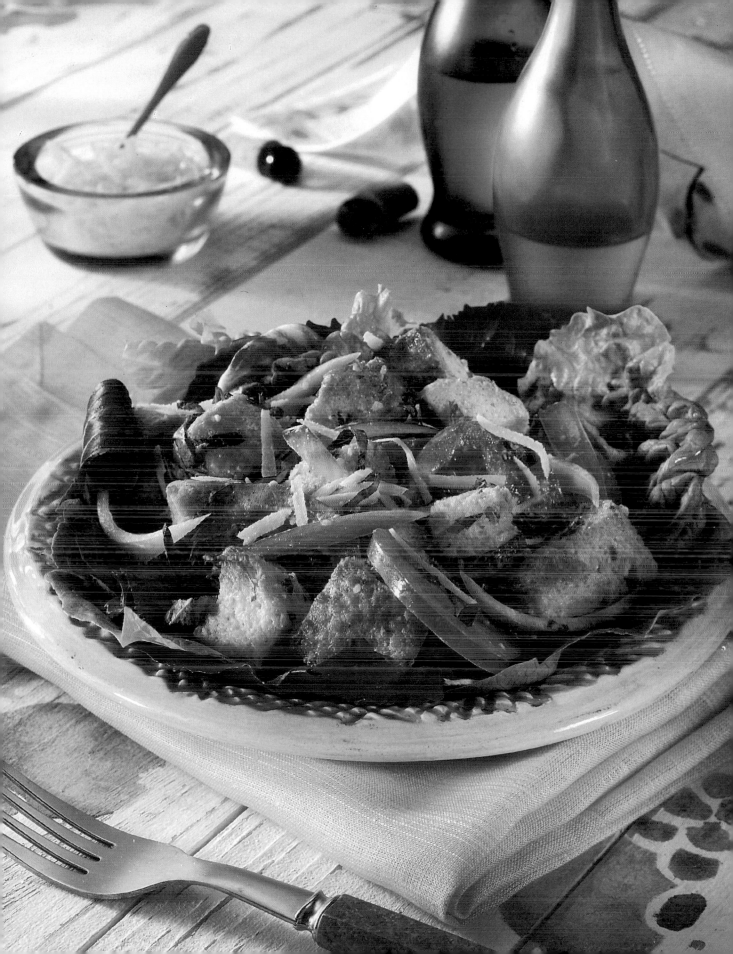

SATISFYING SALADS & SANDWICHES

147 FRESH GREENS WITH HOT BACON DRESSING

3 cups torn spinach leaves
3 cups torn romaine lettuce leaves
2 small tomatoes, cut into wedges
1 cup sliced mushrooms
1 medium carrot, shredded
1 slice bacon, cut into small pieces
3 tablespoons red wine vinegar
1 tablespoon water
¼ teaspoon dried tarragon, crushed
⅛ teaspoon coarsely ground pepper
¼ teaspoon EQUAL® MEASURE™ or
    1 packet EQUAL® sweetener or
    2 teaspoons EQUAL® SPOONFUL™

• Combine spinach, romaine, tomatoes, mushrooms and carrot in large bowl; set aside.

• Cook bacon in 12-inch skillet until crisp. Carefully stir in vinegar, water, tarragon and pepper. Heat to boiling; remove from heat. Stir in Equal®.

• Add spinach mixture to skillet. Toss 30 to 60 seconds or just until greens are wilted. Transfer to serving bowl. Serve immediately.
Makes 4 to 6 (1⅓-cup) servings

Nutrients per Serving: Calories: 51, Fat: 1 g, Protein: 3 g, Carbohydrates: 9 g, Cholesterol: 1 mg, Sodium: 74 mg

Dietary Exchanges: 1½ Vegetable

148 PEAR AND CRANBERRY SALAD

½ cup canned whole berry cranberry sauce
2 tablespoons balsamic vinegar
1 tablespoon olive or canola oil
12 cups (9 ounces) packed assorted bitter or gourmet salad greens
6 small or 4 large pears (about 1¾ pounds)
2 ounces blue or Gorgonzola cheese, crumbled
Freshly ground black pepper

1. Combine cranberry sauce, vinegar and oil in small bowl; mix well. (Dressing may be covered and refrigerated up to 2 days before serving.)

2. Arrange greens on six serving plates. Cut pears lengthwise into ½-inch-thick slices; cut core and seeds from each slice. Arrange pears attractively over greens. Drizzle cranberry dressing over pears and greens; sprinkle with cheese. Sprinkle with pepper to taste. *Makes 6 servings*

Nutrients per Serving: Calories: 161 (29% Calories from Fat), Total Fat: 6 g, Saturated Fat: 2 g, Protein: 4 g, Carbohydrate: 26 g, Cholesterol: 7 mg, Sodium: 165 mg, Fiber: 2 g, Sugar: 1 g

Dietary Exchanges: 2 Fruit, 1 Fat

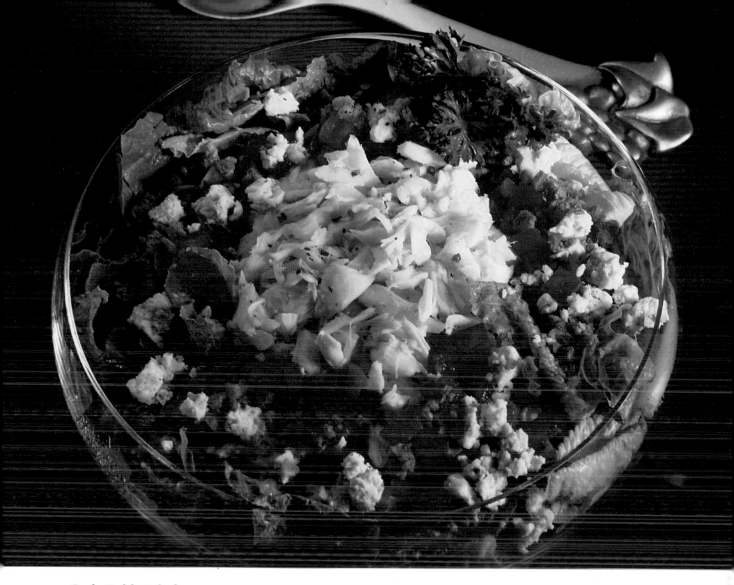

Crab Cobb Salad

149 CRAB COBB SALAD

12 cups washed and torn romaine lettuce
   leaves
 2 cans (6 ounces each) crabmeat, drained
 2 cups diced ripe tomatoes or halved
   cherry tomatoes
¼ cup (1½ ounces) crumbled blue or
   Gorgonzola cheese
¼ cup cholesterol-free bacon bits
¾ cup fat-free Italian or Caesar salad
   dressing
   Freshly ground black pepper

1. Cover large serving platter with lettuce. Arrange crabmeat, tomatoes, blue cheese and bacon bits over lettuce.

2. Just before serving, drizzle dressing evenly over salad; toss well. Transfer to 8 chilled serving plates; season to taste with pepper.   *Makes 8 servings*

Nutrients per Serving: Calories: 110 (27% Calories from Fat), Total Fat: 3 g, Saturated Fat: 1 g, Protein: 12 g, Carbohydrate: 8 g, Cholesterol: 46 mg, Sodium: 666 mg, Fiber: 2 g, Sugar: 3 g

Dietary Exchanges: 1½ Lean Meat, 1½ Vegetable

SATISFYING SALADS & SANDWICHES

150 SWEET AND SOUR BROCCOLI PASTA SALAD

8 ounces uncooked pasta twists
2 cups broccoli florets
2/3 cup shredded carrots
1 medium Red or Golden Delicious apple, cored, seeded and chopped
1/3 cup plain nonfat yogurt
1/3 cup apple juice
3 tablespoons cider vinegar
1 tablespoon olive oil
1 tablespoon Dijon mustard
1 teaspoon honey
1/2 teaspoon dried thyme leaves
   Lettuce leaves

1. Cook pasta according to package directions, omitting salt; add broccoli during the last 2 minutes of cooking. Drain; rinse under cold running water until pasta and broccoli are cool. Drain.

2. Place pasta, broccoli, carrots and apple in medium bowl.

3. Combine yogurt, apple juice, cider vinegar, oil, mustard, honey, and thyme in small bowl. Pour over pasta mixture; toss to coat.

4. Serve on individual dishes lined with lettuce. Garnish with apple slices, if desired.

Makes 6 servings

Nutrients per Serving: Calories: 198 (15% Calories from Fat), Total Fat: 3 g, Saturated Fat: 1 g, Protein: 7 g, Carbohydrate: 36 g, Cholesterol: trace, Sodium: 57 mg, Fiber: 3 g, Sugar: 6 g

Dietary Exchanges: 2 Starch/Bread, 1/2 Fruit, 1/2 Vegetable, 1/2 Fat

151 CHICK–PEA PASTA SALAD

4 ounces uncooked spinach rotini or fusilli
1 can (15 ounces) chick-peas, rinsed and drained
1/3 cup finely chopped carrot
1/3 cup chopped celery
1/2 cup chopped red bell pepper
2 green onions with tops, sliced
3 tablespoons balsamic vinegar
2 tablespoons reduced-calorie mayonnaise
2 teaspoons prepared whole-grain mustard
1/2 teaspoon black pepper
1/4 teaspoon Italian seasoning
   Leaf lettuce

1. Cook pasta according to directions, omitting salt; drain. Rinse under cold running water until cool; drain.

2. Combine pasta, chick-peas, carrot, celery, bell pepper and green onions in medium bowl.

3. Whisk together vinegar, mayonnaise, mustard, black pepper and Italian seasoning in small bowl until blended. Pour over salad; toss to coat evenly. Cover and refrigerate up to 8 hours.

4. Arrange lettuce on individual plates. Spoon salad over lettuce.

Makes 8 servings

Nutrients per Serving: Calories: 129 (16% Calories from Fat), Total Fat: 2 g, Saturated Fat: trace, Protein: 5 g, Carbohydrate: 22 g, Cholesterol: 1 mg, Sodium: 242 mg, Fiber: 3 g, Sugar: trace

Dietary Exchanges: 1½ Starch/Bread, ½ Fat

Sweet and Sour Broccoli Pasta Salad

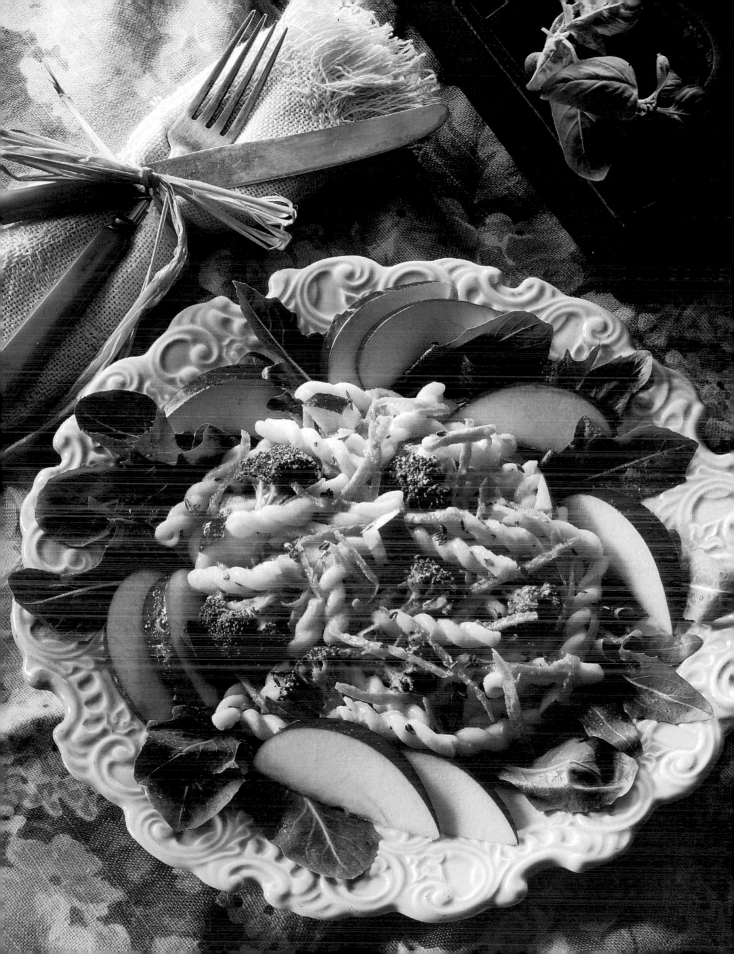

SATISFYING SALADS & SANDWICHES

152 ORIENTAL GARDEN TOSS

⅓ cup thinly sliced green onions
3 tablespoons reduced-sodium soy sauce
3 tablespoons water
1½ teaspoons roasted sesame oil
1 teaspoon EQUAL® MEASURE™ or
    3 packets EQUAL® sweetener or
    2 tablespoons EQUAL® SPOONFUL™
¼ teaspoon garlic powder
⅛ teaspoon crushed red pepper flakes
1 package (3 ounces) low-fat ramen
    noodle soup
2 cups fresh pea pods, halved crosswise
1 cup fresh bean sprouts
1 cup sliced fresh mushrooms
1 can (8¾ ounces) baby corn, drained and
    halved crosswise
1 red bell pepper, cut into bite-size strips
3 cups shredded Chinese cabbage
⅓ cup chopped lightly salted cashews
    (optional)

• Combine green onions, soy sauce, water, sesame oil, Equal®, garlic powder and red pepper flakes in screw-top jar; set aside.

• Break up ramen noodles (discard seasoning packet); combine with pea pods in large bowl. Pour boiling water over mixture to cover. Let stand 1 minute; drain.

• Combine noodles, pea pods, bean sprouts, mushrooms, baby corn and bell pepper in large bowl. Shake dressing and add to noodle mixture; toss to coat. Cover and chill 2 to 24 hours. Just before serving, add shredded cabbage; toss to combine. Sprinkle with cashews, if desired.

Makes 6 (1-cup) servings

Nutrients per Serving: Calories: 124, Fat: 2 g, Protein: 6 g, Carbohydrates: 21 g, Cholesterol: 0 mg, Sodium: 605 mg

Dietary Exchanges: 1 Starch/Bread, 1 Vegetable, ½ Fat

153 GAZPACHO MACARONI SALAD

4 ounces uncooked macaroni
2½ cups chopped and seeded tomatoes
1 cup finely chopped red onion
1 cup finely chopped cucumber
½ cup finely chopped celery
½ cup finely chopped green bell pepper
½ cup finely chopped red bell pepper
2 tablespoons finely chopped black olives
3 tablespoons cider vinegar
1 bay leaf
2 tablespoons minced parsley *or*
    1 teaspoon dried parsley
1 tablespoon fresh thyme *or* ½ teaspoon
    dried thyme leaves
1 clove garlic, minced
3 to 4 dashes hot pepper sauce
¼ teaspoon black pepper

1. Cook pasta according to package directions, omitting salt; drain. Rinse well under cold running water until cool; drain.

2. Combine pasta and remaining ingredients in medium bowl. Cover and refrigerate 4 hours for flavors to blend. Remove bay leaf before serving. Garnish with whole olives, cucumber slices and dill sprigs, if desired. Serve chilled or at room temperature.

Makes 6 servings

Nutrients per Serving: Calories: 136 (11% Calories from Fat), Total Fat: 2 g, Saturated Fat: trace, Protein: 5 g, Carbohydrate: 27 g, Cholesterol: 0 mg, Sodium: 114 mg, Fiber: 3 g, Sugar: 1 g

Dietary Exchanges: 1 Starch/Bread, 2½ Vegetable, ½ Fat

Gazpacho Macaroni Salad

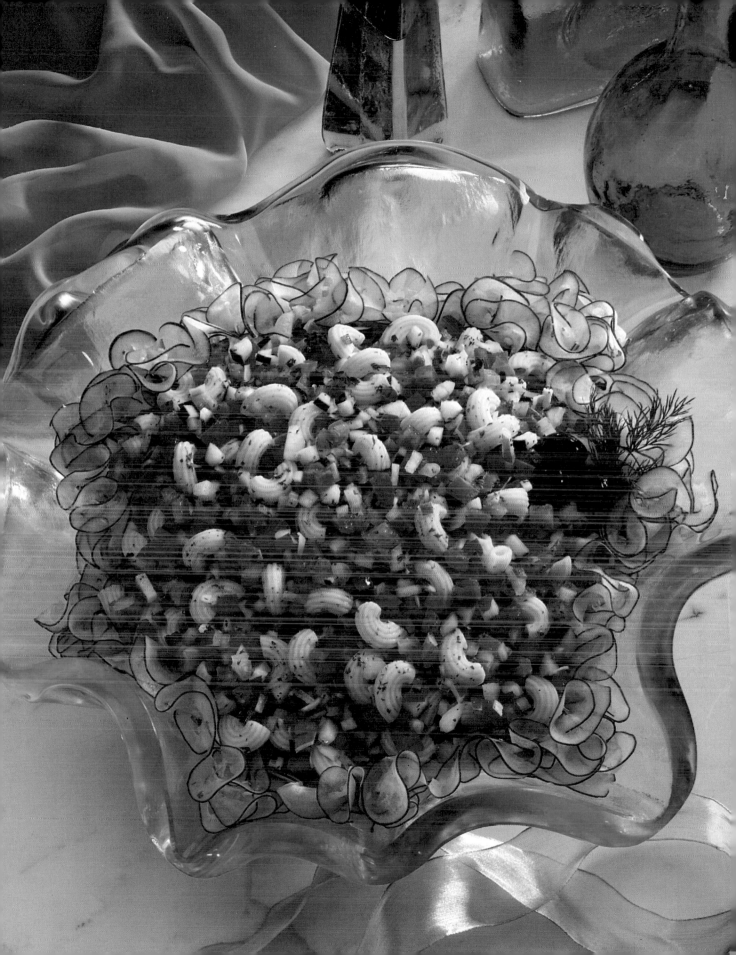

SATISFYING SALADS & SANDWICHES

154 PENNE SALAD WITH SPRING PEAS

1 pound penne or medium pasta shells, cooked and cooled
1½ cups fresh or thawed frozen peas, cooked
1 large yellow or red bell pepper, sliced
½ cup sliced green onions and tops
1 cup skim milk
½ cup fat-free mayonnaise
½ cup red wine vinegar
¼ cup minced parsley
2 teaspoons drained green peppercorns, crushed (optional)
1¾ teaspoons EQUAL® MEASURE™ or
   6 packets EQUAL® sweetener or
   ¼ cup EQUAL® SPOONFUL™
Salt and pepper

• Combine pasta, peas, bell pepper and green onions in salad bowl. Blend milk and mayonnaise in medium bowl until smooth. Stir in vinegar, parsley, peppercorns and Equal®.

• Pour dressing over salad and toss to coat; season to taste with salt and pepper.

Makes 6 (1-cup) servings

Nutrients per Serving: Calories: 190, Fat: 1 g, Protein: 8 g, Carbohydrates: 36 g, Cholesterol: 26 mg, Sodium: 188 mg

Dietary Exchanges: 2 Starch/Bread

155 SALMON AND GREEN BEAN SALAD WITH PASTA

1 can (6 ounces) red salmon
8 ounces small whole wheat or regular pasta shells
¾ cup fresh green beans, cut into 2-inch pieces
⅔ cup finely chopped carrots
½ cup nonfat cottage cheese
3 tablespoons plain nonfat yogurt
1½ tablespoons lemon juice
1 tablespoon chopped fresh dill
2 teaspoons grated onion
1 teaspoon Dijon mustard

1. Drain salmon and separate into chunks; set aside.

2. Cook pasta according to package directions, including ¼ teaspoon salt; add green beans during last 3 minutes of cooking. Drain; rinse under cold running water until pasta and green beans are cool. Drain.

3. Combine pasta, green beans, carrots and salmon in medium bowl.

4. Place cottage cheese, yogurt, lemon juice, dill, onion and mustard in blender or food processor; process until smooth. Pour over pasta mixture; toss to coat evenly.

Makes 6 servings

Nutrients per Serving: Calories: 210 (15% Calories from Fat), Total Fat: 3 g, Saturated Fat: 1 g, Protein: 16 g, Carbohydrate: 29 g, Cholesterol: 15 mg, Sodium: 223 mg, Fiber: 2 g, Sugar: 2 g

Dietary Exchanges: 1½ Starch/Bread, 1½ Lean Meat, ½ Vegetable

Penne Salad with Spring Peas

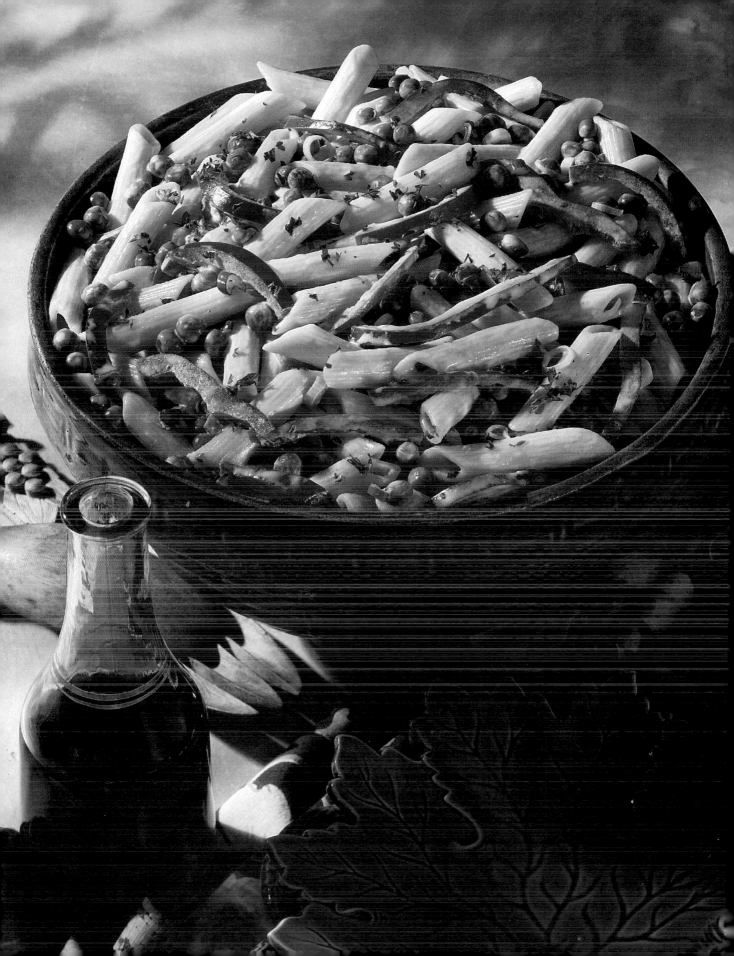

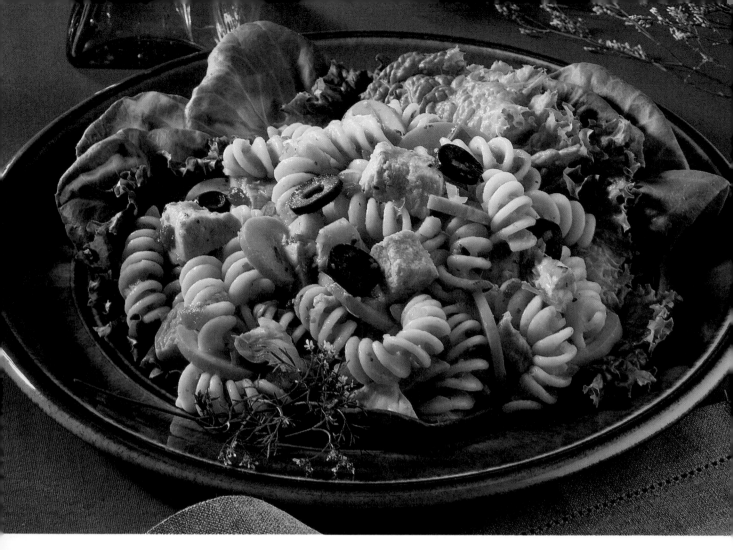

Santa Fe Chicken Pasta Salad

156 SANTA FE CHICKEN PASTA SALAD

12 ounces uncooked spiral pasta
2 cups cooked chicken breast cubes
½ cup chopped green onions
1 medium zucchini or yellow squash, cut in half lengthwise, then sliced crosswise
1 cup GUILTLESS GOURMET® Green Tomatillo Salsa
1 cup drained and coarsely chopped artichoke hearts
½ cup sliced black olives
    Lettuce leaves
    Fresh dill sprigs (optional)

Cook pasta according to package directions; drain. Place pasta in large nonmetal bowl; add chicken, onions, zucchini, tomatillo salsa, artichoke hearts and olives. Toss lightly. Refrigerate at least 6 hours before serving.

To serve, line serving platter with lettuce leaves. Top with pasta mixture. Garnish with dill, if desired.   *Makes 4 servings*

Nutrients per Serving: Calories: 413 (10% Calories from Fat), Total Fat: 5 g, Saturated Fat: trace, Protein: 26 g, Carbohydrate: 66 g, Cholesterol: 45 mg, Sodium: 429 mg, Fiber: 6 g

Dietary Exchanges: 4 Starch/Bread, 2 Lean Meat, 1 Vegetable

SATISFYING SALADS & SANDWICHES

157 PENNE PASTA SALAD

6 cups cooked penne pasta
2 cups shredded cooked skinless chicken breast
1 cup chopped red onion
¾ cup *each* chopped red or green bell pepper and sliced zucchini
1 (4-ounce) can sliced black olives, drained
1 teaspoon crushed red pepper
1 teaspoon salt (optional)
1 HEALTHY CHOICE® RECIPE CREATIONS™ Cream of Roasted Chicken with Herbs Condensed Soup
½ cup *each* lemon juice and fat free shredded Parmesan cheese
½ cup shredded fresh basil (optional)

In large bowl, combine pasta, chicken, onion, bell pepper, zucchini, olives, red pepper and salt; toss lightly. In small bowl, combine soup and lemon juice; mix well. Pour soup mixture over pasta salad; mix well. Sprinkle with Parmesan cheese and basil, if desired. *Makes 8 servings*

Nutrients per Serving: Calories: 258 (22% Calories from Fat), Fat: 6 g, Protein: 21 g, Sodium: 380 mg

Dietary Exchanges: 2½ Starch/Bread, 1 Lean Meat, ½ Fat

158 SMOKED TURKEY PASTA SALAD

8 ounces uncooked ditalini pasta (small tubes)
6 ounces smoked turkey or chicken breast, skin removed, cut into strips
1 can (15 ounces) light kidney beans, rinsed and drained
½ cup thinly sliced celery
¼ cup chopped red onion
⅓ cup reduced-fat mayonnaise
2 tablespoons balsamic vinegar
2 tablespoons chopped fresh chives or green onion
1 tablespoon fresh tarragon *or* 1½ teaspoons dried tarragon leaves
1 teaspoon Dijon mustard
1 clove garlic, minced
¼ teaspoon black pepper
Lettuce leaves (optional)

1. Cook pasta according to package directions, omitting salt; drain. Rinse under cold running water until cool; drain.

2. Combine pasta, turkey, beans, celery and onion in medium bowl. Combine mayonnaise, vinegar, chives, tarragon, mustard, garlic and pepper in small bowl. Pour over pasta mixture; toss to coat. Serve on lettuce leaves, if desired.

Makes 7 servings

Nutrients per Serving: Calories: 233 (19% Calories from Fat), Total Fat: 5 g, Saturated Fat: 1 g, Protein: 13 g, Carbohydrate: 34 g, Cholesterol: 12 mg, Sodium: 249 mg, Fiber: 5 g, Sugar: trace

Dietary Exchanges: 2 Starch/Bread, 1 Lean Meat, ½ Vegetable, ½ Fat

SATISFYING SALADS & SANDWICHES

159 SPICY ORZO AND BLACK BEAN SALAD

2 tablespoons olive oil
2 tablespoons minced jalapeño pepper,* divided
1 teaspoon chili powder
¾ cup uncooked orzo pasta
1 cup frozen mixed vegetables
1 can (16 ounces) black beans, rinsed and drained
2 thin slices red onion
¼ cup chopped fresh cilantro
¼ cup lime juice
¼ cup lemon juice
4 cups washed, stemmed and torn spinach leaves
2 tablespoons crumbled blue cheese (optional)

Jalapeño peppers can sting and irritate the skin; wear rubber gloves when handling peppers and do not touch eyes. Wash hands after handling.

1. Combine oil, 1 tablespoon jalapeño and chili powder in medium bowl; set aside.

2. Bring 6 cups water and remaining 1 tablespoon jalapeño to a boil in large saucepan. Add orzo. Cook 10 to 12 minutes or until tender; drain. Rinse under cold running water until cool; drain.

3. Place frozen vegetables in small microwavable container. Cover; microwave at HIGH 3 minutes or until hot. Cover; let stand 5 minutes.

4. Add orzo, vegetables, black beans, onion, cilantro, lime juice and lemon juice to reserved oil mixture in bowl. Divide spinach evenly among serving plates. Top with orzo and bean mixture. Sprinkle with blue cheese. Garnish with fresh cilantro, if desired.   *Makes 4 servings*

Nutrients per Serving: Calories: 356 (20% Calories from Fat), Total Fat: 9 g, Saturated Fat: 1 g, Protein: 17 g, Carbohydrate: 61 g, Cholesterol: 0 mg, Sodium: 467 mg, Fiber: 10 g, Sugar: 4 g

Dietary Exchanges: 3½ Starch/Bread, 2 Vegetable, 1½ Fat

160 FAR EAST TABBOULEH

¾ cup uncooked bulgur
2 tablespoons reduced-sodium teriyaki sauce
2 tablespoons lemon juice
1 tablespoon olive oil
¾ cup diced seeded cucumber
¾ cup diced seeded tomato
½ cup thinly sliced green onions
½ cup minced fresh cilantro or parsley
1 tablespoon minced fresh ginger
1 clove garlic, crushed

1. Combine bulgur and 1¾ cups boiling water in small bowl. Cover with plastic wrap; let stand 45 minutes or until bulgur is puffed, stirring occasionally. Drain in wire mesh sieve; discard liquid.

2. Combine bulgur, teriyaki sauce, lemon juice and oil in large bowl. Stir in cucumber, tomato, onions, cilantro, ginger and garlic until well blended. Cover; refrigerate 4 hours, stirring occasionally.
          Makes 4 servings

Nutrients per Serving: Calories: 73 (23% Calories from Fat), Total Fat: 2 g, Saturated Fat: trace, Protein: 2 g, Carbohydrate: 13 g, Cholesterol: 0 mg, Sodium: 156 mg, Fiber: 3 g, Sugar: 1 g

Dietary Exchanges: ½ Starch/Bread, 1 Vegetable

Spicy Orzo and Black Bean Salad

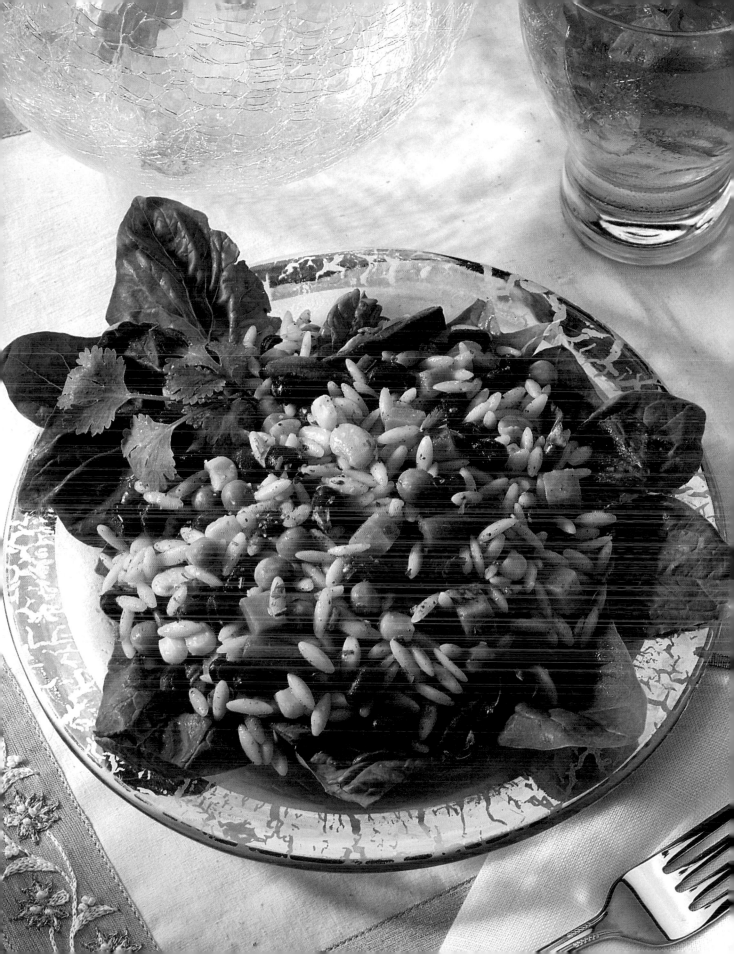

SATISFYING SALADS & SANDWICHES

161 TRIPLE BEAN SALAD

1 can (14½ ounces) green beans, drained
1 can (14½ ounces) wax beans, drained
1 can (15½ ounces) dark kidney beans, drained
¼ cup sliced green onions
¼ cup red wine vinegar
1 tablespoon olive oil
1 teaspoon EQUAL® MEASURE™ or
    3 packets EQUAL® sweetener or
    2 tablespoons EQUAL® SPOONFUL™
1 teaspoon dried basil leaves
1 small clove garlic, minced
¼ teaspoon salt
¼ teaspoon fresh ground pepper

• Combine green beans, wax beans, kidney beans, green onions, vinegar, oil, Equal®, basil, garlic, salt and pepper in large nonmetallic bowl. Mix well. Cover; refrigerate overnight. Serve chilled.

Makes 4 (1-cup) servings

Nutrients per Serving: Calories: 174, Fat: 4 g, Protein: 8 g, Carbohydrates: 29 g, Cholesterol: 0 mg, Sodium: 1025 mg

Dietary Exchanges: 1½ Starch/Bread, 1 Vegetable, ½ Fat

162 MEXICALI BEAN & CHEESE SALAD

1 teaspoon vegetable oil
1 clove garlic, finely chopped
¼ cup finely chopped red onion
1½ teaspoons chili powder
¼ teaspoon ground cumin
⅛ teaspoon red pepper flakes
1 boneless skinless chicken breast (about 6 ounces), cooked and shredded
1 cup frozen corn, thawed
⅓ cup rinsed and drained canned pinto beans
⅓ cup rinsed and drained canned kidney beans
½ cup chopped seeded tomato
2 tablespoons drained canned diced green chilies
1 green onion, finely chopped
1 teaspoon lime juice
2 ounces reduced-fat Monterey Jack cheese, cut into ⅓-inch cubes

1. Heat oil in medium nonstick skillet over medium heat until hot. Add garlic; cook and stir 1 minute. Add red onion, chili powder, cumin and red pepper flakes; cook and stir 3 minutes. Add chicken, corn and beans; cook 5 minutes or until heated through, stirring occasionally.

2. Spoon bean mixture into medium serving bowl. Add tomato, chilies, green onion and lime juice; toss to combine. Add cheese; toss to combine. Refrigerate 2 hours before serving. *Makes 2 servings*

Nutrients per Serving: Calories: 336, (25% Calories from Fat), Total Fat: 10 g, Saturated Fat: 4 g, Protein: 36 g, Carbohydrate: 36 g, Cholesterol: 72 mg, Sodium: 606 mg, Fiber: 6 g, Sugar: 4 g

Dietary Exchanges: 2½ Starch/Bread, 3 Lean Meat, 1 Vegetable

SATISFYING SALADS & SANDWICHES

163 ROASTED RED PEPPER, CORN & GARBANZO BEAN SALAD

2 cans (15 ounces each) garbanzo beans
1 jar (11.5 ounces) GUILTLESS GOURMET® Roasted Red Pepper Salsa
1 cup frozen whole kernel corn, thawed and drained
½ cup GUILTLESS GOURMET® Green Tomatillo Salsa
2 green onions, thinly sliced
8 lettuce leaves
   Fresh tomato wedges and sunflower sprouts (optional)

Rinse and drain beans well; place in 2-quart casserole dish. Add roasted red pepper salsa, corn, tomatillo salsa and onions; stir to combine. Cover and refrigerate 1 hour or up to 24 hours.

To serve, line serving platter with lettuce. Spoon bean mixture over top. Garnish with tomatoes and sprouts, if desired.

Makes 8 servings

Nutrients per Serving: Calories: 174 (9% Calories from Fat), Total Fat: 2 g, Saturated Fat: 0 g, Protein: 9 g, Carbohydrate: 32 g, Cholesterol: 0 mg, Sodium: 268 mg, Fiber: 1 g

Dietary Exchanges: 2 Starch/Bread, ½ Vegetable

Roasted Red Pepper, Corn & Garbanzo Bean Salad

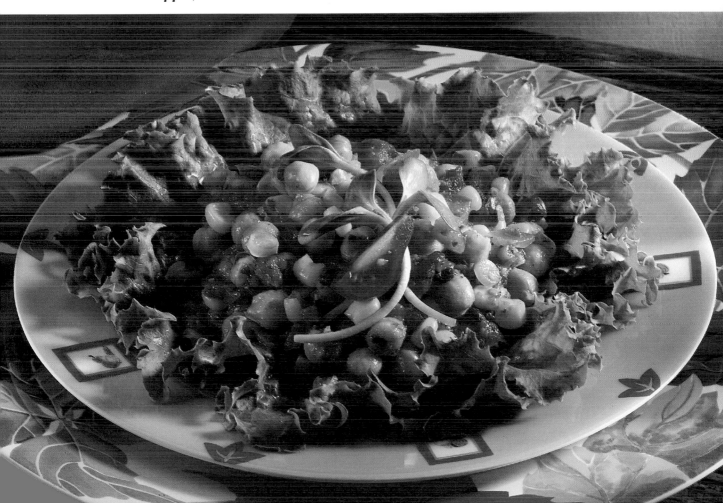

SATISFYING SALADS & SANDWICHES

164 SANTA FE GRILLED VEGETABLE SALAD

1 medium yellow summer squash, cut into halves
1 medium zucchini, cut into halves
1 green bell pepper, cut into quarters
1 red bell pepper, cut into quarters
2 baby eggplants (6 ounces each), cut into halves
1 small onion, peeled and cut into halves
½ cup orange juice
2 tablespoons lime juice
1 tablespoon olive oil
2 cloves garlic, minced
1 teaspoon dried oregano leaves
¼ teaspoon salt
¼ teaspoon ground red pepper
¼ teaspoon black pepper
2 tablespoons chopped fresh cilantro

1. Combine all ingredients except cilantro in large bowl; toss to coat.

2. To prevent sticking, spray grid with nonstick cooking spray. Prepare coals for grilling. Place vegetables on grid, 2 to 3 inches from hot coals; reserve marinade. Grill 3 to 4 minutes per side or until tender and lightly charred; cool 10 minutes. Or, place vegetables on rack of broiler pan coated with nonstick cooking spray; reserve marinade. Broil 2 to 3 inches from heat, 3 to 4 minutes per side or until tender; cool 10 minutes.

3. Remove peel from eggplants, if desired. Slice vegetables into bite-sized pieces; return to reserved marinade. Stir in cilantro; toss to coat.   *Makes 8 servings*

Nutrients per Serving: Calories: 63 (27% Calories from Fat), Total Fat: 2 g, Saturated Fat: trace, Protein: 2 g, Carbohydrate: 11 g, Cholesterol: 0 mg, Sodium: 70 mg, Fiber: 1 g, Sugar: 2 g

Dietary Exchanges: 2 Vegetable, ½ Fat

165 MARINATED TOMATO SALAD

MARINADE
1½ cups tarragon or white wine vinegar
½ teaspoon salt
¼ cup finely chopped shallots
2 tablespoons finely snipped chives
2 tablespoons lemon juice
¼ teaspoon white pepper
2 tablespoons olive oil

SALAD
6 plum tomatoes, quartered vertically
2 large yellow tomatoes, sliced horizontally into ½-inch slices
16 red cherry tomatoes, halved vertically
16 small yellow pear tomatoes, halved vertically

1. To prepare marinade, combine vinegar and salt in large bowl; stir until salt is completely dissolved. Add shallots, chives, lemon juice and white pepper; mix well. Slowly whisk in oil until well blended.

2. Add tomatoes to marinade; toss well. Cover and let stand at room temperature 2 to 3 hours.   *Makes 8 servings*

Nutrients per Serving: Calories: 56 (24% Calories from Fat), Total Fat: 2 g, Saturated Fat: trace, Protein: 2 g, Carbohydrate: 10 g, Cholesterol: 0 mg, Sodium: 64 mg, Fiber: 2 g, Sugar: 5 g

Dietary Exchanges: 2 Vegetable

Marinated Tomato Salad

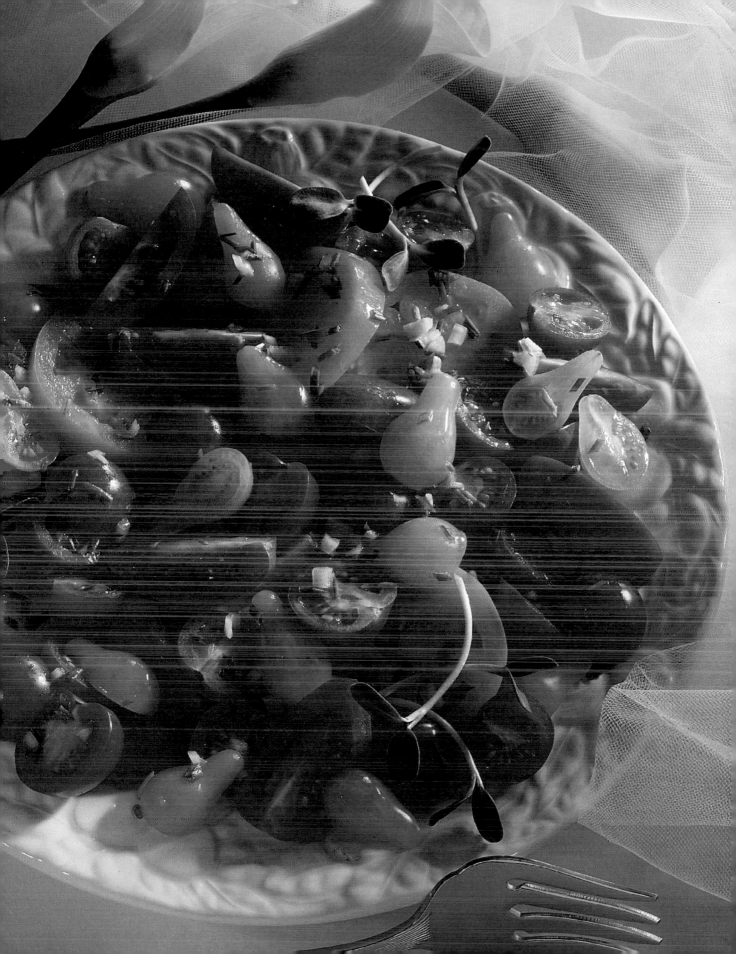

SATISFYING SALADS & SANDWICHES

166 FESTIVE POTATO SALAD

1 can HEALTHY CHOICE® RECIPE CREATIONS™ Cream of Celery with Sautéed Onion & Garlic Condensed Soup
½ cup plain nonfat yogurt
3 tablespoons *each* red wine vinegar and sweet relish
1 tablespoon Dijon mustard
1 clove garlic, minced
½ teaspoon salt (optional)
¼ teaspoon black pepper
4 russet potatoes, peeled, cooked and cut into 1-inch cubes
¾ cup sliced green onions
½ cup *each* diced red bell pepper and thinly sliced celery
3 hard-boiled egg whites, chopped
½ teaspoon dry mustard

In small bowl, combine soup, yogurt, vinegar, relish, mustard, garlic, salt and black pepper. Using wire whisk, blend until smooth. Set aside.

In large bowl, combine potatoes, green onions, bell pepper, celery, egg whites and mustard. Add soup mixture and toss gently until well coated. Refrigerate at least 1 hour to blend flavors.   *Makes 8 servings*

Nutrients per Serving: Calories: 110 (8% Calories from Fat), Fat: 1 g, Protein: 4 g, Sodium: 240 mg

Dietary Exchanges: 2 Starch/Bread

167 CARIBBEAN COLE SLAW

Orange-Mango Dressing (recipe follows)
8 cups shredded green cabbage
1½ large mangoes, peeled, pitted and diced
½ medium red bell pepper, thinly sliced
½ medium yellow bell pepper, thinly sliced
6 green onions, thinly sliced
¼ cup chopped cilantro

1. Prepare Orange-Mango Dressing.

2. Combine cabbage, mangoes, bell peppers, green onions and cilantro in large bowl; stir gently to mix evenly. Pour in Orange-Mango Dressing; toss gently to coat. Serve, or store in refrigerator up to 1 day.
Makes 6 servings

ORANGE–MANGO DRESSING
½ mango, peeled, pitted and cubed
1 carton (6 ounces) plain nonfat yogurt
¼ cup frozen orange juice concentrate
3 tablespoons lime juice
½ to 1 jalapeño pepper,* stemmed, seeded and minced
1 teaspoon finely minced fresh ginger

*Jalapeño peppers can sting and irritate the skin; wear rubber gloves when handling peppers and do not touch eyes. Wash hands after handling.

1. Place mango in food processor; process until smooth. Add remaining ingredients; process until smooth.
Makes about 1 cup

Nutrients per Serving: Calories: 124 (4% Calories from Fat), Total Fat: 1 g, Saturated Fat: trace, Protein: 4 g, Carbohydrate: 28 g, Cholesterol: 1 mg, Sodium: 52 mg, Fiber: 4 g, Sugar: 16 g

Dietary Exchanges: 2 Fruit

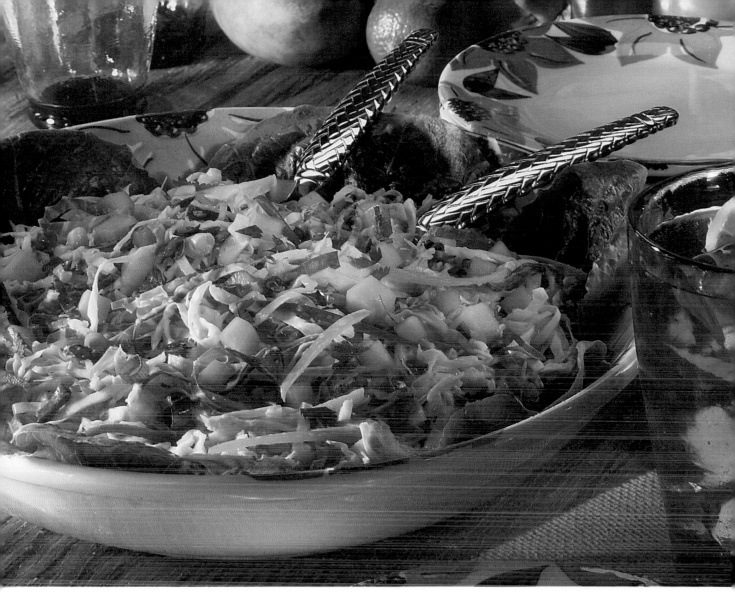

Caribbean Cole Slaw

168 SHREDDED CARROT AND RAISIN SALAD

1 pound carrots, peeled and shredded
1½ cups thinly sliced, cored, peeled apples
¼ cup dark raisins
½ cup plain low-fat yogurt or sour cream
⅓ cup skim milk
1 tablespoon lemon juice
1½ teaspoons EQUAL® MEASURE™ or
    5 packets EQUAL® sweetener or
    3½ tablespoons EQUAL® SPOONFUL™
¼ teaspoon ground nutmeg
¼ teaspoon ground cinnamon

• Combine carrots, apples and raisins in large bowl. Combine remaining ingredients; spoon over carrot mixture and toss to coat. Refrigerate until chilled.

Makes 6 servings

Nutrients per Serving: Calories: 90, Fat: 0 g, Protein: 3 g, Carbohydrate: 20 g, Cholesterol: 1 mg, Sodium: 48 mg

Dietary Exchanges: 1 Vegetable, 1 Fruit

SATISFYING SALADS & SANDWICHES

169 TURKEY BURGERS

1 pound ground turkey breast
1 cup whole wheat bread crumbs
1 egg white
$\frac{1}{2}$ teaspoon dried sage leaves
$\frac{1}{2}$ teaspoon dried marjoram leaves
$\frac{1}{4}$ teaspoon salt
$\frac{1}{4}$ teaspoon black pepper
1 teaspoon vegetable oil
4 whole grain sandwich rolls, split in half
$\frac{1}{4}$ cup Cowpoke Barbecue Sauce (page 162) or prepared barbecue sauce

1. Combine turkey, bread crumbs, egg white, sage, marjoram, salt and pepper in large bowl until well blended. Shape into 4 patties.

2. Heat oil in large nonstick skillet over medium-high heat until hot. Add patties; cook 10 minutes or until patties are no longer pink in center, turning once.

3. Place one patty on bottom half of each roll. Spoon 1 tablespoon Cowpoke Barbecue Sauce over top of each burger. Place tops of rolls over burgers. Serve with lettuce and tomato and garnish with carrot slices, if desired. *Makes 4 burgers*

Nutrients per Serving: Calories: 319 (17% Calories from Fat), Total Fat: 6 g, Saturated Fat: 1 g, Protein: 26 g, Carbohydrate: 40 g, Cholesterol: 41 mg, Sodium: 669 mg, Fiber: 2 g, Sugar: 2 g

Dietary Exchanges: 2 Starch/Bread, 3 Lean Meat

170 PITA POCKETS

1 can HEALTHY CHOICE® RECIPE CREATIONS™ Tomato with Garden Herbs Condensed Soup
$\frac{1}{4}$ cup fat free sour cream
Vegetable cooking spray
1 pound ground turkey
$\frac{1}{2}$ cup each HEALTHY CHOICE® Fat Free Shredded Cheddar Cheese and sliced green onions
$\frac{1}{2}$ teaspoon salt (optional)
3 pita bread rounds, cut in half to form pockets
1 cup *each* shredded lettuce and diced tomato

In small bowl, combine soup and sour cream; mix well. Set aside. In large nonstick skillet sprayed with vegetable cooking spray, cook turkey over medium-high heat until no longer pink; drain.

Add soup mixture, cheese, onions and salt to skillet; mix well. Reduce heat; cover and simmer 5 minutes or until cheese is melted. Fill pita bread pockets with turkey mixture. Garnish with lettuce and tomato.

Makes 6 servings

Nutrients per Serving: Calories: 270 (24% Calories from Fat), Fat: 7 g, Protein: 21 g, Sodium: 430 mg

Dietary Exchanges: 2 Starch/Bread, 2 Lean Meat, $\frac{1}{2}$ Fat

Turkey Burger

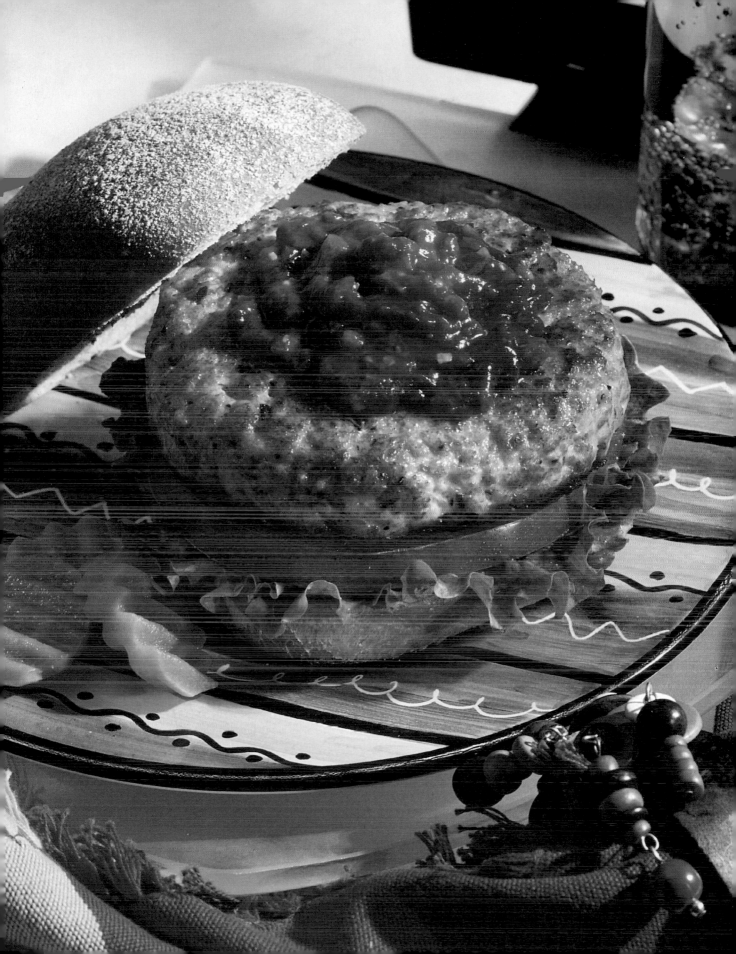

SATISFYING SALADS & SANDWICHES

171 ITALIAN MEATBALL SUBS

Nonstick cooking spray
½ cup chopped onion
3 teaspoons finely chopped garlic, divided
1 can (14½ ounces) Italian-style crushed tomatoes, undrained
2 bay leaves
2½ teaspoons dried basil leaves, divided
2 teaspoons dried oregano leaves, divided
¾ teaspoon black pepper, divided
¼ teaspoon red pepper flakes
½ pound lean ground beef
⅓ cup chopped green onions
⅓ cup dry bread crumbs
¼ cup chopped parsley
1 egg white
½ teaspoon dried marjoram leaves
½ teaspoon ground mustard
4 French bread rolls, warmed and halved

1. Spray large nonstick saucepan with cooking spray; heat over medium heat. Add onion and 2 teaspoons garlic; cook and stir 5 minutes. Add tomatoes with liquid, bay leaves, 2 teaspoons basil, 1 teaspoon oregano, ½ teaspoon black pepper and red pepper; simmer, covered, 30 minutes, stirring occasionally. Discard bay leaves.

2. Combine beef, green onions, bread crumbs, parsley, egg white, 2 tablespoons water, remaining 1 teaspoon garlic, ½ teaspoon basil, 1 teaspoon oregano, ¼ teaspoon black pepper, marjoram and mustard in medium bowl. Shape into 16 meatballs.

3. Spray large nonstick skillet with cooking spray; heat over medium heat. Add meatballs; cook 5 minutes or until no longer pink in centers. Add meatballs to tomato sauce; cook and stir 5 minutes. Place 4 meatballs in each roll; spoon sauce over meatballs. *Makes 4 servings*

Nutrients per Serving: Calories: 282 (30% Calories from Fat), Total Fat: 9 g, Saturated Fat: 3 g, Protein: 18 g, Carbohydrate: 32 g, Cholesterol: 35 mg, Sodium: 497 mg, Fiber: 1 g, Sugar: 6 g

Dietary Exchanges: 2 Starch/Bread, 2 Lean Meat, 1 Vegetable

172 SOUTHWESTERN SLOPPY JOES

1 pound lean ground round
1 cup chopped onion
¼ cup chopped celery
¼ cup water
1 can (10 ounces) diced tomatoes and green chilies
1 can (8 ounces) no-salt-added tomato sauce
4 teaspoons brown sugar
½ teaspoon ground cumin
¼ teaspoon salt
9 whole wheat hamburger buns

1. Heat large nonstick skillet over high heat. Add beef, onion, celery and water. Reduce heat to medium; cook and stir 5 minutes or until meat is no longer pink. Drain fat.

2. Stir in tomatoes and green chilies, tomato sauce, brown sugar, cumin and salt; bring to a boil over high heat. Reduce heat; simmer 20 minutes or until mixture thickens. Serve on whole wheat buns. *Makes 9 servings*

Nutrients per Serving: Calories: 190 (19% Calories from Fat), Total Fat: 4 g, Saturated Fat: 1 g, Protein: 13 g, Carbohydrate: 26 g, Cholesterol: 15 mg, Sodium: 413 mg, Fiber: 1 g, Sugar: 1 g

Dietary Exchanges: 1½ Starch/Bread, 1 Lean Meat, 1 Vegetable

Southwestern Sloppy Joe

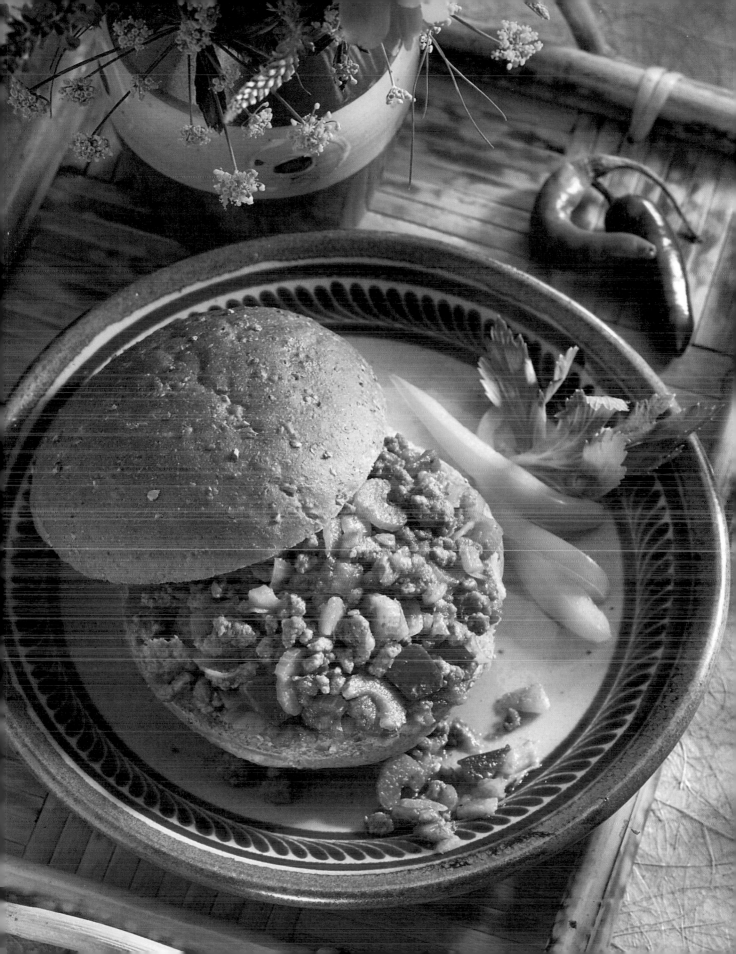

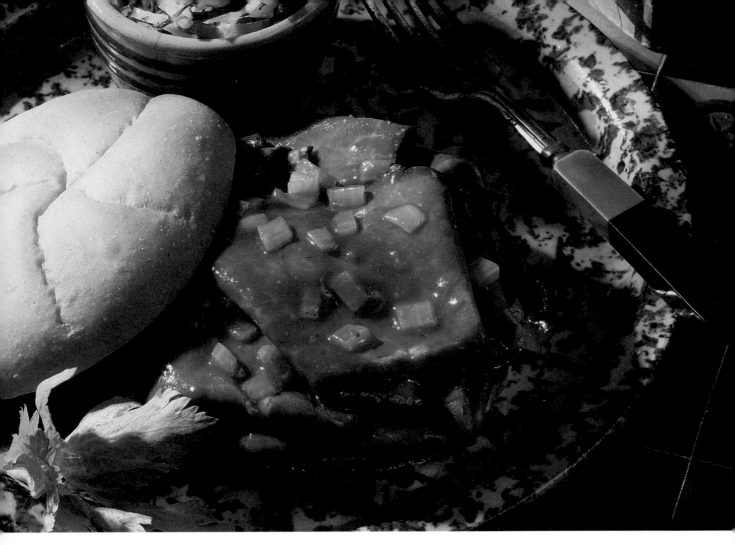

Down Home Barbecued Beef

173 DOWN HOME BARBECUED BEEF

1 slice bacon
½ cup chopped onion
½ cup ketchup
½ cup apple juice
1 tablespoon white vinegar
1 teaspoon prepared mustard
1 teaspoon Worcestershire sauce
⅛ teaspoon salt
⅛ teaspoon ground black pepper
2½ teaspoons EQUAL® MEASURE™ or
    8 packets EQUAL® sweetener or
    ⅓ cup EQUAL® SPOONFUL™
12 ounces thinly sliced roast beef
4 kaiser rolls (optional)

• Cut bacon into 1-inch pieces; cook in medium saucepan over medium-high heat 3 to 4 minutes or until almost cooked. Add onion; cook 3 to 5 minutes or until bacon is crisp and onion is tender, stirring occasionally.

• Combine ketchup, apple juice, vinegar, mustard, Worcestershire sauce, salt and pepper; add to bacon mixture. Reduce heat; cover and simmer until flavors are blended, 15 to 20 minutes.

• Stir in Equal® and sliced beef. Serve warm on rolls, if desired.   *Makes 4 servings*

MICROWAVE DIRECTIONS: Cut bacon into 1-inch pieces and place in 1½-quart microwavable casserole. Cook, uncovered,

SATISFYING SALADS & SANDWICHES

at HIGH 1 minute. Add onion and cook at HIGH for 2½ to 3 minutes or until bacon is crisp and onion is tender, stirring once. Combine ketchup, apple juice, vinegar, mustard, Worcestershire sauce, salt and pepper; add to bacon mixture. Cook, covered, at HIGH 4 to 5 minutes or until boiling. Cook at MEDIUM 8 to 10 minutes or until flavors are blended, stirring twice. Stir in Equal® and sliced beef. Serve warm.

Nutrients per Serving: Calories: 223, Fat: 6 g, Protein: 26 g, Carbohydrates: 16 g, Cholesterol: 70 mg, Sodium: 542 mg,

Dietary Exchanges: 1 Starch/Bread, 3 Lean Meat

174 BARBECUED PORK SANDWICHES

2 pork tenderloins (about 1½ pounds total)
⅓ cup prepared barbecue sauce
½ cup prepared horseradish
4 rounds pita bread, halved
1 onion, thinly sliced
4 romaine lettuce leaves
1 red bell pepper, cut lengthwise into ¼-inch-thick slices
1 green bell pepper, cut lengthwise into ¼-inch-thick slices

1. Preheat oven to 400°F. Place pork tenderloins in roasting pan; brush with barbecue sauce.

2. Bake tenderloins 15 minutes; turn and bake 15 minutes or until internal temperature reaches 155°F. Cover with foil; let stand 15 minutes.

3. Slice pork across grain. Spread horseradish on pitas; stuff with pork, onion, lettuce and bell peppers.

Makes 4 servings

Nutrients per Serving: Calories: 440 (17% Calories from Fat), Total Fat: 9 g, Saturated Fat: 2 g, Protein: 46 g, Carbohydrate: 46 g, Cholesterol: 121 mg, Sodium: 628 mg, Fiber: 2 g, Sugar: 2 g

Dietary Exchanges: 2½ Starch/Bread, 4 Lean Meat, 1 Vegetable

175 MEATLESS SLOPPY JOES

2 cups thinly sliced onions
2 cups chopped green peppers
2 cloves garlic, finely chopped
2 tablespoons ketchup
1 tablespoon mustard
1 can (15 ounces) kidney beans, rinsed, drained and slightly mashed
1 can (8 ounces) tomato sauce
1 teaspoon chili powder
  Cider vinegar
2 sandwich rolls, halved

Spray skillet with cooking spray. Add onions, peppers and garlic. Cook and stir 5 minutes over medium heat. Stir in ketchup and mustard. Add beans, sauce and chili powder. Cook 5 minutes, stirring frequently. Add ⅓ cup vinegar if dry. Serve on halves.

Makes 4 servings

Nutrients per Serving: Calories: 242 (7% Calories from Fat), Total Fat: 2 g, Saturated Fat: trace, Protein: 10 g, Carbohydrate: 48 g, Cholesterol: 0 mg, Sodium: 994 mg, Fiber: 10 g, Sugar: 6 g

Dietary Exchanges: 2 Starch/Bread, 3 Vegetable, ½ Fat

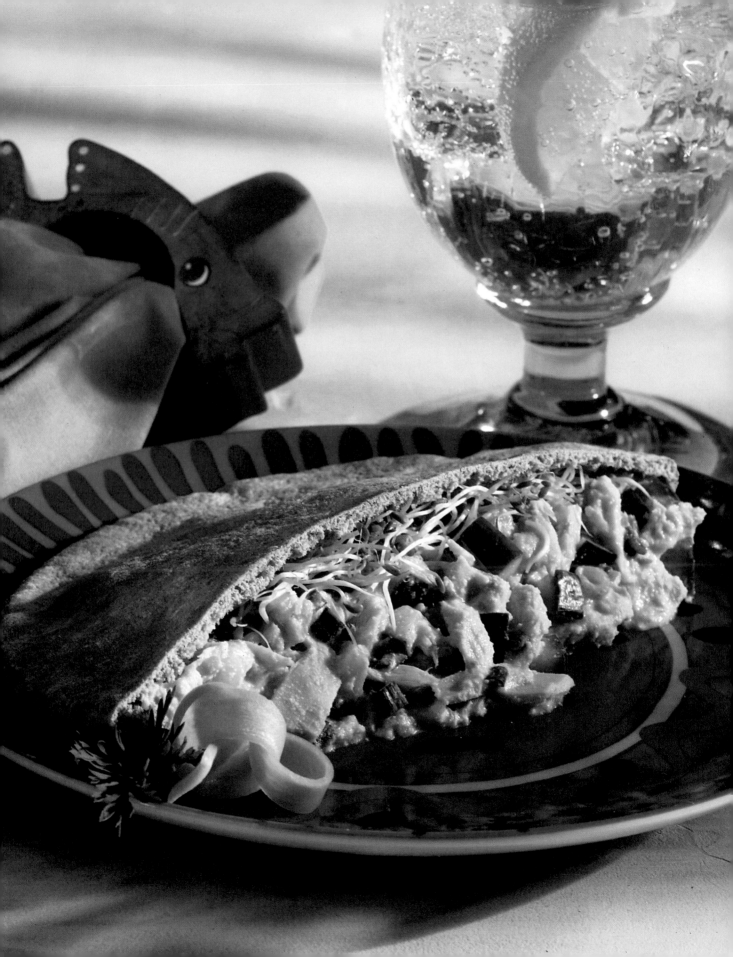

SATISFYING SALADS & SANDWICHES

176 TUNA SALAD PITA POCKETS

1 can (9 ounces) tuna packed in water, drained
1 cup chopped cucumber
¼ cup part-skim ricotta cheese
2 tablespoons reduced-fat mayonnaise
2 tablespoons red wine vinegar
2 green onions, chopped
1 tablespoon sweet pickle relish
2 cloves garlic, finely chopped
½ teaspoon salt
¼ teaspoon black pepper
2 rounds pita bread, halved
1 cup alfalfa sprouts

Combine tuna, cucumber, ricotta cheese, mayonnaise, vinegar, onions, relish, garlic, salt and pepper in medium bowl. Fill pitas with sprouts and tuna.

Makes 4 servings

Nutrients per Serving: Calories: 209 (18% Calories from Fat), Total Fat: 4 g, Saturated Fat: 1 g, Protein: 22 g, Carbohydrate: 22 g, Cholesterol: 22 mg, Sodium: 752 mg, Fiber: trace, Sugar: trace

Dietary Exchanges: 1½ Starch/Bread, 2 Lean Meat

177 OPEN–FACED EGGPLANT MELT

1 can HEALTHY CHOICE® RECIPE CREATIONS™ Tomato with Garden Herbs Condensed Soup
¼ cup fat free, low sodium chicken broth
3 sandwich-size English muffins, split and toasted
  Vegetable cooking spray
1 small eggplant, cut crosswise into 1-inch slices and grilled
½ cup roasted red bell pepper strips, drained (6 strips)
6 slices HEALTHY CHOICE® Low Fat Smoked Ham
½ cup HEALTHY CHOICE® Fat Free Shredded Mozzarella Cheese

In small bowl, combine soup and chicken broth; mix well. Set aside. Place toasted muffin halves in single layer in shallow baking dish sprayed with vegetable cooking spray. Spread 1 tablespoon soup mixture on each muffin half. Top each muffin half with 1 slice eggplant, 1 bell pepper strip and 1 slice ham.

Pour remaining soup mixture evenly over sandwiches and sprinkle with cheese. Cover and bake at 350°F 10 minutes or until cheese is melted and sandwiches are heated through.

Makes 6 servings

Nutrients per Serving: Calories: 100 (9% Calories from Fat), Fat: 1 g, Protein: 7 g, Sodium: 360 mg

Dietary Exchanges: 1 Starch/Bread, 1 Meat, 1 Vegetable

Tuna Salad Pita Pocket

178 GRILLED VEGETABLE MUFFULETTA

10 cloves garlic, peeled
   Nonstick cooking spray
 1 tablespoon balsamic vinegar
 1 tablespoon lemon juice
 1 tablespoon olive oil
¼ teaspoon black pepper
 1 round whole wheat sourdough bread
    loaf (1½ pounds)
 1 medium eggplant, cut crosswise into
    eight ¼-inch-thick slices
 2 small yellow squash, cut lengthwise into
    thin slices
 1 small red onion, thinly sliced
 1 large red bell pepper, quartered
 2 slices (1 ounce each) reduced-fat Swiss
    cheese
 8 spinach leaves

1. Preheat oven to 350°F. Place garlic in ovenproof dish; spray with cooking spray. Cover with foil; bake 30 to 35 minutes or until garlic is very soft and golden brown.

2. Place garlic, vinegar, lemon juice, olive oil and black pepper in food processor; process using on/off pulsing action until smooth. Set aside.

3. Slice top off bread loaf; hollow out loaf, leaving ½-inch-thick shell. Reserve bread for another use.

4. Prepare coals for grilling. Brush vegetables with garlic mixture; arrange on grid over medium coals. Grill 10 to 12 minutes or until crisp-tender, turning once. Separate onion slices into rings.

5. Layer half of eggplant, squash, onion, bell pepper, cheese and spinach in hollowed bread, pressing gently after each layer. Repeat layers with remaining vegetables, cheese and spinach. Replace bread top;

serve immediately or wrap tightly with plastic wrap and refrigerate for up to 4 hours. *Makes 6 servings*

Nutrients per Serving: Calories: 422 (17% Calories from Fat), Total Fat: 8 g, Saturated Fat: 2 g, Protein: 16 g, Carbohydrate: 73 g, Cholesterol: 7 mg, Sodium: 721 mg, Fiber: 1 g, Sugar: trace

Dietary Exchanges: 4 Starch/Bread, ½ Lean Meat, 2 Vegetable, 1½ Fat

179 HUEVOS RANCHWICH

¼ cup EGG BEATERS® Healthy Real Egg
    Substitute
 1 teaspoon diced green chiles
 1 whole wheat hamburger roll, split and
    toasted
 1 tablespoon thick and chunky salsa
 1 tablespoon shredded reduced-fat
    Cheddar and Monterey Jack cheese
    blend

On lightly greased griddle or skillet, pour Egg Beaters into lightly greased 4-inch egg ring or biscuit cutter. Sprinkle with chiles. Cook 2 to 3 minutes or until bottom of egg patty is set. Remove egg ring and turn egg patty over. Cook 1 to 2 minutes longer or until done.

To serve, place egg patty on bottom of roll. Top with salsa, cheese and roll top.
Makes 1 sandwich

Prep Time: 10 minutes
Cook Time: 5 minutes

Nutrients per Serving: Calories: 143, Cholesterol: 6 mg, Total Fat: 2 g, Saturated Fat: 1 g, Sodium: 411 mg, Fiber: 0 g

Dietary Exchanges: 1½ Starch/Bread, 1 Lean Meat

Grilled Vegetable Muffuletta

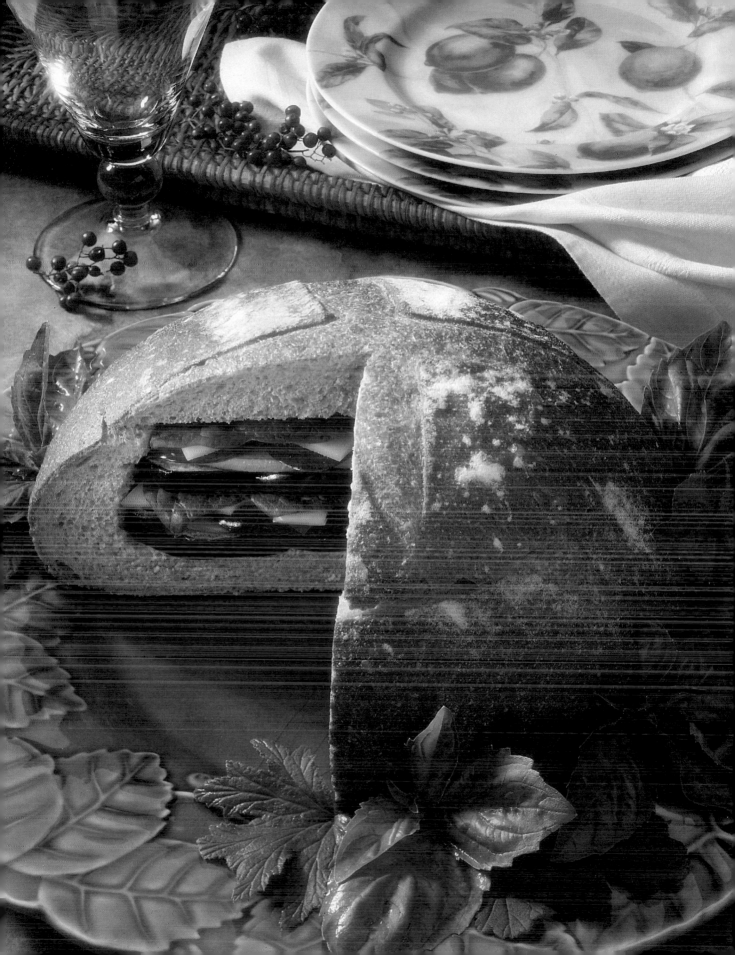

SATISFYING SALADS & SANDWICHES

180 MEDITERRANEAN VEGETABLE SANDWICHES

1 small eggplant, peeled, halved and cut into ¼-inch-thick slices
  Salt
1 small zucchini, halved and cut lengthwise into ¼-inch-thick slices
1 green or red bell pepper, sliced
3 tablespoons balsamic vinegar
½ teaspoon salt
½ teaspoon garlic powder
2 French bread rolls, halved

1. Place eggplant in nonaluminum colander; sprinkle eggplant with salt. Let stand 30 minutes to drain. Rinse eggplant; pat dry with paper towels.

2. Preheat broiler. Spray rack of broiler pan with nonstick cooking spray; place vegetables on rack. Broil 4 inches from heat, 8 to 10 minutes or until vegetables are browned, turning once.

3. Combine vinegar, ½ teaspoon salt and garlic powder in medium bowl until well blended. Add vegetables; toss to coat. Divide vegetable mixture evenly between rolls. Serve immediately.   *Makes 2 servings*

Nutrients per Serving: Calories: 178, (10% Calories from Fat), Total Fat: 2 g, Saturated Fat: trace, Protein: 5 g, Carbohydrate: 36 g, Cholesterol: 0 mg, Sodium: 775 mg, Fiber: 1 g, Sugar: 2 g

Dietary Exchanges: 1½ Starch/Bread, 3 Vegetable

181 HUMMUS PITA SANDWICHES

2 tablespoons sesame seeds
1 can (15 ounces) chick-peas, undrained
1 to 2 cloves garlic, peeled
¼ cup loosely packed parsley
3 tablespoons lemon juice
1 tablespoon olive oil
¼ teaspoon black pepper
4 rounds pita bread, halved
2 tomatoes, thinly sliced
1 cucumber, sliced
1 cup alfalfa sprouts, rinsed and drained
2 tablespoons crumbled feta cheese

1. Toast sesame seeds in small nonstick skillet over medium heat until lightly browned, stirring frequently. Remove from skillet; cool. Drain chick-peas; reserve liquid.

2. Place garlic in food processor; process until minced. Add chick-peas, parsley, lemon juice, olive oil and pepper; process until almost smooth, scraping sides of bowl once. If mixture is very thick, add 1 to 2 tablespoons reserved chick-pea liquid. Pour hummus into medium bowl; stir in sesame seeds.

3. Spread about 3 tablespoons hummus in each pita. Divide tomatoes, cucumber and alfalfa sprouts evenly among pitas; sprinkle with feta cheese.   *Makes 4 servings*

Nutrients per Serving: (2 pita bread halves), Calories: 364 (21% Calories from Fat), Total Fat: 9 g, Saturated Fat: 2 g, Protein: 18 g, Carbohydrate: 59 g, Cholesterol: 7 mg, Sodium: 483 mg, Fiber: 8 g, Sugar: 2 g

Dietary Exchanges: 3½ Starch/Bread, 1 Vegetable, 2 Fat

182 GRILLED CHEESE 'N' TOMATO SANDWICHES

8 slices whole wheat bread, divided
6 ounces part-skim mozzarella cheese, cut into 4 slices
1 large tomato, cut into 8 thin slices
⅓ cup yellow cornmeal
2 tablespoons grated Parmesan cheese
1 teaspoon dried basil leaves
½ cup EGG BEATERS® Healthy Real Egg Substitute
¼ cup skim milk
2 tablespoons FLEISCHMANN'S® 70% Corn Oil Spread, divided
1 cup low-salt tomato sauce, heated

On each of 4 bread slices, place 1 cheese slice and 2 tomato slices; top with remaining bread slices. Combine cornmeal, Parmesan cheese and basil on waxed paper. In shallow bowl, combine Egg Beaters and milk. Melt 1 tablespoon spread in large nonstick griddle or skillet. Dip sandwiches in egg mixture; coat with cornmeal mixture. Transfer 2 sandwiches to griddle. Cook sandwiches for 3 minutes on each side or until golden. Repeat using remaining spread and sandwiches. Cut sandwiches in half; serve warm with tomato sauce for dipping.

Makes 4 servings

Prep Time: 20 minutes
Cook Time: 14 minutes

Nutrients per Serving: Calories: 420, Total Fat: 18 g, Saturated Fat: 8 g, Cholesterol: 35 mg, Sodium: 657 mg, Fiber: 6 g

Dietary Exchanges: 2 Starch/Bread, 2 Lean Meat, 1 Vegetable, 2 Fat

Grilled Cheese 'n' Tomato Sandwich

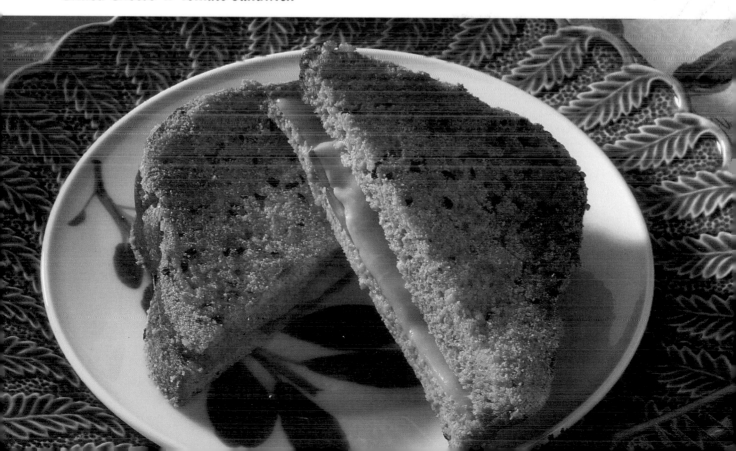

Mouthwatering
Main Dishes

183 CHICKEN FAJITAS WITH COWPOKE BARBECUE SAUCE

1 cup Cowpoke Barbecue Sauce (recipe follows), divided
Nonstick cooking spray
10 ounces boneless skinless chicken breasts, cut lengthwise into 1×½-inch pieces
2 green or red bell peppers, thinly sliced
1 cup sliced onion
2 cups tomato wedges
4 (6-inch) warm flour tortillas

1. Prepare Cowpoke Barbecue Sauce.

2. Spray large nonstick skillet with cooking spray; heat over medium-high heat until hot. Brush chicken with ¼ cup barbecue sauce. Add to skillet; cook and stir 3 minutes or until chicken is browned. Add peppers and onion; cook and stir 3 minutes or until vegetables are crisp-tender and chicken is no longer pink. Add tomatoes; cook 2 minutes or until heated through, stirring occasionally.

3. Serve with warm flour tortillas and remaining ¾ cup Cowpoke Barbecue Sauce. Garnish with fresh cilantro, if desired.

Makes 4 servings

COWPOKE BARBECUE SAUCE
1 teaspoon vegetable oil
¾ cup chopped green onions
3 cloves garlic, finely chopped
1 can (14½ ounces) crushed tomatoes
½ cup ketchup
¼ cup water
¼ cup orange juice
2 tablespoons cider vinegar
2 teaspoons chili sauce
Dash Worcestershire sauce

Heat oil in large nonstick saucepan over medium heat until hot. Add onions and garlic; cook and stir 5 minutes or until onions are tender. Stir in remaining ingredients; reduce heat to medium-low. Cook 15 minutes, stirring occasionally.

Makes 2 cups

Nutrients per Serving: Calories: 310 (18% Calories from Fat), Total Fat: 6 g, Saturated Fat: 1 g, Protein: 20 g, Carbohydrate: 47 g, Cholesterol: 36 mg, Sodium: 736 mg, Fiber: 4 g, Sugar: 9 g

Dietary Exchanges per Serving:
1½ Starch/Bread, 2 Lean Meat, 2½ Vegetable

Chicken Fajitas with Cowpoke Barbecue Sauce

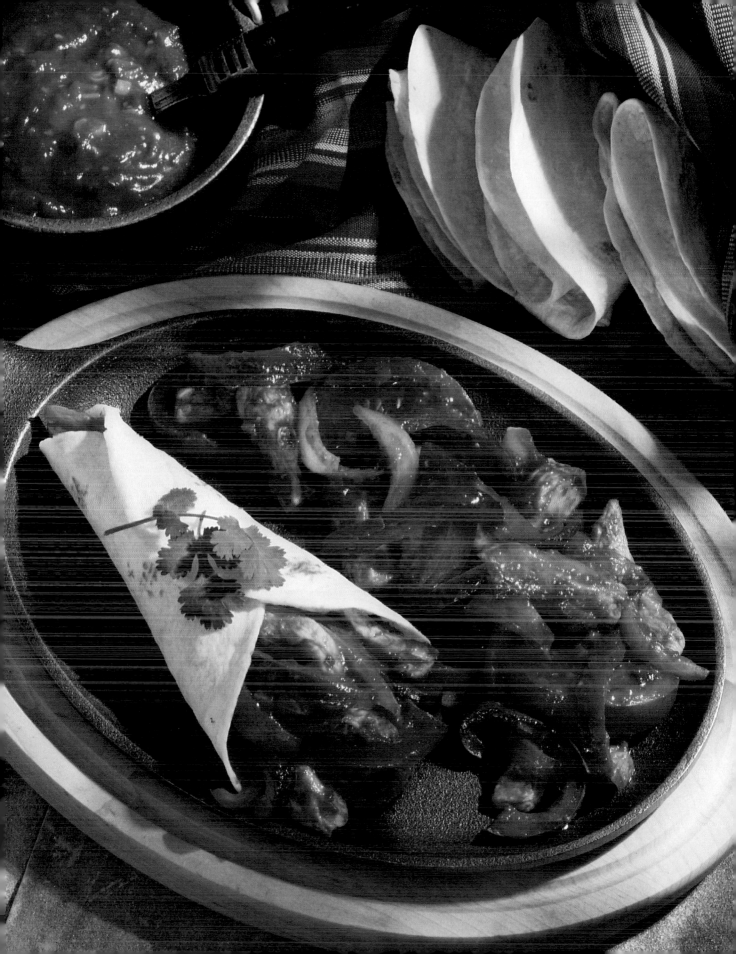

MOUTHWATERING MAIN DISHES

184 CHICKEN FLORENTINE WITH LEMON–MUSTARD SAUCE

2 whole boneless skinless chicken breasts, halved (1 pound)
¼ cup EGG BEATERS® Healthy Real Egg Substitute
½ cup plain dry bread crumbs
1 teaspoon dried basil leaves
1 teaspoon garlic powder
2 tablespoons FLEISCHMANN'S® Sweet Unsalted 70% Corn Oil Spread, divided
⅓ cup water
2 tablespoons GREY POUPON® Dijon Mustard
2 tablespoons lemon juice
1 tablespoon sugar
1 (10-ounce) package frozen chopped spinach, cooked, well drained and kept warm

Pound chicken breasts to ¼-inch thickness. Pour Egg Beaters into shallow bowl. Combine bread crumbs, basil and garlic. Dip chicken breasts into Egg Beaters, then coat with bread crumb mixture.

In large nonstick skillet, over medium-high heat, melt 1 tablespoon spread. Add chicken; cook for 5 to 7 minutes on each side or until browned and no longer pink in center. Remove chicken from skillet; keep warm. In same skillet, melt remaining spread; stir in water, mustard, lemon juice and sugar. Simmer 1 minute or until thickened. To serve, arrange chicken on serving platter. Top with spinach; drizzle with lemon-mustard sauce. *Makes 4 servings*

Prep Time: 25 minutes
Cook Time: 15 minutes

Nutrients per Serving: Calories: 278, Total Fat: 8 g, Saturated Fat: 2 g, Cholesterol: 69 mg, Sodium: 468 mg, Fiber: 0 g

Dietary Exchanges: 1 Starch/Bread, 4 Lean Meat

185 CHICKEN DIVAN

1 can HEALTHY CHOICE® RECIPE CREATIONS™ Cream of Broccoli with Cheddar and Onion Condensed Soup
¼ cup nonfat milk
½ teaspoon salt (optional)
Vegetable cooking spray
4 slices reduced fat white bread, toasted
4 boneless, skinless chicken breast halves, cooked
1 (10-ounce) box frozen broccoli spears, thawed and drained
2 tablespoons fat-free shredded Parmesan cheese

In medium bowl, combine soup, milk and salt; mix well. In 1½-quart baking dish sprayed with vegetable cooking spray, place toast slices; top each slice with chicken breast half. Arrange broccoli spears over chicken. Pour soup mixture evenly over broccoli and sprinkle with Parmesan cheese. Cover and bake at 350°F 15 minutes or until hot and bubbly. *Makes 4 servings*

Nutrients per Serving: Calories: 270 (17% Calories from Fat), Protein: 34 g, Fat: 5 g, Sodium: 530 mg

Dietary Exchanges: 1½ Starch/Bread, 3 Lean Meat

Chicken Florentine with Lemon-Mustard Sauce

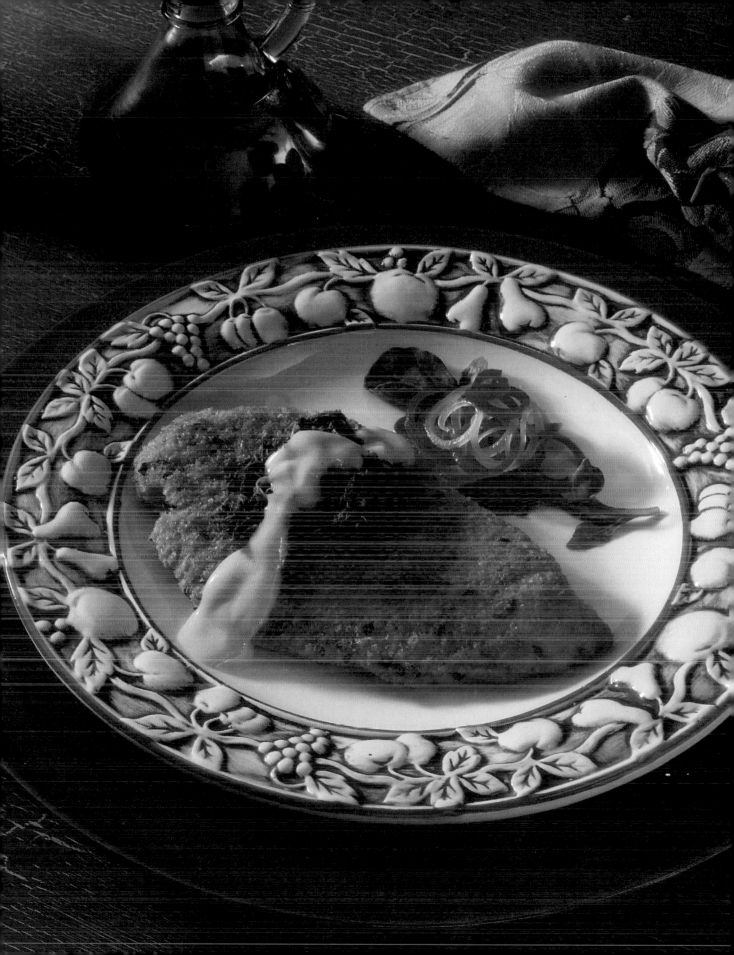

MOUTHWATERING MAIN DISHES

186 CAJUN–STYLE CHICKEN GUMBO

1 pound boneless skinless chicken breasts
1 teaspoon Cajun or Creole seasoning
1 teaspoon dried thyme leaves
2 tablespoons vegetable oil
1 medium onion, coarsely chopped
1 green bell pepper, coarsely chopped
1 cup thinly sliced carrots
½ cup thinly sliced celery
4 cloves garlic, minced
2 tablespoons all-purpose flour
1 can (about 14 ounces) fat-free reduced-sodium chicken broth
1 can (14½ ounces) no-salt-added stewed tomatoes, undrained
½ teaspoon hot pepper sauce
2 cups hot cooked rice
¼ cup chopped parsley (optional)
Additional hot pepper sauce (optional)

1. Cut chicken into 1-inch pieces; place in medium bowl. Sprinkle with seasoning and thyme; toss well. Set aside.

2. Heat oil in large saucepan over medium-high heat. Add onion, bell pepper, carrots, celery and garlic to saucepan; cover and cook 10 minutes or until vegetables are crisp-tender, stirring once. Add chicken; cook 3 minutes, stirring occasionally. Sprinkle mixture with flour; cook 1 minute, stirring frequently.

3. Add chicken broth, tomatoes and pepper sauce; bring to a boil over high heat. Reduce heat to medium; simmer, uncovered, 10 minutes or until chicken is no longer pink in center, vegetables are tender and sauce is slightly thickened.

4. Ladle gumbo into 4 shallow bowls; top each with a scoop of rice. Sprinkle with parsley and serve with additional pepper sauce, if desired. *Makes 4 servings*

Nutrients per Serving: Calories: 378 (26% Calories from Fat), Total Fat: 11 g, Saturated Fat: 2 g, Protein: 31 g, Carbohydrate: 39 g, Cholesterol: 69 mg, Sodium: 176 mg, Fiber: 3 g, Sugar: 6 g

Dietary Exchanges: 2 Starch/Bread, 3 Lean Meat, 2 Vegetable, ½ Fat

187 LEMON CHICKEN WITH HERBS

1 can HEALTHY CHOICE® RECIPE CREATIONS™ Cream of Roasted Chicken with Herbs Condensed Soup
¼ cup nonfat milk
2 tablespoons lemon juice
2 tablespoons minced fresh parsley
Vegetable cooking spray
4 boneless, skinless chicken breast halves
½ cup sliced mushrooms
¼ cup chopped red onion

In small bowl, mix soup, milk, lemon juice and parsley; set aside. Heat large nonstick skillet sprayed with vegetable cooking spray over medium heat 1 minute. Add chicken; brown 5 minutes on each side. Remove from skillet. Add mushrooms and onion to skillet; sauté 2 to 3 minutes. Stir in soup mixture.

Return chicken to skillet; reduce heat to low. Cover and simmer 5 to 10 minutes or until chicken is no longer pink in center.

Makes 4 servings

Nutrients per Serving: Calories: 209 (22% Calories from Fat), Fat: 5 g, Protein: 29 g, Sodium: 290 mg

Dietary Exchanges: 3 Lean Meat, 2 Vegetable

MOUTHWATERING MAIN DISHES

188 TUSCAN CHICKEN BREASTS WITH POLENTA

4 cups fat-free reduced-sodium chicken broth
1 cup yellow cornmeal
　Tuscan Tomato Sauce (recipe follows)
½ teaspoon garlic powder
½ teaspoon dried Italian seasoning
¼ teaspoon salt
¼ teaspoon pepper
8 skinless bone-in chicken breast halves (3 pounds)
　Nonstick cooking spray
　Fresh spinach leaves, steamed (optional)

1. Heat chicken broth in large nonstick saucepan; bring to a boil. Slowly stir in cornmeal. Reduce heat to low; cook, stirring frequently, 15 to 20 minutes or until mixture is very thick and pulls away from side of pan. (Mixture may be lumpy.) Pour polenta into greased 9×5-inch loaf pan. Cool; refrigerate 2 to 3 hours or until firm.

2. Prepare Tuscan Tomato Sauce; set aside.

3. Heat oven to 350°F. Combine garlic powder, Italian seasoning, salt and pepper in small bowl; rub on all surfaces of chicken. Arrange chicken, breast side up, in single layer in 13×9-inch baking pan. Bake, uncovered, about 45 minutes or until chicken is no longer pink in center and juices run clear.

4. Remove polenta from pan; transfer to cutting board. Cut polenta crosswise into 16 slices. Cut slices into triangles, if desired. Spray large nonstick skillet with cooking spray; heat over medium heat until hot. Cook polenta about 4 minutes per side or until lightly browned.

5. Place spinach leaves, if desired, on serving plates. Arrange polenta slices and chicken over spinach; top with Tuscan Tomato Sauce. *Makes 8 servings*

Nutrients per Serving: Calories: 240 (16% Calories from Fat), Total Fat: 4 g, Saturated Fat: 1 g, Protein: 29 g, Carbohydrate: 22 g, Cholesterol: 69 mg, Sodium: 345 mg, Fiber: 5 g, Sugar: trace

Dietary Exchanges: 1 Starch/Bread, 2½ Lean Meat, 1½ Vegetable

TUSCAN TOMATO SAUCE

　Nonstick cooking spray
½ cup chopped onion
2 cloves garlic, minced
8 plum tomatoes, coarsely chopped
1 can (8 ounces) tomato sauce
2 teaspoons dried basil leaves
2 teaspoons dried oregano leaves
2 teaspoons dried rosemary
½ teaspoon pepper

1. Spray medium nonstick saucepan with cooking spray; heat over medium heat until hot. Add onion and garlic; cook and stir about 5 minutes or until tender.

2. Stir in tomatoes, tomato sauce, basil, oregano, rosemary and pepper; heat to a boil. Reduce heat to low and simmer, uncovered, about 6 minutes or until desired consistency, stirring occasionally. *Makes about 3 cups*

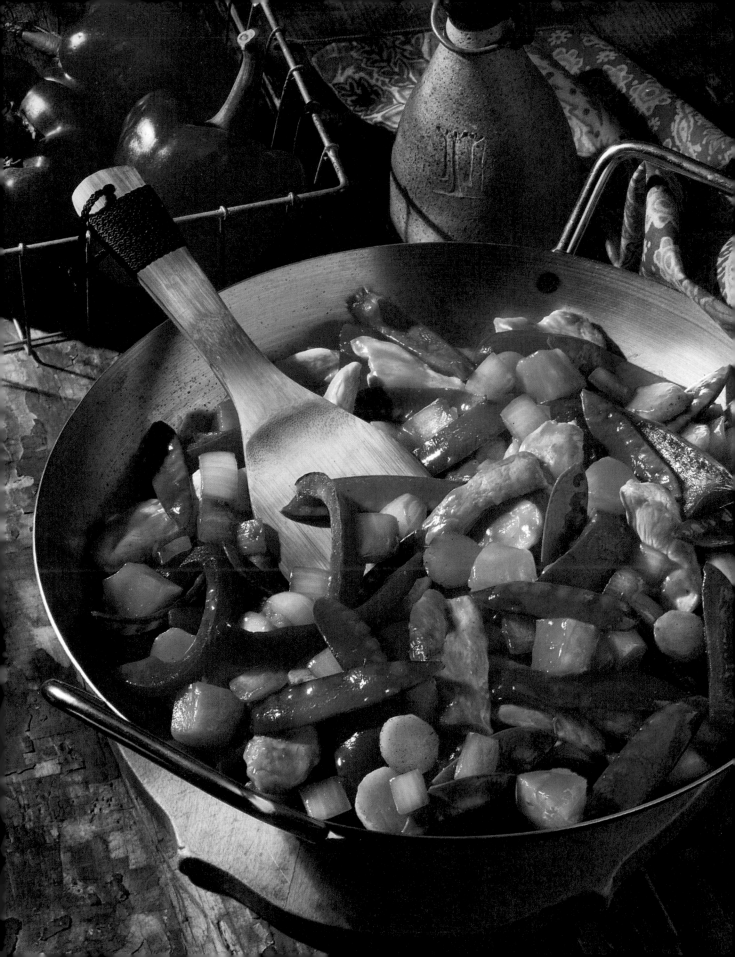

MOUTHWATERING MAIN DISHES

189 HEALTHY CHOICE® TANGY OVEN–FRIED BBQ CHICKEN

1 cup all-purpose flour
1 tablespoon *each* garlic powder, onion powder and poultry seasoning
6 boneless, skinless chicken breast halves
½ teaspoon salt (optional)
   Vegetable cooking spray
1 can HEALTHY CHOICE® RECIPE CREATIONS™ Tomato with Garden Herbs Condensed Soup
¼ cup *each* low sodium Worcestershire sauce and packed brown sugar
2 tablespoons cider vinegar
½ cup chopped onion

In large bowl, combine flour, garlic powder, onion powder and poultry seasoning. Season chicken with salt. Coat chicken pieces with flour mixture and place on foil-lined baking sheet sprayed with vegetable cooking spray. Bake chicken at 350°F 20 minutes.

Meanwhile, in small saucepan, combine soup, Worcestershire sauce, brown sugar, vinegar and onion; bring to a boil over medium heat. Reduce heat to low; simmer 10 minutes. Baste chicken generously with 1 cup sauce, reserving remaining sauce. Continue baking 20 minutes or until no longer pink in center. Serve with remaining sauce for dipping.

Makes 4 to 6 servings

Nutrients per Serving: Calories: 310 (11% Calories from Fat), Fat: 4 g, Protein: 30 g, Sodium: 230 mg

Dietary Exchanges: 2 Starch/Bread, 4 Lean Meat

190 SWEET AND SOUR STIR–FRY

1 tablespoon vegetable oil
1 pound boneless skinless chicken breasts, cut into 3-inch strips
1 can (8 ounces) sliced water chestnuts, drained
1 cup 2×½-inch red bell pepper strips
¼ cup chopped onion
2 tablespoons cornstarch
2 tablespoons soy sauce
1 tablespoon white vinegar
1 can (8 ounces) pineapple chunks, packed in juice, undrained
¼ teaspoon ground ginger
¼ teaspoon salt
1¾ teaspoons EQUAL® MEASURE™ or
   6 packets EQUAL® sweetener or
   ¼ cup EQUAL® SPOONFUL™
1 package (6 ounces) frozen pea pods

• Heat oil in wok or skillet. Add chicken; cook until chicken is no longer pink, 5 to 6 minutes. Remove and set aside. Add water chestnuts, pepper and onion to wok; cook until vegetables are tender, 3 to 4 minutes, stirring constantly.

• Combine cornstarch, soy sauce and vinegar in small bowl; stir to dissolve cornstarch. Add pineapple with juice, ginger and salt. Add to vegetable mixture; cook until sauce thickens, 2 to 3 minutes, stirring constantly.

• Stir in Equal®. Add pea pods and chicken; cook until pea pods and chicken are heated through, 2 to 3 minutes.

Makes 4 servings

Nutrients per Serving: Calories: 272, Fat: 5 g, Protein: 29 g, Carbohydrates: 27 g, Cholesterol: 66 mg, Sodium: 620 mg

Dietary Exchanges: 1 Starch/Bread, 3 Lean Meat, 2 Vegetable

Sweet and Sour Stir-Fry

MOUTHWATERING MAIN DISHES

191 ROAST CHICKEN & POTATOES CATALAN

2 tablespoons olive oil
2 tablespoons lemon juice
1 teaspoon dried thyme leaves
½ teaspoon salt
¼ teaspoon ground red pepper
¼ teaspoon ground saffron *or* ½ teaspoon crushed saffron threads or turmeric
2 large baking potatoes (about 1½ pounds), cut into 1½-inch chunks
4 skinless bone-in chicken breast halves (about 2 pounds)
1 cup sliced red bell pepper
1 cup frozen peas, thawed
  Lemon wedges

1. Preheat oven to 400°F. Spray large shallow roasting pan or 15×10-inch jelly-roll pan with nonstick cooking spray.

2. Combine oil, lemon juice, thyme, salt, ground red pepper and saffron in large bowl; mix well. Add potatoes; toss to coat.

3. Arrange potatoes in single layer around edges of pan. Place chicken in center of pan; brush both sides of chicken with remaining oil mixture in bowl.

4. Bake 20 minutes. Turn potatoes; baste chicken with pan juices. Add bell pepper; continue baking 20 minutes or until chicken is no longer pink in center, juices run clear and potatoes are browned. Stir peas into potato mixture; bake 5 minutes or until heated through. Garnish with lemon wedges.

Makes 4 servings

Nutrients per Serving: Calories: 541 (18% Calories from Fat), Total Fat: 11 g, Saturated Fat: 2 g, Protein: 42 g, Carbohydrate: 69 g, Cholesterol: 91 mg, Sodium: 132 mg, Fiber: 3 g, Sugar: 2 g

Dietary Exchanges: 4 Starch/Bread, 4 Lean Meat, 1 Vegetable

192 SKILLET CHICKEN WITH GARLIC & SUN–DRIED TOMATOES

  Vegetable cooking spray
4 boneless, skinless chicken breast halves
1½ cups thinly sliced onions
½ cup finely chopped sun-dried tomatoes
1 can HEALTHY CHOICE® RECIPE CREATIONS™ Cream of Roasted Garlic Condensed Soup
¾ cup fat free, low sodium chicken broth
¼ cup white wine
½ teaspoon salt (optional)
¼ teaspoon pepper

In large skillet sprayed with vegetable cooking spray, cook chicken until brown on both sides. Arrange onions and tomatoes over chicken.

In small bowl, combine soup, chicken broth, wine, salt and pepper; mix well. Pour mixture over chicken. Cover and simmer 20 to 25 minutes or until chicken is no longer pink in center. *Makes 4 servings*

Nutrients per Serving: Calories: 230 (16% Calories from Fat), Fat: 4 g, Protein: 29 g, Sodium: 450 mg

Dietary Exchanges: 1 Starch/Bread, 3 Lean Meat

Roast Chicken & Potatoes Catalan

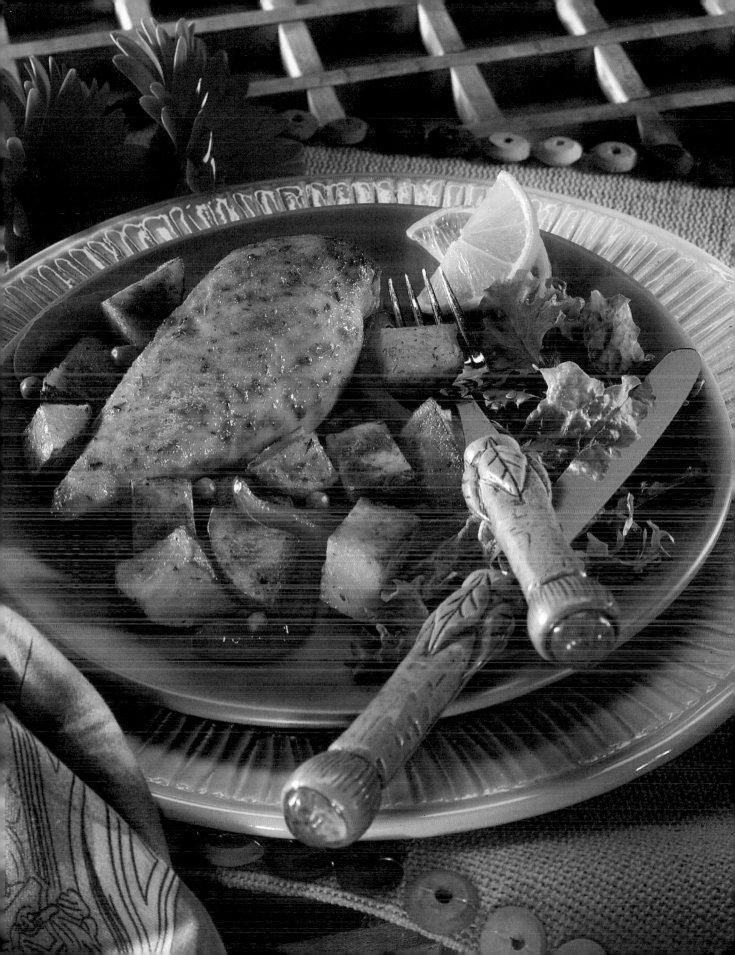

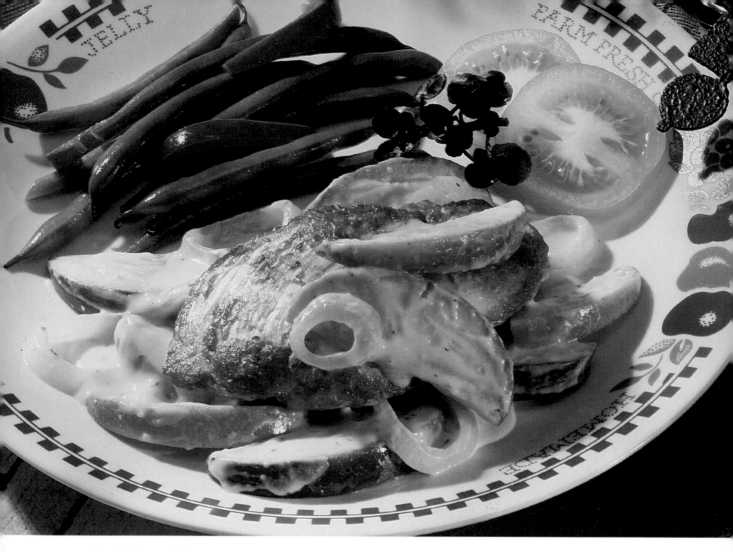

Herb Chicken with Apples

193 HERB CHICKEN WITH APPLES

1 can HEALTHY CHOICE® RECIPE
  CREATIONS™ Cream of Roasted
  Chicken with Herbs Condensed Soup
½ cup nonfat milk
½ teaspoon Italian seasoning
  Vegetable cooking spray
4 boneless, skinless chicken breast halves
2 medium red or green apples, cored and
  sliced
1 small onion, thinly sliced into rings

In small bowl, mix soup, milk and Italian
seasoning; set aside. Heat large nonstick
skillet sprayed with vegetable cooking spray
over medium heat 1 minute. Add chicken;
brown 5 minutes on each side. Remove from
skillet.

Add apples and onion to skillet; cook until
onion is tender. Stir in soup mixture. Return
chicken to skillet; reduce heat to low. Cover
and simmer 5 to 10 minutes or until chicken
is no longer pink in center.

Makes 4 servings

Nutrients per Serving: Calories: 242
(20% Calories from Fat), Fat: 5 g, Protein: 29 g,
Sodium: 297 mg

Dietary Exchanges: ½ Starch/Bread,
3 Lean Meat, 1 Fruit

MOUTHWATERING MAIN DISHES

194 CASHEW CHICKEN

10 ounces boneless skinless chicken
    breasts, cut into 1×½-inch pieces
1 tablespoon cornstarch
1 tablespoon dry white wine
1 tablespoon reduced-sodium soy sauce
½ teaspoon garlic powder
1 teaspoon vegetable oil
6 green onions, cut into 1-inch pieces
2 cups sliced mushrooms
1 red or green bell pepper, thinly sliced
1 can (6 ounces) sliced water chestnuts,
    rinsed and drained
2 tablespoons hoisin sauce (optional)
2 cups hot cooked white rice
¼ cup roasted cashews

1. Place chicken in large resealable plastic food storage bag. Blend cornstarch, wine, soy sauce and garlic powder in small bowl. Pour over chicken pieces. Seal bag; turn to coat. Marinate in refrigerator 1 hour. Drain chicken; discard marinade.

2. Heat oil in wok or large nonstick skillet over medium-high heat until hot. Add onions; stir-fry 1 minute. Add chicken; stir-fry 2 minutes or until browned. Add mushrooms, pepper and water chestnuts; stir-fry 3 minutes or until vegetables are crisp-tender and chicken is no longer pink in center. Stir in hoisin sauce; cook and stir 1 minute or until heated through.

3. Serve chicken and vegetables over rice. Top servings evenly with cashews.

Makes 4 servings

Nutrients per Serving: Calories: 274 (23% Calories from Fat), Total Fat: 7 g, Saturated Fat: 1 g, Protein: 18 g, Carbohydrate: 34 g, Cholesterol: 36 mg, Sodium: 83 mg, Fiber: 3 g, Sugar: 2 g

Dietary Exchanges: 1½ Starch/Bread, 2 Lean Meat, 1½ Vegetable, ½ Fat

195 PAELLA

Nonstick cooking spray
10 ounces boneless skinless chicken breasts
1 teaspoon vegetable oil
½ cup uncooked white rice
4 cloves garlic, finely chopped
½ cup sliced onion
½ cup sliced green bell pepper
1 cup fat-free reduced-sodium chicken
    broth
½ teaspoon ground turmeric
¼ teaspoon salt
¼ teaspoon paprika
¼ teaspoon black pepper
½ cup frozen green peas
½ cup drained canned diced tomatoes
8 ounces medium shrimp, peeled and
    deveined

1. Preheat oven to 350°F. Spray large skillet with cooking spray; heat over medium-high heat until hot. Add chicken; cook 10 minutes or until chicken is no longer pink in center, turning once. Remove chicken from skillet; cool 10 minutes. Cut into 1-inch pieces.

2. Heat oil in large ovenproof skillet or paella pan over medium heat until hot. Add rice and garlic; cook 5 minutes or until rice is browned, stirring occasionally. Add onion and bell pepper; stir in chicken broth, turmeric, salt, paprika and black pepper. Stir in peas and tomatoes; place chicken and shrimp on top of rice mixture.

3. Bake 20 minutes or until heated through. Let stand 5 minutes before serving.

Makes 4 servings

Nutrients per Serving: Calories: 258 (14% Calories from Fat), Total Fat: 4 g, Saturated Fat: 1 g, Protein: 27 g, Carbohydrate: 28 g, Cholesterol: 123 mg, Sodium: 371 mg, Fiber: 2 g, Sugar: 3 g

Dietary Exchanges: 1½ Starch/Bread, 3 Lean Meat, 1 Vegetable

MOUTHWATERING MAIN DISHES

196 TURKEY JAMBALAYA

1 teaspoon vegetable oil
1 cup chopped onion
1 green bell pepper, chopped
½ cup chopped celery
3 cloves garlic, finely chopped
1¾ cups fat-free reduced-sodium chicken broth
1 cup chopped seeded tomato
¼ pound cooked ground turkey breast
¼ pound cooked turkey sausage
3 tablespoons tomato paste
1 bay leaf
1 teaspoon dried basil leaves
¼ teaspoon ground red pepper
1 cup uncooked white rice
¼ cup chopped parsley

1. Heat oil in large nonstick skillet over medium-high heat until hot. Add onion, bell pepper, celery and garlic; cook and stir 5 minutes or until vegetables are tender.

2. Add chicken broth, tomato, ground turkey, turkey sausage, tomato paste, bay leaf, basil and red pepper. Stir in rice; bring to a boil over high heat, stirring occasionally. Reduce heat to medium-low; simmer, covered, 20 minutes or until rice is tender.

3. Remove skillet from heat; remove and discard bay leaf. Top servings with parsley.
Makes 4 servings

Nutrients per Serving: Calories: 416 (18% Calories from Fat), Total Fat: 9 g, Saturated Fat: 2 g, Protein: 28 g, Carbohydrate: 51 g, Cholesterol: 74 mg, Sodium: 384 mg, Fiber: 3 g, Sugar: 6 g

Dietary Exchanges: 2½ Starch/Bread, 2 Lean Meat, 2½ Vegetable, ½ Fat

197 SOUTHWESTERN TURKEY

1 can HEALTHY CHOICE® RECIPE CREATIONS™ Tomato with Herbs Condensed Soup
½ cup fat free sour cream
Vegetable cooking spray
1 cup sliced green onions or yellow onion
½ cup *each* diced green chiles, frozen whole kernel yellow corn and chopped red bell pepper
2 cloves garlic, minced
1 pound turkey tenderloins, cut into thin 2-inch strips
½ teaspoon salt (optional)
Hot cooked rice (optional)

In small bowl, combine soup and sour cream; mix well. Set aside. In large nonstick skillet sprayed with vegetable cooking spray, sauté onions, chiles, corn, pepper and garlic over medium-high heat until onions and pepper are tender.

Add turkey strips to skillet and brown evenly. Add soup mixture and salt, if desired, blending well; bring to a simmer. Reduce heat to low; cover and simmer 5 minutes. Serve with rice, if desired. *Makes 4 servings*

Nutrients per Serving: Calories: 261 (16% Calories from Fat), Fat: 5 g, Protein: 28 g, Sodium: 301 mg

Dietary Exchanges: 1½ Starch/Bread, 2 Lean Meat

Southwestern Turkey

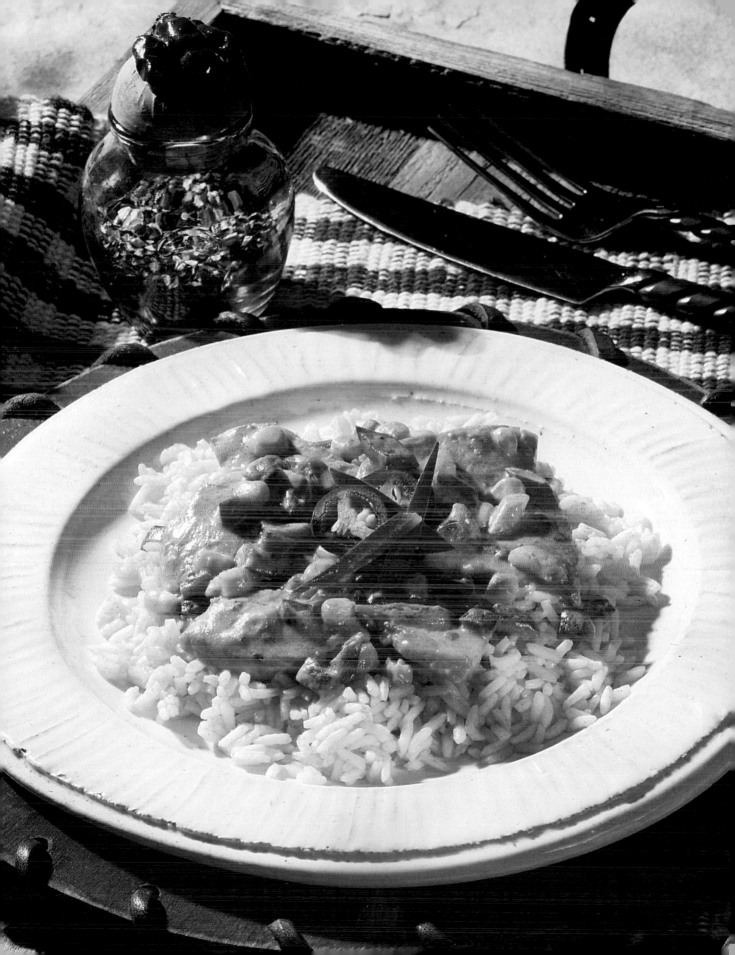

MOUTHWATERING MAIN DISHES

198 CHIPOTLE TAMALE PIE

¾ **pound ground turkey breast**
1 **cup chopped onion**
¾ **cup diced green bell pepper**
¾ **cup diced red bell pepper**
4 **cloves garlic, minced**
2 **teaspoons ground cumin**
1 **can (15 ounces) pinto or red beans, rinsed and drained**
1 **can (8 ounces) no-salt-added stewed tomatoes, undrained**
2 **canned chipotle chilies in adobo sauce, minced (about 1 tablespoon)**
1 **to 2 teaspoons adobo sauce from canned chilies (optional)**
1 **cup (4 ounces) low-sodium reduced-fat shredded Cheddar cheese**
½ **cup chopped fresh cilantro**
1 **package (8½ ounces) corn bread mix**
⅓ **cup 1% low-fat milk**
1 **large egg white**

1. Preheat oven to 400°F.

2. Cook and stir turkey, onion, bell peppers and garlic in large nonstick skillet over medium heat 8 minutes or until turkey is no longer pink. Drain fat; sprinkle with cumin.

3. Add beans, tomatoes, chilies and adobo sauce; bring to a boil over high heat. Reduce heat to medium; simmer, uncovered, 5 minutes. Remove from heat; stir in cheese and cilantro.

4. Spray 8-inch square baking dish with nonstick cooking spray. Spoon turkey mixture evenly into prepared dish. Combine corn bread mix, milk and egg white in bowl; mix just until dry ingredients are moistened. Spoon batter evenly over turkey mixture. Bake 20 to 22 minutes or until corn bread is golden brown. Let stand 5 minutes before serving.   *Makes 6 servings*

Nutrients per Serving: Calories: 396 (23% Calories from Fat), Total Fat: 10 g, Saturated Fat: 3 g, Protein: 26 g, Carbohydrate: 52 g, Cholesterol: 32 mg, Sodium: 733 mg, Fiber: 2 g, Sugar: 3 g

Dietary Exchanges: 3 Starch/Bread, 2 Lean Meat, 1½ Vegetable, ½ Fat

199 TURKEY & CHEESE STUFFED POTATOES

6 **baking potatoes, washed and pierced**
2 **cups frozen vegetables (such as broccoli, cauliflower, zucchini, carrots), thawed and drained**
1½ **cups ½-inch reduced fat cooked turkey breast cubes**
1 **can HEALTHY CHOICE® RECIPE CREATIONS™ Cream of Broccoli with Cheddar and Onion Condensed Soup**
½ **cup *each* reduced fat sour cream and nonfat milk**
¼ **teaspoon *each* garlic powder and pepper**
½ **cup sliced green onions**

Bake or microwave potatoes to desired doneness. In medium saucepan, combine vegetables, turkey, soup, sour cream, milk, garlic powder and pepper; mix well. Simmer 5 minutes, stirring occasionally.

Cut warm potatoes lengthwise and squeeze potatoes to open. Spoon equal portions of soup mixture down centers of potatoes. Sprinkle with green onions.

Makes 6 servings

Nutrients per Serving: Calories: 210 (17% Calories from Fat), Fat: 4 g, Protein: 17 g, Sodium: 240 mg

Dietary Exchanges: 4 Starch/Bread, 1 Lean Meat

Chipotle Tamale Pie

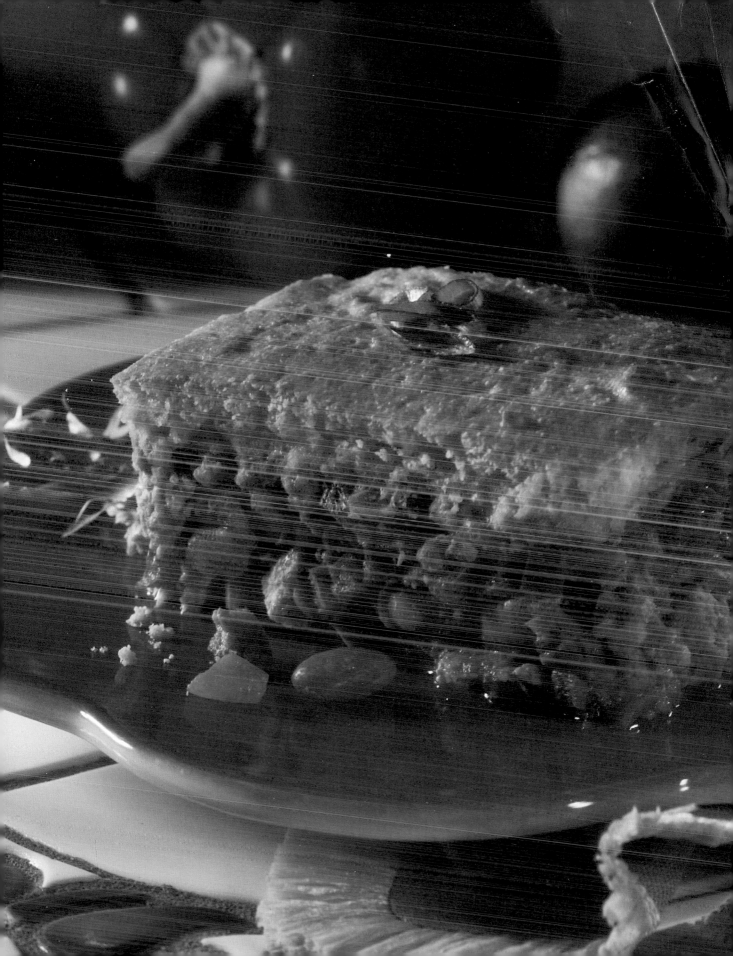

MOUTHWATERING MAIN DISHES

200 BEEF AND CARAMELIZED ONIONS

1 can HEALTHY CHOICE® RECIPE
  CREATIONS™ Cream of Mushroom
  with Cracked Pepper & Herbs
  Condensed Soup
¾ cup nonfat milk
½ cup fat free sour cream
½ teaspoon salt (optional)
1 (14-ounce) can pearl onions, drained *or*
  2 cups thinly sliced onions
1 clove garlic, minced
1 tablespoon low fat margarine
1 teaspoon sugar
1 tablespoon vinegar
1 cup sliced mushrooms
12 ounces sirloin steak, cut into 2×¼-inch
  slices
4 cups hot cooked yolk free egg noodles
1 tablespoon minced fresh parsley

In small bowl, mix soup, milk, sour cream and salt; set aside. In nonstick skillet, sauté onions and garlic in hot margarine over medium heat until lightly brown. Add sugar; cook until golden, stirring constantly. Stir in vinegar; cook 1 minute. Remove from skillet; set aside.

Add mushrooms to skillet; sauté mushrooms until lightly brown. Remove from skillet; set aside. Add steak; sauté over high heat until browned on both sides. Remove from skillet; drain skillet. Add soup mixture to skillet; cook over low heat until heated through. Return onions, mushrooms and steak to skillet. Heat 2 minutes. *(Do not boil.)* Serve over hot cooked noodles; garnish with parsley.   *Makes 6 servings*

Nutrients per Serving: Calories: 305 (16% Calories from Fat), Fat: 5 g, Protein: 21 g, Sodium: 495 mg

Dietary Exchanges: 3 Starch/Bread, 2 Lean Meat

Beef and Carmelized Onions

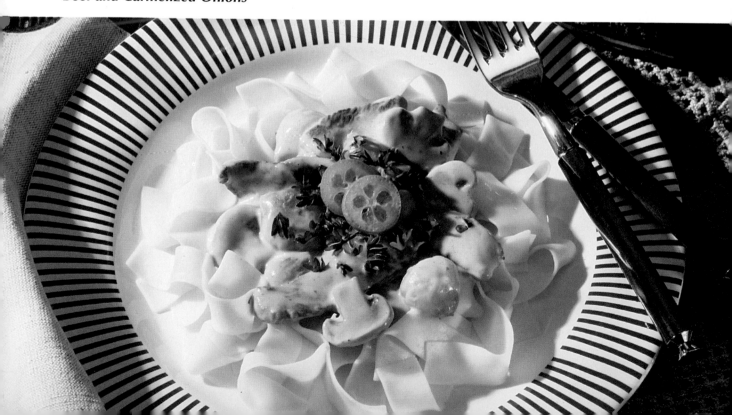

201 BEEF & VEGETABLE STIR-FRY

½ cup fat-free reduced-sodium beef broth
3 tablespoons reduced-sodium soy sauce
2 teaspoons cornstarch
1 teaspoon sugar
½ teaspoon ground ginger
½ teaspoon garlic powder
½ teaspoon dark sesame oil
¼ teaspoon salt
¼ teaspoon black pepper
1 teaspoon vegetable oil
½ pound beef flank steak, cut diagonally
    into 1 inch slices
2 green bell peppers, thinly sliced
1 tomato, cut into wedges
8 green onions, cut into 1-inch pieces
4 cups hot cooked white rice (optional)

1. Blend beef broth, soy sauce, cornstarch, sugar, ginger, garlic powder, sesame oil, salt and black pepper in medium bowl.

2. Heat vegetable oil in wok or nonstick skillet over medium-high heat until hot. Add beef; stir-fry 3 minutes or until beef is browned. Add bell peppers, tomato and onions; stir-fry 2 minutes or until vegetables are crisp-tender.

3. Stir beef broth mixture; add to wok. Cook and stir 3 minutes or until sauce boils and thickens.

4. Serve beef mixture over hot cooked white rice, if desired.   *Makes 4 servings*

Nutrients per Serving: Calories: 357 (15% Calories from Fat), Total Fat: 6 g, Saturated Fat: 2 g, Protein: 19 g, Carbohydrate: 54 g, Cholesterol: 23 mg, Sodium: 614 mg, Fiber: 2 g, Sugar: 4 g

Dietary Exchanges: 2½ Starch/Bread, 2 Lean Meat, 2 Vegetable

202 BEEF & BEAN BURRITOS

Nonstick cooking spray
½ pound beef top round steak, cut into
    ½-inch strips
3 cloves garlic, minced
1 can (about 15 ounces) pinto beans,
    rinsed and drained
1 can (4 ounces) diced green chilies,
    drained
¼ cup finely chopped fresh cilantro
6 (6-inch) flour tortillas
½ cup (2 ounces) shredded reduced-fat
    Cheddar cheese
Salsa (optional)
Nonfat sour cream (optional)

1. Spray nonstick skillet with cooking spray; heat over medium heat. Add steak and garlic; cook and stir 5 minutes or to desired doneness.

2. Add beans, chilies and cilantro; cook and stir 5 minutes or until heated through.

3. Spoon steak mixture evenly down center of each tortilla; sprinkle cheese evenly over each tortilla. Fold bottom of each tortilla up over filling, then fold sides over filling. Garnish with salsa and nonfat sour cream, if desired.   *Makes 6 servings*

Nutrients per Serving: Calories: 278 (22% Calories from Fat), Total Fat: 7 g, Saturated Fat: 2 g, Protein: 19 g, Carbohydrate: 36 g, Cholesterol: 31 mg, Sodium: 956 mg, Fiber: 1 g, Sugar: trace

Dietary Exchanges: 2 Starch/Bread, 1½ Lean Meat, 1 Vegetable, ½ Fat

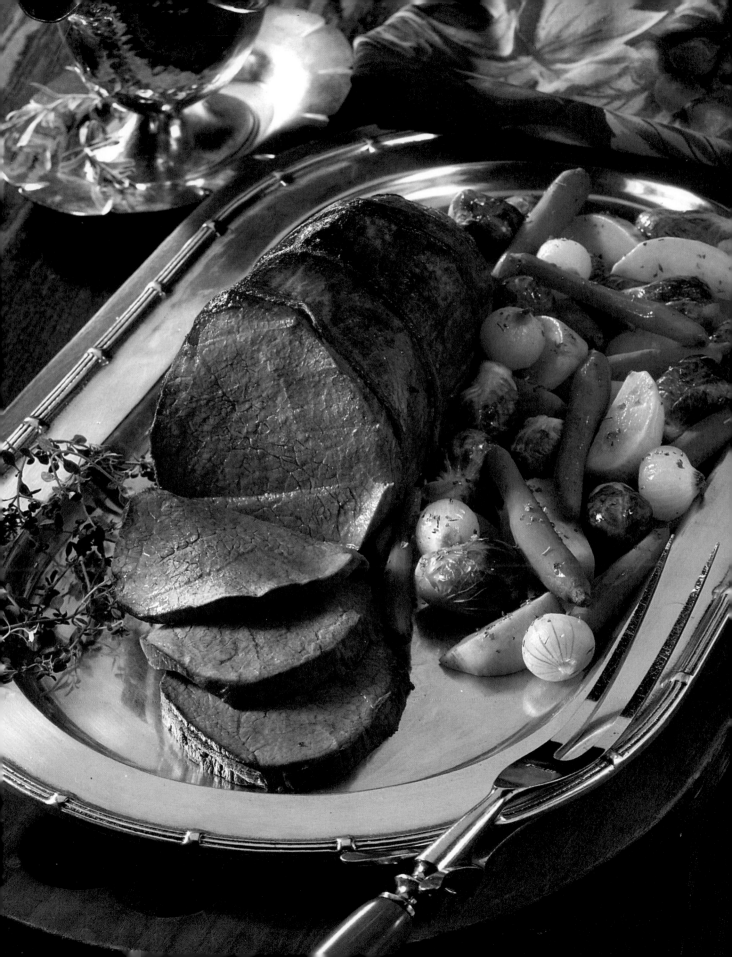

MOUTHWATERING MAIN DISHES

203 SHANGHAI BEEF

1 can HEALTHY CHOICE® RECIPE CREATIONS™ Cream of Mushroom with Cracked Pepper & Herbs Condensed Soup

⅓ cup nonfat milk

1½ teaspoons teriyaki sauce

¼ teaspoon garlic powder

⅛ teaspoon crushed red pepper (optional) Vegetable cooking spray

12 ounces sirloin steak,* cut into 2×¼-inch slices

¾ cup julienne-cut carrots

1 (8-ounce) can sliced water chestnuts, drained

3 dried shiitake mushrooms, soaked, drained and sliced *or* 1 (4-ounce) can sliced mushrooms, drained

Pork or chicken may be substituted for steak.

In medium bowl, mix soup, milk, teriyaki sauce, garlic powder and red pepper; set aside. Heat large nonstick skillet sprayed with vegetable cooking spray over medium high heat 1 minute. Add steak; sauté until brown on both sides. Remove from skillet.

Add carrots, water chestnuts and mushrooms to skillet; sauté 2 to 3 minutes. Stir in soup mixture; reduce heat and cook until heated through. Return steak to skillet; heat 1 minute. *Makes 4 servings*

Nutrients per Serving: Calories: 226, Fat: 6 g (23% Calories from Fat), Protein: 22 g, Sodium: 490 mg

Dietary Exchanges: ½ Starch/Bread, 2 Lean Meat, 2 Vegetable

204 BEEF POT ROAST

3 pounds beef eye of round roast

1 can (14 ounces) fat-free reduced-sodium beef broth

2 cloves garlic

1 teaspoon herbs de Provence

4 small turnips, peeled and cut into wedges

10 ounces fresh brussels sprouts, trimmed

20 baby carrots

4 ounces pearl onions, outer skins removed

2 teaspoons cornstarch mixed with 1 tablespoon water

1. Heat large nonstick skillet over medium-high heat. Place roast, fat side down, in skillet; cook until evenly browned. Remove roast from skillet; place in Dutch oven.

2. Pour broth into Dutch oven; bring to a boil over high heat. Add garlic and herbs de Provence; cover tightly. Reduce heat; cook 1½ hours.

3. Add turnips, brussels sprouts, carrots and onions to Dutch oven. Cover; cook 25 to 30 minutes or until vegetables are tender. Remove roast and vegetables from Dutch oven; arrange on serving platter. Cover with foil to keep warm.

4. Strain broth; return to Dutch oven. Stir blended cornstarch mixture into broth. Bring to a boil over medium-high heat; cook and stir 1 minute or until thick and bubbly. Serve over pot roast and vegetables. *Makes 6 servings*

Nutrients per Serving: Calories: 299 (20% Calories from Fat), Total Fat: 7 g, Saturated Fat: 2 g, Protein: 46 g, Carbohydrate: 14 g, Cholesterol: 79 mg, Sodium: 287 mg, Fiber: 3 g, Sugar: 4 g

Dietary Exchanges: 4 Lean Meat, 3 Vegetable

Beef Pot Roast

MOUTHWATERING MAIN DISHES

205 BEEF STROGANOFF

1 large onion, cut lengthwise and thinly sliced
½ cup plain nonfat yogurt
½ cup reduced-fat sour cream
3 tablespoons snipped chives, divided
1 tablespoon all-purpose flour
2 teaspoons Dijon mustard
¼ teaspoon salt
⅛ teaspoon white pepper
1 teaspoon olive oil
1 pound boneless sirloin steak, cut in half lengthwise and sliced into ¼-inch pieces
6 ounces portabella mushrooms or other fresh mushrooms, sliced
8 ounces cooked mafalda or other wide noodles
12 ounces steamed baby carrots

1. Heat large nonstick skillet over low heat; add onion. Cover; cook, stirring occasionally, 10 minutes or until tender. Remove onion from skillet; set aside.

2. Combine yogurt, sour cream, 2 tablespoons chives, flour, mustard, salt and pepper in small bowl; set aside.

3. Heat oil in skillet over medium-high heat. Add beef and mushrooms; cook and stir 3 to 4 minutes or until beef is lightly browned. Return onion to skillet. Reduce heat to low; stir in yogurt mixture until well blended and slightly thickened, about 2 minutes. Serve over noodles and carrots. Sprinkle with remaining 1 tablespoon chives.

Makes 6 servings

Nutrients per Serving: Calories: 179 (24% Calories from Fat), Total Fat: 5 g, Saturated Fat: 1 g, Protein: 20 g, Carbohydrate: 14 g, Cholesterol: 45 mg, Sodium: 190 mg, Fiber: 2 g, Sugar: 7 g

Dietary Exchanges: 2½ Lean Meat, 2 Vegetable

206 ITALIAN–STYLE MEAT LOAF

1 can (6 ounces) no-salt-added tomato paste
½ cup dry red wine plus ½ cup water *or* 1 cup water
1 teaspoon minced garlic
½ teaspoon dried basil leaves
½ teaspoon dried oregano leaves
¼ teaspoon salt
12 ounces lean ground round
12 ounces ground turkey breast
1 cup fresh whole wheat bread crumbs (2 slices whole wheat bread)
½ cup shredded zucchini
¼ cup cholesterol-free egg substitute *or* 2 egg whites

1. Preheat oven to 350°F. Combine tomato paste, wine, water, garlic, basil, oregano and salt in small saucepan. Bring to a boil; reduce heat to low. Simmer, uncovered, 15 minutes. Set aside.

2. Combine beef, turkey, bread crumbs, zucchini, egg substitute and ½ cup reserved tomato mixture in large bowl; mix well. Shape into loaf; place into ungreased 9×5×3-inch loaf pan. Bake 45 minutes. Discard any drippings. Pour ½ cup remaining tomato mixture over top of loaf; return to oven for 15 minutes. Place on serving platter. Cool 10 minutes before slicing. *Makes 8 servings*

Nutrients per Serving: Calories: 144 (11% Calories from Fat), Total Fat: 2 g, Saturated Fat: 1 g, Protein: 19 g, Carbohydrate: 7 g, Cholesterol: 41 mg, Sodium: 171 mg, Fiber: 1 g, Sugar: 2 g

Dietary Exchanges: 2½ Lean Meat, 1 Vegetable

Italian-Style Meat Loaf

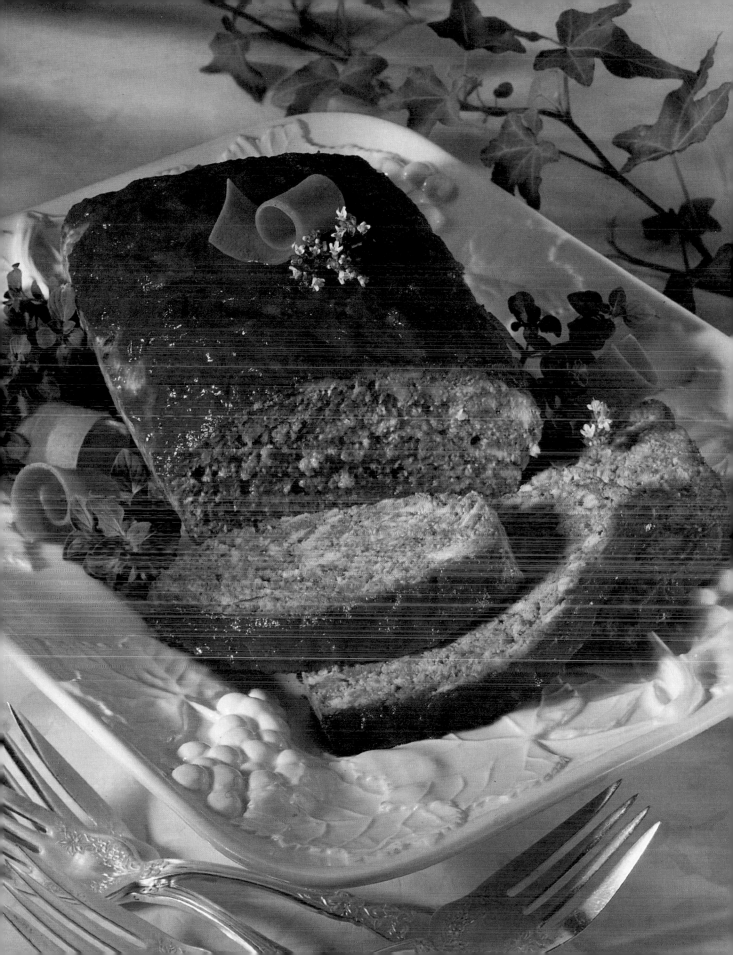

MOUTHWATERING MAIN DISHES

207 MEATLOAF RING WITH GARLIC MASHED POTATOES

4 large red potatoes, cubed
1 pound extra-lean ground beef
1 can HEALTHY CHOICE® RECIPE
   CREATIONS™ Cream of Roasted
   Garlic Condensed Soup, divided
3 slices fresh reduced fat white bread,
   processed to form crumbs
½ cup fat free egg substitute (equivalent to
   2 eggs)
½ cup *each* shredded carrots and shredded
   zucchini
¼ cup *each* minced red bell pepper and
   minced onion
2 tablespoons minced fresh parsley,
   divided
1 teaspoon Italian seasoning
   Vegetable cooking spray
⅓ cup fat free cream cheese
½ teaspoon salt (optional)

In medium saucepan, combine potatoes and enough water to cover potatoes. Bring to a boil; cover and reduce heat to medium-high. Cook 20 to 25 minutes or until tender.

Meanwhile, combine beef, ⅓ cup soup, bread crumbs, egg substitute, carrots, zucchini, pepper, onion, 1 tablespoon parsley and Italian seasoning; mix well. In shallow round 2-quart baking dish sprayed with vegetable cooking spray, form beef mixture into ring around outer edge of dish, leaving center open. Bake at 400°F 20 to 25 minutes.

Drain potatoes; mash with potato masher. Add remaining soup, cream cheese and salt; mash until well mixed. Remove meatloaf from oven; mound potatoes in center. Place under broiler 5 minutes or until lightly browned. Sprinkle with remaining 1 tablespoon parsley.   *Makes 6 servings*

Nutrients per Serving: Calories: 317 (21% Calories from Fat), Fat: 6 g, Protein: 9 g, Sodium: 452 mg

Dietary Exchanges: 2 Starch/Bread, 2 Lean Meat

208 FESTIVE STUFFED PEPPERS

1 can HEALTHY CHOICE® RECIPE
   CREATIONS™ Tomato with Garden
   Herbs Condensed Soup, divided
¼ cup water
8 ounces extra-lean ground beef or turkey
1 cup cooked rice
½ cup frozen corn, thawed
¼ cup *each* sliced celery and chopped red
   bell pepper
½ teaspoon Italian seasoning
2 green, yellow or red bell peppers, cut in
   half lengthwise, seeds removed

In small bowl, mix ¼ cup soup and water. Pour into 8×8-inch baking dish; set aside. In large skillet, brown beef over medium-high heat; drain well. In large bowl, combine remaining soup with cooked beef, rice, corn, celery, chopped pepper and Italian seasoning; mix well.

Fill pepper halves equally with beef mixture. Place stuffed peppers on top of soup mixture in baking dish. Cover and bake at 350°F 35 to 40 minutes. Place peppers on serving dish and spoon remaining sauce from baking dish over peppers.
                              Makes 4 servings

Nutrients per Serving: Calories: 260 (29% Calories from Fat), Fat: 8 g, Protein: 15 g, Sodium: 215 mg

Dietary Exchanges: 2 Starch/Bread, 2 Lean Meat, ½ Fat

Festive Stuffed Peppers

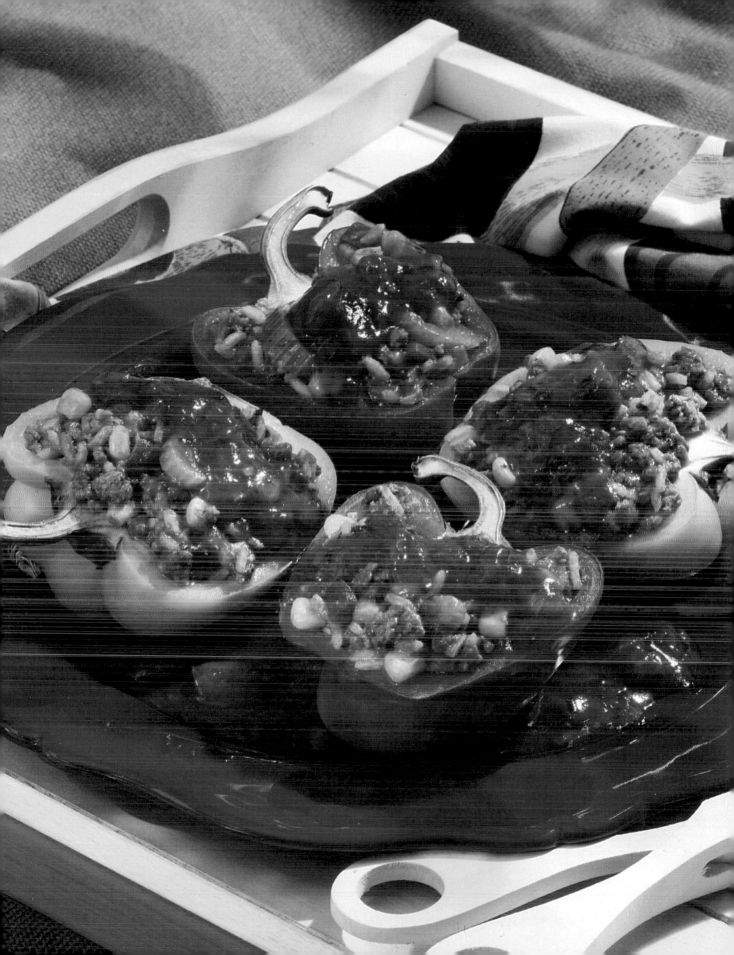

MOUTHWATERING MAIN DISHES

209 THAI–STYLE PORK KABOBS

⅓ cup reduced-sodium soy sauce
2 tablespoons lime juice
2 tablespoons water
2 teaspoons hot chili oil*
2 cloves garlic, minced
1 teaspoon minced fresh ginger
12 ounces well-trimmed pork tenderloin
1 red or yellow bell pepper, cut into ½-inch chunks
1 red or sweet onion, cut into ½-inch chunks
2 cups hot cooked rice

*If hot chili oil is not available, combine 2 teaspoons vegetable oil and ½ teaspoon red pepper flakes in small microwavable cup. Microwave at HIGH 1 minute. Let stand 5 minutes to infuse flavor.

1. Combine soy sauce, lime juice, water, chili oil, garlic and ginger in medium bowl; reserve ⅓ cup mixture for dipping sauce. Set aside.

2. Cut pork tenderloin lengthwise in half; cut crosswise into 4-inch slices. Cut slices into ½-inch strips. Add to bowl with soy sauce mixture; toss to coat. Cover; refrigerate at least 30 minutes or up to 2 hours, turning once.

3. To prevent sticking, spray grid with nonstick cooking spray. Prepare coals for grilling.

4. Remove pork from marinade; discard marinade. Alternately weave pork strips and thread bell pepper and onion chunks onto eight 8- to 10-inch metal skewers.

Thai-Style Pork Kabobs

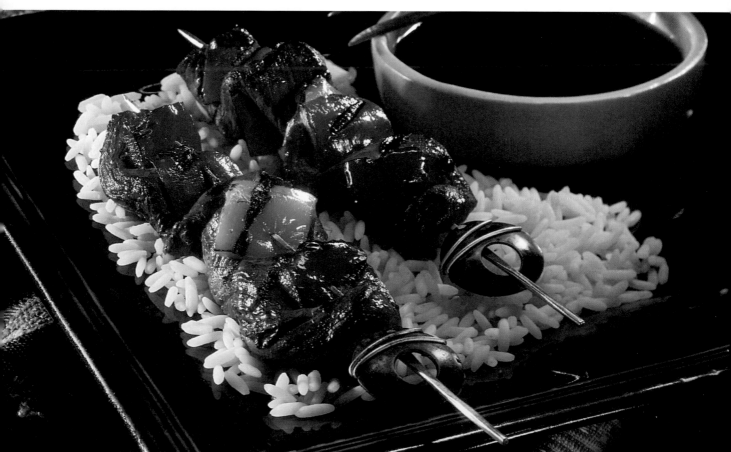

MOUTHWATERING MAIN DISHES

5. Grill, covered, over medium-hot coals 6 to 8 minutes or until pork is no longer pink in center, turning halfway through grilling time. Serve with rice and reserved dipping sauce.

Makes 4 servings

Nutrients per Serving: Calories: 248 (16% Calories from Fat), Total Fat: 4 g, Saturated Fat: 1 g, Protein: 22 g, Carbohydrate: 30 g, Cholesterol: 49 mg, Sodium: 271 mg, Fiber: 2 g, Sugar: 1 g

Dietary Exchanges: 1½ Starch/Bread, 2 Lean Meat, 1 Vegetable

210 MUSTARD–CRUSTED ROAST PORK

3 tablespoons Dijon mustard
4 teaspoons minced garlic, divided
2 tablespoons dried thyme
1 teaspoon black pepper
¼ teaspoon salt
2 whole well-trimmed pork tenderloins, about 1 pound each
1 pound asparagus spears, ends trimmed
2 red or yellow bell peppers (or one of each), cut lengthwise into ½-inch-wide strips
1 cup fat-free reduced-sodium chicken broth, divided

1. Preheat oven to 375°F. Combine mustard and 3 teaspoons garlic in small bowl. Spread mustard mixture evenly over top and sides of both tenderloins. Combine thyme, black pepper and salt in small bowl; reserve 1 teaspoon mixture. Sprinkle remaining mixture evenly over tenderloins, patting so that seasoning adheres to mustard. Place tenderloins on rack in shallow roasting pan. Roast 25 minutes.

2. Arrange asparagus and bell peppers in single layer in shallow casserole or 13×9-inch baking pan. Add ¼ cup broth, reserved thyme mixture and remaining 1 teaspoon garlic; toss to coat.

3. Roast vegetables in oven alongside tenderloins 15 to 20 minutes or until thermometer inserted into center of pork registers 160°F and vegetables are tender. Transfer tenderloins to carving board; tent with foil and let stand 5 minutes. Arrange vegetables on serving platter, reserving juices in dish; cover and keep warm. Add remaining ¾ cup broth and juices in dish to roasting pan. Place over range top burner(s); simmer 3 to 4 minutes over medium-high heat or until juices are reduced to ¾ cup, stirring frequently. Carve tenderloins crosswise into ¼-inch slices; arrange on serving platter. Spoon juices over pork and vegetables. *Makes 8 servings*

Nutrients per Serving: Calories: 182 (23% Calories from Fat), Total Fat: 5 g, Saturated Fat: 2 g, Protein: 27 g, Carbohydrate: 8 g, Cholesterol: 65 mg, Sodium: 304 mg, Fiber: 1 g, Sugar: trace

Dietary Exchanges: 3 Lean Meat, 1 Vegetable

MOUTHWATERING MAIN DISHES

211 PORK CHOPS IN CREAMY GARLIC SAUCE

1 cup fat-free reduced-sodium chicken broth
¼ cup garlic cloves, peeled and crushed
½ teaspoon olive oil
4 boneless pork loin chops, about ¼ inch thick each
1 tablespoon minced parsley
½ teaspoon tarragon
¼ teaspoon salt
¼ teaspoon black pepper
1 tablespoon all-purpose flour
2 tablespoons water
1 tablespoon dry sherry
2 cups hot cooked white rice

1. Place chicken broth and garlic in small saucepan. Bring to a boil over high heat. Reduce heat to low; simmer, covered, 25 to 30 minutes or until garlic mashes easily with fork. Cool. Purée in food processor until smooth.

2. Heat olive oil in large nonstick skillet over medium-high heat. Add pork; cook 1 to 1½ minutes on each side or until browned. Pour garlic purée into skillet; sprinkle with parsley, tarragon, salt and pepper. Bring to a boil. Reduce heat to low; simmer, covered, 10 to 15 minutes or until pork is barely pink in center. Remove from skillet; keep warm.

3. Combine flour and water in small cup. Slowly pour flour mixture into skillet; bring to a boil. Cook and stir until mixture thickens. Stir in sherry. Serve sauce over pork and rice. *Makes 4 servings*

Nutrients per Serving: Calories: 188 (28% Calories from Fat), Total Fat: 9 g, Saturated Fat: 3 g, Protein: 20 g, Carbohydrate: 5 g, Cholesterol: 40 mg, Sodium: 260 mg, Fiber: 0 g, Sugar: trace

Dietary Exchanges: 3 Lean Meat, ½ Vegetable

212 PORK WITH COUSCOUS & ROOT VEGETABLES

1 teaspoon vegetable oil
½ pound pork tenderloin, thinly sliced
2 sweet potatoes, peeled and chopped
2 medium turnips, peeled and chopped
1 carrot, sliced
3 cloves garlic, finely chopped
1 can (about 15 ounces) chick-peas, rinsed and drained
1 cup fat-free reduced-sodium vegetable broth
½ cup pitted prunes, cut into thirds
1 teaspoon ground cumin
½ teaspoon ground cinnamon
¼ teaspoon ground allspice
¼ teaspoon ground nutmeg
¼ teaspoon black pepper
1 cup uncooked quick-cooking couscous, cooked
2 tablespoons dried currants

1. Heat oil in large nonstick skillet over medium-high heat until hot. Add pork, sweet potatoes, turnips, carrot and garlic; cook and stir 5 minutes. Stir in chick-peas, vegetable broth, prunes, cumin, cinnamon, allspice, nutmeg and pepper. Cover; bring to a boil over high heat. Reduce heat to medium-low; simmer 30 minutes.

2. Serve pork and vegetables on couscous. Top servings with currants.
Makes 4 servings

Nutrients per Serving: Calories: 508 (11% Calories from Fat), Total Fat: 6 g, Saturated Fat: 1 g, Protein: 26 g, Carbohydrate: 88 g, Cholesterol: 30 mg, Sodium: 500 mg, Fiber: 17 g, Sugar: 18 g

Dietary Exchanges: 4 Starch/Bread, 2 Lean Meat, 1 Fruit, 2 Vegetable

Pork with Couscous & Root Vegetables

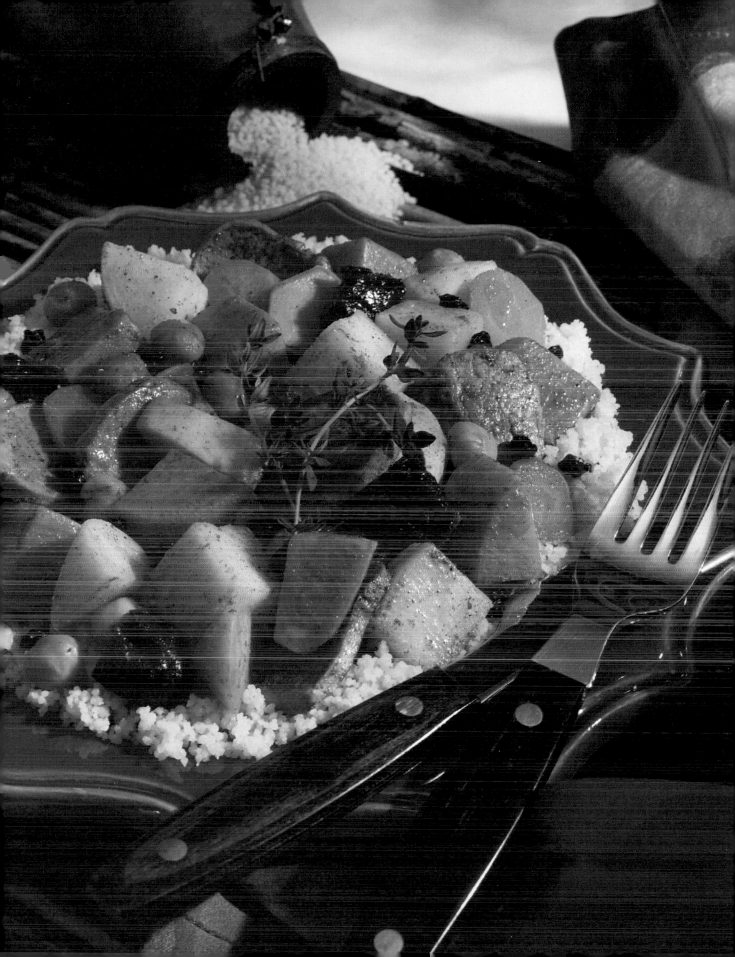

MOUTHWATERING MAIN DISHES

213 MOROCCAN PORK TAGINE

1 pound well-trimmed pork tenderloin, cut into ¾-inch medallions
1 tablespoon all-purpose flour
1 teaspoon ground cumin
1 teaspoon paprika
¼ teaspoon powdered saffron
¼ teaspoon ground red pepper
¼ teaspoon ground ginger
1 tablespoon olive oil
1 medium onion, chopped
3 cloves garlic, minced
2½ cups canned chicken broth, divided
⅓ cup golden or dark raisins
1 cup quick-cooking couscous
¼ cup chopped fresh cilantro
¼ cup sliced toasted almonds (optional)

1. Toss pork with flour, cumin, paprika, saffron, pepper and ginger in medium bowl.

2. Heat oil in large nonstick skillet over medium heat. Add onion; cook 5 minutes, stirring occasionally. Add pork and garlic; cook and stir 4 to 5 minutes or until pork is no longer pink. Add ¾ cup chicken broth and raisins; bring to a boil over high heat. Reduce heat to medium; simmer, 7 to 8 minutes, stirring occasionally.

3. Meanwhile, bring remaining 1¾ cups chicken broth to a boil in medium saucepan. Stir in couscous. Cover; remove from heat. Let stand 5 minutes. Serve pork atop couscous. Sprinkle with cilantro and almonds, if desired.   *Makes 4 servings*

Nutrients per Serving: Calories: 435 (20% Calories from Fat), Total Fat: 10 g, Saturated Fat: 2 g, Protein: 33 g, Carbohydrate: 53 g, Cholesterol: 70 mg, Sodium: 686 mg, Fiber: 8 g, Sugar: 10 g

Dietary Exchanges: 2½ Starch/Bread, 3½ Lean Meat, 1 Fruit

214 HOPPIN' JOHN SUPPER

1 cup uncooked white rice
1 can (about 14 ounces) fat-free reduced-sodium chicken broth
¼ cup water
1 package (16 ounces) frozen black-eyed peas, thawed
1 tablespoon vegetable oil
1 cup chopped onion
1 cup diced carrots
¾ cup thinly sliced celery with tops
3 cloves garlic, minced
12 ounces reduced-sodium lean ham, cut into ¾-inch pieces
¾ teaspoon hot pepper sauce
½ teaspoon salt

1. Combine rice, chicken broth and water in large saucepan; bring to a boil over high heat. Reduce heat; cover and simmer 10 minutes. Stir in black-eyed peas; cover and simmer 10 minutes or until rice and peas are tender and liquid is absorbed.

2. Meanwhile, heat oil in large skillet over medium heat. Add onion, carrots, celery and garlic; cook and stir 15 minutes or until vegetables are tender. Add ham; heat through. Add hot rice mixture, pepper sauce and salt; mix well. Cover; cook over low heat 10 minutes. Sprinkle with parsley and serve with additional pepper sauce, if desired.   *Makes 8 servings*

Nutrients per Serving: Calories: 245 (13% Calories from Fat), Total Fat: 3 g, Saturated Fat: 1 g, Protein: 16 g, Carbohydrate: 38 g, Cholesterol: 20 mg, Sodium: 624 mg, Fiber: 4 g, Sugar: 3 g

Dietary Exchanges: 2 Starch/Bread, 1 Lean Meat, 1½ Vegetable

Moroccan Pork Tagine

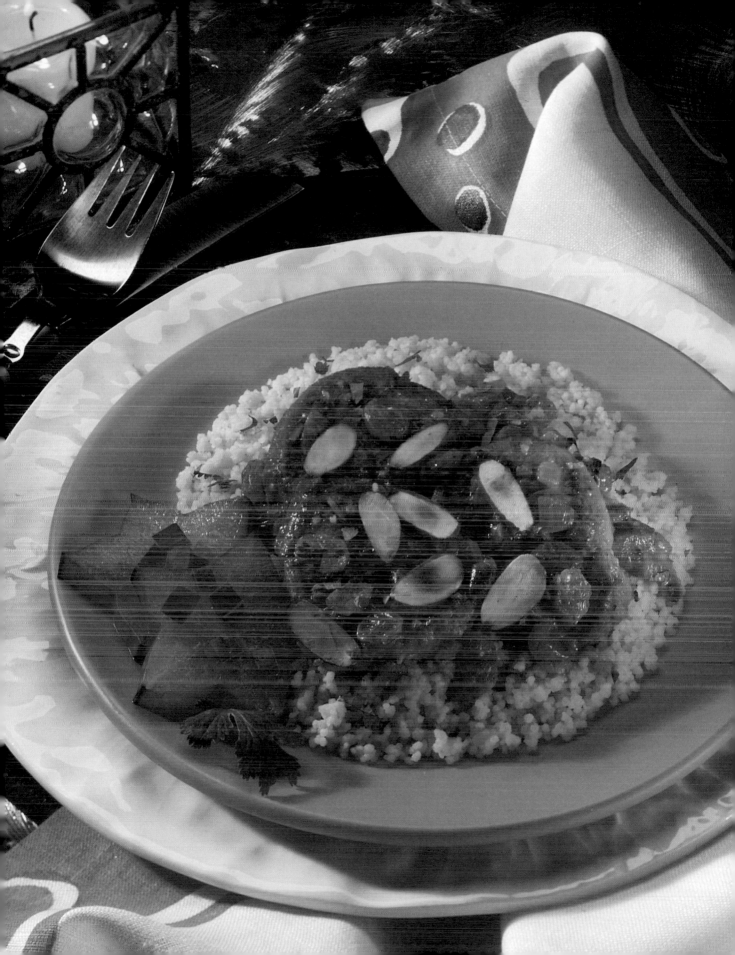

MOUTHWATERING MAIN DISHES

215 GRILLED FISH WITH PINEAPPLE–CILANTRO SAUCE

1 medium pineapple (about 2 pounds), peeled, cored and cut into scant 1-inch chunks
¾ cup unsweetened pineapple juice
2 tablespoons lime juice
2 cloves garlic, minced
½ to 1 teaspoon minced jalapeño pepper
2 tablespoons minced cilantro
2 tablespoons cold water
1 tablespoon cornstarch
1 to 1½ teaspoons EQUAL® MEASURE™ or
  3 to 4 packets EQUAL® sweetener or
  2 to 3 tablespoons EQUAL® SPOONFUL™
Salt and pepper
6 halibut, haddock or salmon steaks or fillets (about 4 ounces each), grilled

• Heat pineapple, pineapple juice, lime juice, garlic and jalapeño pepper to boiling in medium saucepan. Reduce heat and simmer, uncovered, 5 minutes. Stir in cilantro; heat to boiling.

• Mix cold water and cornstarch; stir into boiling mixture. Boil, stirring constantly, until thickened. Remove from heat; cool 2 to 3 minutes.

• Stir in Equal®; season to taste with salt and pepper. Serve warm sauce over fish.

Makes 6 servings

NOTE: Pineapple-cilantro sauce is also excellent served with pork or lamb.

Nutrients per Serving: Calories: 185, Fat: 3 g, Protein: 24 g, Carbohydrates: 16 g, Cholesterol: 36 mg, Sodium: 159 mg

Dietary Exchanges: 2½ Lean Meat, 1 Fruit

216 SNAPPER VERACRUZ

Nonstick cooking spray
1 teaspoon olive oil
¼ large onion, thinly sliced
⅓ cup low sodium fish or vegetable broth, defatted and divided
2 cloves garlic, minced
1 cup GUILTLESS GOURMET® Salsa (medium)
20 ounces fresh red snapper, tilapia, sea bass or halibut fillets

Preheat oven to 400°F. Coat baking dish with cooking spray. (Dish needs to be large enough for fish to fit snugly together.) Heat oil in large nonstick skillet over medium heat until hot. Add onion; cook and stir until onion is translucent. Stir in 3 tablespoons broth. Add garlic; cook and stir 1 minute more. Stir in remaining broth and salsa. Bring mixture to a boil. Reduce heat to low; simmer about 2 minutes or until heated through.

Wash fish thoroughly; pat dry with paper towels. Place in prepared baking dish, overlapping thin edges to obtain an overall equal thickness. Pour and spread salsa mixture over fish.

Bake 15 minutes or until fish turns opaque and flakes easily when tested with fork. Serve hot. *Makes 4 servings*

Nutrients per Serving: Calories: 184 (16% Calories from Fat), Total Fat: 3 g, Saturated Fat: trace, Protein: 30 g, Cholesterol: 52 mg, Sodium: 353 mg, Carbohydrate: 6 g, Fiber: 0 g

Dietary Exchanges: 4 Lean Meat, ½ Vegetable

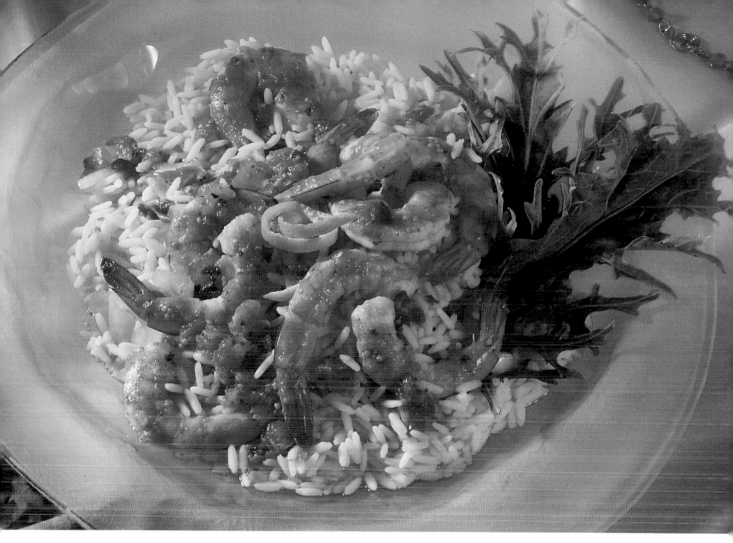

Shrimp in Tomatillo Sauce Over Rice

217 SHRIMP IN TOMATILLO SAUCE OVER RICE

1 teaspoon olive oil
¼ cup chopped onion
1 cup GUILTLESS GOURMET® Green Tomatillo Salsa
¾ cup white wine
Juice of ½ lemon
12 ounces medium-size raw shrimp, peeled and deveined
4 cups hot cooked white rice
Lemon peel strip (optional)

Heat oil in large nonstick skillet over medium-high heat until hot. Add onion; cook and stir until onion is translucent. Add salsa, wine and juice, stirring just until mixture begins to boil. Reduce heat to medium-low; simmer 10 minutes. Add shrimp; cook about 2 minutes or until shrimp turn pink and opaque, stirring occasionally. To serve, place 1 cup rice in each of 4 individual serving bowls. Pour shrimp mixture evenly over rice. Garnish with lemon peel, if desired.

Makes 4 servings

Nutrients per Serving: Calories: 274 (7% Calories from Fat), Total Fat: 2 g, Saturated Fat: trace, Protein: 18 g, Carbohydrate: 41 g, Cholesterol: 130 mg, Sodium: 479 mg, Fiber: 3 g,

Dietary Exchanges: 2 Starch/Bread, 1½ Lean Meat, 1 Vegetable

MOUTHWATERING MAIN DISHES

218 OVEN–ROASTED BOSTON SCROD

½ cup seasoned dry bread crumbs
1 teaspoon grated fresh lemon peel
1 teaspoon dill weed
1 teaspoon paprika
3 tablespoons all-purpose flour
2 egg whites
1 tablespoon water
1½ pounds Boston scrod or orange roughy
        fillets, cut into 6 (4-ounce) pieces
2 tablespoons margarine, melted
  Tartar Sauce (recipe follows)
  Lemon wedges

1. Preheat oven to 400°F. Spray 15×10-inch jelly-roll pan with nonstick cooking spray. Combine bread crumbs, lemon peel, dill and paprika in shallow bowl or pie plate. Place flour in resealable plastic food storage bag. Beat egg whites and water together in another shallow bowl or pie plate.

2. Add fish, one fillet at a time, to bag. Seal bag; turn to coat fish lightly. Dip fish into egg white mixture, letting excess drip off. Roll fish in bread crumb mixture; place in prepared jelly-roll pan. Repeat with remaining fish fillets; brush margarine evenly over fish. Bake 15 to 18 minutes or until fish begins to flake when tested with fork.

3. Prepare Tartar Sauce while fish is baking. Serve fish with lemon wedges and Tartar Sauce.   *Makes 6 servings*

TARTAR SAUCE
½ cup nonfat or reduced-fat mayonnaise
¼ cup sweet pickle relish
2 teaspoons Dijon mustard
¼ teaspoon hot pepper sauce (optional)

1. Combine all ingredients in small bowl; mix well.   *Makes ⅔ cup*

Nutrients per Serving: Calories: 215 (21% Calories from Fat), Total Fat: 5 g, Saturated Fat: 1 g, Protein: 23 g, Carbohydrate: 18 g, Cholesterol: 49 mg, Sodium: 754 mg, Fiber: trace, Sugar: trace

Dietary Exchanges: 1 Starch/Bread, 2½ Lean Meat

219 HAZELNUT–COATED SALMON STEAKS

¼ cup hazelnuts
4 salmon steaks, about 5 ounces each
1 tablespoon apple butter
1 tablespoon Dijon mustard
¼ teaspoon dried thyme leaves
⅛ teaspoon black pepper
2 cups hot cooked white rice

1. Preheat oven to 375°F. Place hazelnuts on baking sheet; bake 8 minutes or until lightly browned. Quickly transfer nuts to clean dry dish towel. Fold towel; rub vigorously to remove as much of the skins as possible. Finely chop hazelnuts using food processor.

2. *Increase oven temperature to 450°F.* Place salmon in baking dish. Combine apple butter, mustard, thyme and pepper in small bowl. Brush on salmon; top each steak with nuts. Bake 14 to 16 minutes or until salmon flakes easily with fork. Serve with rice and steamed snow peas, if desired.

Makes 4 servings

Nutrients per Serving: Calories: 329 (30% Calories from Fat), Total Fat: 11 g, Saturated Fat: 1 g, Protein: 31 g, Carbohydrate: 26 g, Cholesterol: 72 mg, Sodium: 143 mg, Fiber: 1 g, Sugar: trace

Dietary Exchanges: 1½ Starch/Bread, 4 Lean Meat

MOUTHWATERING MAIN DISHES

220 ORIENTAL–STYLE SEA SCALLOPS

2 tablespoons sesame or vegetable oil
1½ cups broccoli flowerets
1 cup thinly sliced onion
1 pound sea scallops
3 cups thinly sliced napa cabbage
    or bok choy
2 cups snow peas, ends trimmed
1 cup shiitake or button mushrooms,
    sliced
2 cloves garlic, minced
2 teaspoons ground star anise*
¼ teaspoon ground coriander
½ cup chicken broth
¼ cup rice wine vinegar
2 to 3 teaspoons reduced-sodium soy
    sauce
¼ cup cold water
2 tablespoons cornstarch
1 to 1½ teaspoons EQUAL® MEASURE™ or
    3 to 4 packets EQUAL® sweetener or
    2 to 3 tablespoons EQUAL®
    SPOONFUL™
4 cups hot cooked rice

Or, substitute 2 teaspoons five-spice powder for star anise and coriander; amounts of vinegar and soy sauce may need to be adjusted to taste.

• Heat oil in wok or large skillet. Stir-fry broccoli and onion 3 to 4 minutes. Add scallops, cabbage, snow peas, mushrooms, garlic, anise and coriander; stir-fry 2 to 3 minutes.

• Add chicken broth, vinegar and soy sauce; heat to boiling. Reduce heat and simmer, uncovered, until scallops are cooked and vegetables are tender, about 5 minutes. Heat to boiling.

• Mix cold water and cornstarch. Stir cornstarch mixture into boiling mixture; boil, stirring constantly, until thickened. Remove from heat; let stand 2 to 3 minutes. Stir in Equal®. Serve over rice.

Makes 6 servings

Nutrients per Serving: (2 ounces scallops and ⅔ cup rice), Calories: 330, Fat: 6 g, Protein: 20 g, Carbohydrates: 49 g, Cholesterol: 26 mg, Sodium: 276 mg

Dietary Exchanges: 2½ Starch/Bread, 2 Lean Meat, 1 Vegetable

221 SHRIMP AND PINEAPPLE KABOBS

8 ounces medium shrimp, peeled and
    deveined
½ cup pineapple juice
¼ teaspoon garlic powder
12 chunks canned pineapple
1 green bell pepper, cut into 1-inch pieces
¼ cup prepared chili sauce

1. Combine shrimp, juice and garlic powder in bowl; toss to coat. Marinate in refrigerator 30 minutes. Drain shrimp; discard marinade.

2. Alternately thread pineapple, pepper and shrimp onto 4 (10-inch) skewers. Brush with chili sauce. Grill, 4 inches from hot coals, 5 minutes or until shrimp are opaque, turning once and basting with chili sauce.

Makes 4 servings

Nutrients per Serving: Calories: 100 (7% Calories from Fat), Total Fat: trace, Saturated Fat: trace, Protein: 10 g, Carbohydrate: 14 g, Cholesterol: 87 mg, Sodium: 302 mg, Fiber: 1 g, Sugar: 1 g

Dietary Exchanges: 1 Lean Meat, ½ Fruit, 1 Vegetable

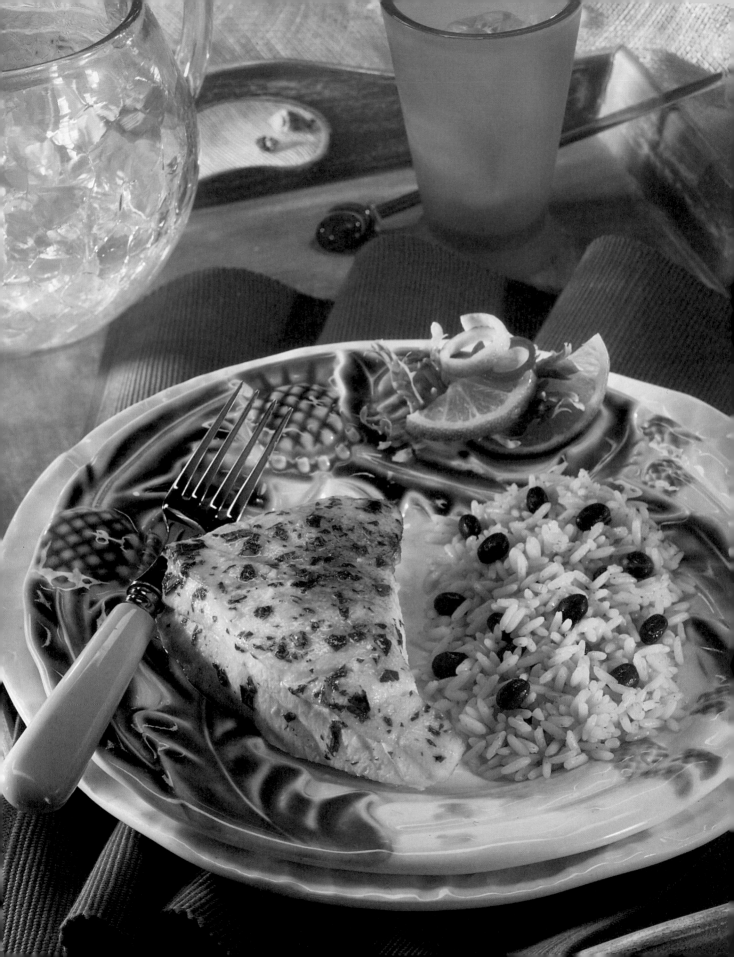

MOUTHWATERING MAIN DISHES

222 BROILED CARIBBEAN SEA BASS

6 skinless sea bass or striped bass fillets
    (5 to 6 ounces each), about ½ inch
    thick
⅓ cup chopped fresh cilantro
2 tablespoons olive oil
2 tablespoons lime juice
2 teaspoons hot pepper sauce
2 cloves garlic, minced
1 package (7 ounces) black bean and rice
    mix
  Lime wedges

1. Place fish in shallow dish. Combine cilantro, oil, lime juice, pepper sauce and garlic in small bowl; pour over fish. Cover; marinate in refrigerator 30 minutes or up to 2 hours.

2. Prepare black bean and rice mix according to package directions; keep warm.

3. Preheat broiler. Remove fish from marinade. Place fish on rack of broiler pan; drizzle with any remaining marinade in dish. Broil, 4 to 5 inches from heat, 8 to 10 minutes or until fish is opaque. Serve with black beans and rice and lime wedges.

Makes 6 servings

Nutrients per Serving: Calories: 307 (23% Calories from Fat), Total Fat: 8 g, Saturated Fat: 1 g, Protein: 33 g, Carbohydrate: 30 g, Cholesterol: 59 mg, Sodium: 432 mg, Fiber: 5 g, Sugar: 5 g

Dietary Exchanges: 2 Starch/Bread, 3 Lean Meat

223 SHRIMP ÉTOUFFÉE

3 tablespoons vegetable oil
¼ cup all-purpose flour
1 cup chopped onion
1 cup chopped green bell pepper
½ cup chopped carrots
½ cup chopped celery
4 cloves garlic, minced
1 can (about 14 ounces) vegetable broth
1 bottle (8 ounces) clam juice
½ teaspoon salt
2½ pounds large shrimp, peeled and
    deveined
1 teaspoon red pepper flakes
1 teaspoon hot pepper sauce
4 cups hot cooked rice
½ cup chopped parsley

1. Heat oil in Dutch oven over medium heat. Add flour; cook and stir 10 to 15 minutes or until flour mixture is deep golden brown. Add onion, bell pepper, carrots, celery and garlic; cook and stir 5 minutes.

2. Stir in vegetable broth, clam juice and salt; bring to a boil. Simmer, uncovered, 10 minutes or until vegetables are tender. Stir in shrimp, red pepper flakes and pepper sauce; simmer 6 to 8 minutes or until shrimp are opaque.

3. Ladle into eight shallow bowls; top each with ½ cup rice. Sprinkle with parsley. Serve with additional pepper sauce, if desired.

Makes 8 servings

Nutrients per Serving: Calories: 306 (20% Calories from Fat), Total Fat: 7 g, Saturated Fat: 1 g, Protein: 27 g, Carbohydrate: 32 g, Cholesterol: 219 mg, Sodium: 454 mg, Fiber: 1 g, Sugar: 2 g

Dietary Exchanges: 1½ Starch/Bread, 3 Lean Meat, 1 Vegetable

Broiled Caribbean Sea Bass

MOUTHWATERING MAIN DISHES

224 STACKED BURRITO PIE

½ cup GUILTLESS GOURMET® Mild Black
    Bean Dip
2 teaspoons water
5 low fat flour tortillas (6 inches each)
½ cup nonfat sour cream or plain yogurt
½ cup GUILTLESS GOURMET® Roasted
    Red Pepper Salsa
1¼ cups (5 ounces) shredded low fat
    Monterey Jack cheese
4 cups shredded iceberg or romaine
    lettuce
½ cup GUILTLESS GOURMET® Salsa
    (medium)
    Lime slices and chili pepper (optional)

Preheat oven to 350°F. Combine bean dip and 2 teaspoons water in small bowl; mix well. Line 7½-inch springform pan with 1 tortilla. Spread 2 tablespoons bean dip mixture over tortilla, then spread with 2 tablespoons sour cream and 2 tablespoons red pepper salsa. Sprinkle with ¼ cup cheese. Repeat layers 3 more times. Place remaining tortilla on top and sprinkle with remaining ¼ cup cheese.

Bake 40 minutes or until heated through. (Place sheet of foil under springform pan to catch any juices that may seep through the bottom.) Cool slightly before unmolding. To serve, cut into 4 quarters. Place 1 cup lettuce on 4 serving plates. Top each serving with 1 quarter burrito pie and 2 tablespoons salsa. Garnish with lime slices and pepper, if desired. *Makes 4 servings*

Nutrients per Serving: (1 quarter),
Calories: 302 (21% Calories from Fat),
Total Fat: 7 g, Saturated Fat: 2 g, Protein: 22 g,
Carbohydrate: 36 g, Cholesterol: 12 mg,
Sodium: 650 mg, Fiber: 1 g

Dietary Exchanges: 2 Starch/Bread,
2 Lean Meat, 1 Vegetable

225 PINTO BEAN & ZUCCHINI BURRITOS

6 flour tortillas (6 inches each)
¾ cup GUILTLESS GOURMET® Pinto Bean
    Dip (spicy)
2 teaspoons water
1 teaspoon olive oil
1 medium zucchini, chopped
¼ cup chopped green onions
¼ cup GUILTLESS GOURMET® Green
    Tomatillo Salsa
1 cup GUILTLESS GOURMET® Salsa
    (medium), divided
1½ cups shredded lettuce
    Fresh cilantro leaves (optional)

Preheat oven to 300°F. Wrap tortillas in foil. Bake 10 minutes or until softened and heated through. Meanwhile, combine bean dip and water in small bowl. Heat oil in large skillet over medium-high heat until hot. Add zucchini and onions. Cook and stir until zucchini is crisp-tender; stir in bean dip mixture and tomatillo salsa.

Fill each tortilla with zucchini mixture, dividing evenly. Roll up tortillas; place on 6 individual serving plates. Top with salsa. Serve hot with lettuce. Garnish with cilantro, if desired. *Makes 6 servings*

Nutrients per Serving: (1 burrito),
Calories: 176 (18% Calories from Fat),
Total Fat: 3 g, Saturated Fat: trace, Protein: 5 g,
Carbohydrate: 29 g, Cholesterol: 0 mg,
Sodium: 515 mg, Fiber: 2 g

Dietary Exchanges: 1½ Starch/Bread,
½ Lean Meat, 1 Vegetable

Stacked Burrito Pie

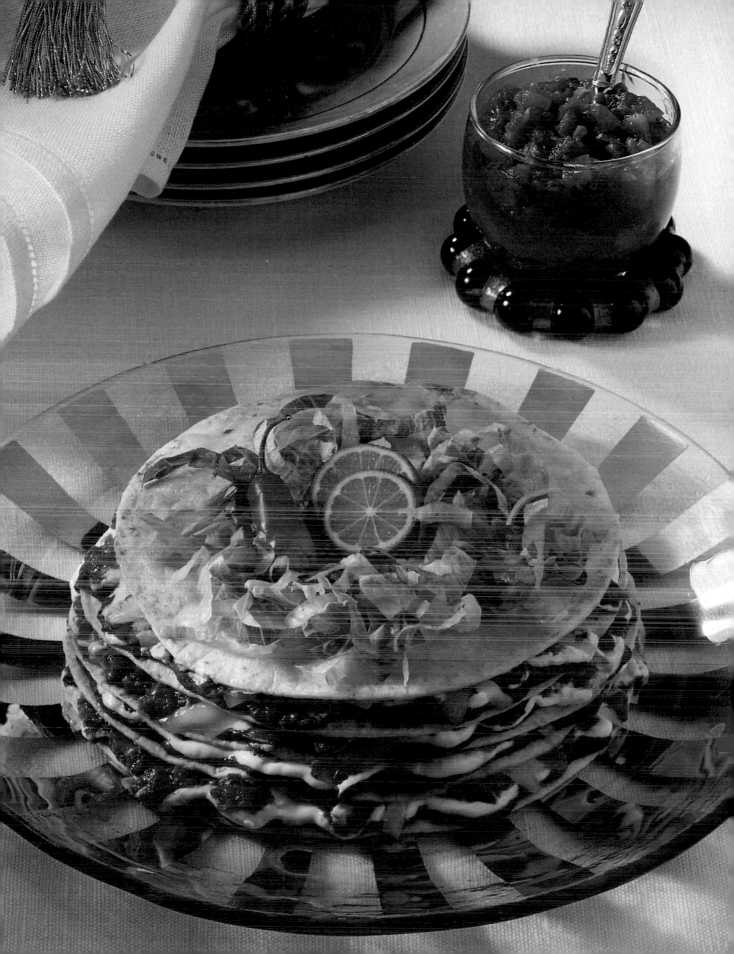

MOUTHWATERING MAIN DISHES

226 MUSHROOM RAGOÛT WITH POLENTA

1 package (about ½ ounce) dried porcini
  mushrooms
½ cup boiling water
1 can (about 14 ounces) vegetable broth
½ cup yellow cornmeal
1 tablespoon olive oil
⅓ cup sliced shallots or chopped onion
1 package (4 ounces) sliced mixed fresh
  exotic mushrooms or sliced cremini
  mushrooms
4 cloves garlic, minced
1 can (14½ ounces) Italian-style diced
  tomatoes, undrained
¼ teaspoon red pepper flakes
¼ cup chopped fresh basil or parsley
½ cup grated fat-free Parmesan cheese

1. Soak porcini mushrooms in boiling water
10 minutes.

2. Meanwhile, whisk together vegetable
broth and cornmeal in large microwavable
bowl. Cover with waxed paper; microwave
at HIGH 5 minutes. Whisk well; cook at
HIGH 3 to 4 minutes or until polenta is very
thick. Whisk again; cover. Set aside.

3. Heat oil in large nonstick skillet over
medium-high heat. Add shallots; cook and
stir 3 minutes. Add fresh mushrooms and
garlic; cook and stir 3 to 4 minutes. Add
tomatoes and red pepper flakes.

4. Drain porcini mushrooms; add liquid to
skillet. If mushrooms are large, cut into ½-
inch pieces; add to skillet. Bring to a boil
over high heat. Reduce heat to medium;
simmer, uncovered, 5 minutes or until
slightly thickened. Stir in basil.

5. Spoon polenta onto 4 plates; top with
mushroom mixture. Sprinkle with cheese.

Makes 4 servings

Nutrients per Serving: Calories: 184
(25% Calories from Fat), Total Fat: 5 g,
Saturated Fat: 1 g, Protein: 6 g,
Carbohydrate: 30 g, Cholesterol: 0 mg,
Sodium: 572 mg, Fiber: 3 g, Sugar: 6 g

Dietary Exchanges: 1 Starch/Bread,
½ Lean Meat, 2½ Vegetable, ½ Fat

227 BLACK BEAN & RICE BURRITOS

½ cup nonfat cottage cheese
2 tablespoons soft fresh goat cheese
1½ cups cooked brown rice or long-grain
  rice, kept warm
3 tablespoons minced red onion
3 tablespoons chopped fresh cilantro
¼ teaspoon ground cumin
¼ cup low sodium chicken broth, defatted
8 whole wheat tortillas (6 inches each)
¾ cup GUILTLESS GOURMET® Spicy Black
  Bean Dip
½ cup (2 ounces) shredded low fat
  Monterey Jack cheese
3 cups finely shredded lettuce
½ cup GUILTLESS GOURMET® Salsa
  (medium)
  Fresh cilantro sprigs (optional)

Preheat oven to 350°F. Place cottage and
goat cheeses in medium bowl; blend with
fork until smooth. Add rice, onion, chopped
cilantro and cumin. Mix well; set aside.

MOUTHWATERING MAIN DISHES

Place broth in shallow bowl. Working with 1 tortilla at a time, dip tortilla in broth to moisten each side. Spread 1 heaping tablespoonful bean dip on tortilla, then top with 1 heaping tablespoonful rice mixture. Roll up tortilla and place in 12×8-inch baking dish, seam side down. Repeat with remaining tortillas, bean dip and rice mixture. Cover with foil.

Bake about 25 to 30 minutes or until heated through. Remove foil; top with shredded cheese. Return to oven until cheese melts. To serve, arrange burritos on plate. Top with lettuce and salsa. Garnish with cilantro sprigs, if desired. *Makes 8 servings*

Nutrients per Serving: Calories: 224 (20% Calories from Fat), Total Fat: 5 g, Saturated Fat: 2 g, Protein: 11 g, Carbohydrate: 34 g, Cholesterol: 7 mg, Sodium: 425 mg, Fiber: 1 g

Dietary Exchanges: 2 Starch/Bread, 1 Lean Meat, ½ Fat

Mushroom Ragoût with Polenta

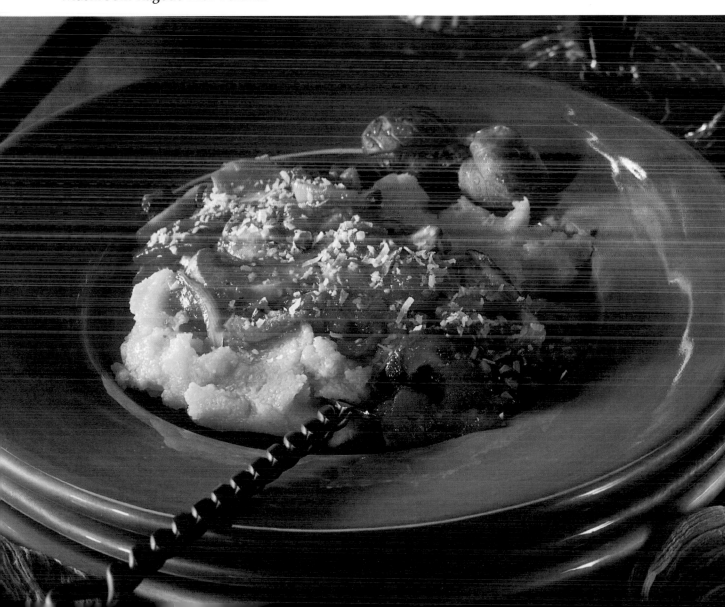

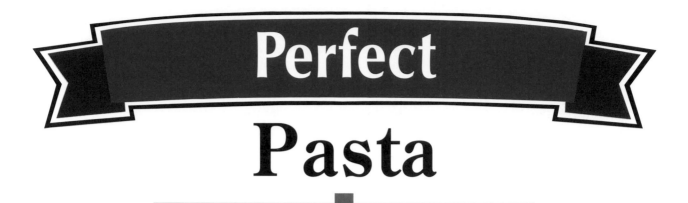

Perfect
Pasta

228 ORANGE BEEF AND BROCCOLI

1 pound lean boneless beef, cut 1 inch thick
½ cup orange juice
2 teaspoons reduced-sodium soy sauce
1 teaspoon sugar
3 teaspoons vegetable oil, divided
¾ pound broccoli, coarsely chopped
1 cup diagonally sliced carrots
½ cup thinly sliced red bell pepper
1 green onion, diagonally sliced
¾ cup cold water
2 teaspoons cornstarch
1 tablespoon grated orange peel
6 ounces uncooked yolk-free wide noodles

1. Slice beef across grain into ⅛-inch slices; place beef in nonmetallic bowl. Add orange juice, soy sauce and sugar; toss to coat evenly. Let stand 30 minutes, or cover and refrigerate overnight.

2. Heat 2 teaspoons oil in large nonstick skillet or wok over medium-high heat until hot. Add broccoli, carrots, bell pepper and green onion; cook and stir 2 minutes. Remove vegetables to large bowl.

3. Drain beef; reserve marinade. Heat remaining 1 teaspoon oil in same skillet over medium-high heat until hot. Add beef to skillet; cook 1 to 2 minutes or until no longer pink. Add vegetables and reserved marinade to skillet; bring to a boil. Stir water into cornstarch until smooth; add to skillet. Cook until thickened, stirring constantly. Sprinkle with grated orange peel.

4. Cook noodles according to package directions, omitting salt; drain. Spoon beef mixture over noodles; serve immediately.

Makes 4 servings

Nutrients per Serving: Calories: 424 (27% Calories from Fat), Total Fat: 13 g, Saturated Fat: 3 g, Protein: 35 g, Carbohydrate: 43 g, Cholesterol: 77 mg, Sodium: 169 mg, Fiber: 6 g, Sugar: 9 g

Dietary Exchanges: 2 Starch/Bread, 3½ Lean Meat, 2½ Vegetables, ½ Fat

Orange Beef and Broccoli

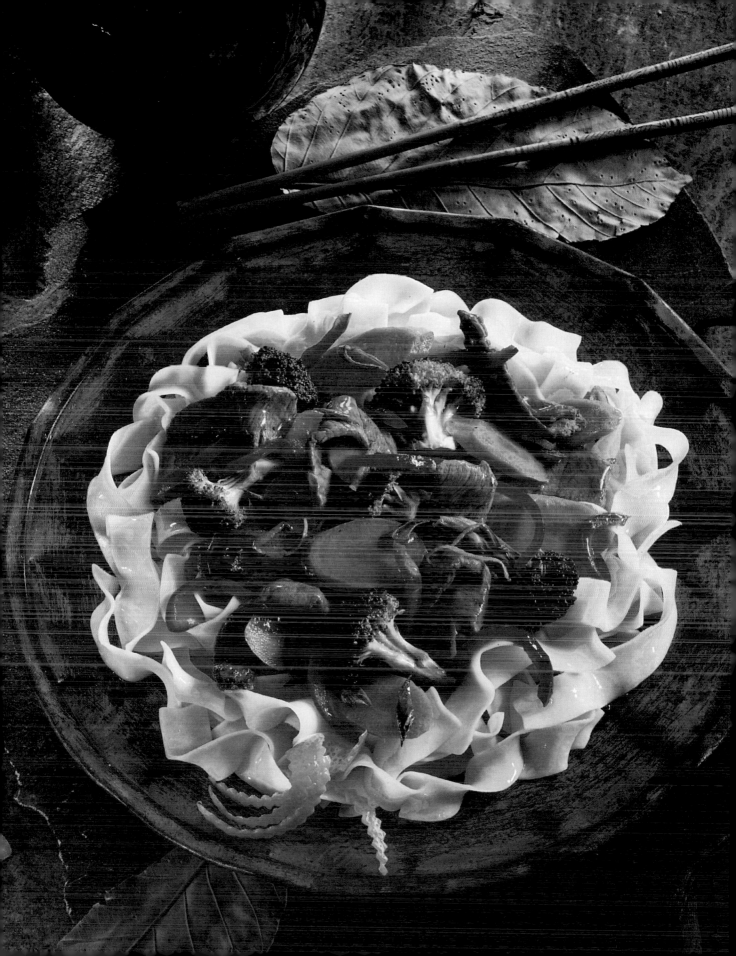

PERFECT PASTA

229 PASTITSO

8 ounces uncooked elbow macaroni
½ cup cholesterol-free egg substitute
¼ teaspoon ground nutmeg
¾ pound lean ground lamb, beef or turkey
½ cup chopped onion
1 clove garlic, minced
1 can (8 ounces) tomato sauce
¾ teaspoon dried mint leaves
½ teaspoon dried oregano leaves
½ teaspoon black pepper
⅛ teaspoon ground cinnamon
2 teaspoons reduced-calorie margarine
3 tablespoons all-purpose flour
1½ cups skim milk
2 tablespoons grated Parmesan cheese

1. Cook pasta according to package directions, omitting salt; drain. Transfer to bowl; stir in egg substitute and nutmeg.

2. Spray bottom of 9-inch square baking dish with nonstick cooking spray. Spread pasta mixture in baking dish; set aside.

3. Preheat oven to 350°F. Cook ground lamb, onion and garlic in large nonstick skillet over medium heat until lamb is no longer pink. Stir in tomato sauce, mint, oregano, pepper and cinnamon. Reduce heat and simmer 10 minutes; spread over pasta.

4. Melt margarine in small saucepan. Add flour; stir constantly for 1 minute. Whisk in milk; cook and stir until thickened, about 6 minutes. Spread over meat mixture; sprinkle with Parmesan cheese. Bake 30 to 40 minutes or until set.   *Makes 6 servings*

Nutrients per Serving: Calories: 280 (15% Calories from Fat), Total Fat: 5 g, Saturated Fat: 2 g, Protein: 20 g, Carbohydrate: 39 g, Cholesterol: 31 mg, Sodium: 366 mg, Fiber: 1 g, Sugar: 3 g

Dietary Exchanges: 2½ Starch/Bread, 1½ Lean Meat, ½ Vegetable

230 PASTA PICADILLO

12 ounces uncooked medium shell pasta
   Nonstick cooking spray
1 pound lean ground sirloin
⅔ cup finely chopped green bell pepper
½ cup finely chopped onion
2 cloves garlic, minced
1 can (8 ounces) tomato sauce
½ cup water
⅓ cup raisins
3 tablespoons sliced pimiento-stuffed green olives
2 tablespoons drained capers
2 tablespoons vinegar
½ teaspoon black pepper
¼ teaspoon salt

1. Cook pasta according to package directions, omitting salt. Drain; set aside.

2. Spray large nonstick skillet with cooking spray; add beef, bell pepper, onion and garlic. Brown beef mixture over medium-high heat 5 minutes or until no longer pink, stirring to separate beef; drain fat. Stir in tomato sauce, water, raisins, olives, capers, vinegar, pepper and salt. Reduce heat to medium-low; cook, covered, 15 minutes, stirring occasionally.

3. Add pasta to skillet; toss to coat. Cover and heat through, about 2 minutes.
Makes 6 servings

Nutrients per Serving: Calories: 366 (13% Calories from Fat), Total Fat: 5 g, Saturated Fat: 2 g, Protein: 23 g, Carbohydrate: 56 g, Cholesterol: 43 mg, Sodium: 568 mg, Fiber: 2 g, Sugar: 6 g

Dietary Exchanges: 3 Starch/Bread, 2 Lean Meat, 1½ Vegetable

Pasta Picadillo

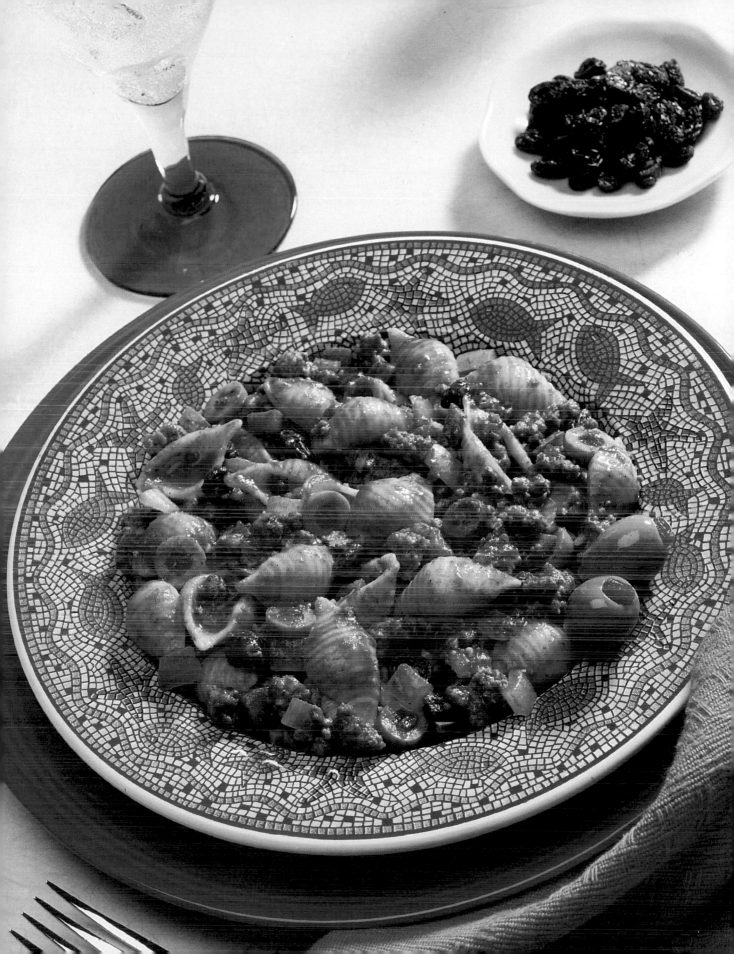

PERFECT PASTA

231 BEEF BURGUNDY AND MUSHROOMS

8 ounces uncooked yolk-free egg noodles
¼ cup water
2 tablespoons all-purpose flour
1 can (10 ounces) beef broth
2 tablespoons dry red wine
½ teaspoon Worcestershire sauce
1 bay leaf
¾ teaspoon sugar
   Nonstick cooking spray
1½ teaspoons olive oil
1 package (16 ounces) sliced fresh
   mushrooms
4 cloves garlic, minced
1 pound beef sirloin, cut into thin strips
½ cup chopped green onions, with tops
¼ cup chopped parsley
   Black pepper

1. Cook noodles according to package directions, omitting salt. Drain; set aside.

2. Meanwhile, combine water and flour in small bowl; whisk until smooth. Slowly whisk in beef broth, wine, Worcestershire sauce, bay leaf and sugar; set aside.

3. Spray large nonstick skillet with cooking spray; add oil. Heat over high heat until hot. Add mushrooms and garlic; cook 2 minutes. Reduce heat to medium-high; cook 3 to 4 minutes or until tender. Place in separate bowl; set aside.

4. Spray same skillet with nonstick cooking spray; brown sirloin strips over high heat 2 to 3 minutes. Add green onions, reserved mushrooms and broth mixture; bring to a boil. Reduce heat to medium-low; simmer, uncovered, 30 minutes or until meat is tender. Remove from heat; remove and

discard bay leaf. Add parsley; season with pepper to taste. Let stand 10 minutes before serving. Spoon over egg noodles.

Makes 4 servings

Nutrients per Serving: Calories: 417 (16% Calories from Fat), Total Fat: 8 g, Saturated Fat: 2 g, Protein: 31 g, Carbohydrate: 56 g, Cholesterol: 65 mg, Sodium: 298 mg, Fiber: 2 g, Sugar: 3

Dietary Exchanges: 3 Starch/Bread, 3 Lean Meat, 1 Vegetable

232 SZECHWAN BEEF LO MEIN

1 pound well-trimmed boneless beef top
   sirloin steak, 1 inch thick
4 cloves garlic, minced
2 teaspoons minced fresh ginger
¾ teaspoon red pepper flakes, divided
1 tablespoon vegetable oil
1 can (about 14 ounces) vegetable broth
1 cup water
2 tablespoons reduced-sodium soy sauce
1 package (8 ounces) frozen mixed
   vegetables for stir-fry
1 package (9 ounces) refrigerated angel
   hair pasta
¼ cup chopped fresh cilantro (optional)

1. Cut steak crosswise into ⅛-inch strips; cut strips into 1½-inch pieces. Toss steak with garlic, ginger and ½ teaspoon red pepper flakes.

2. Heat oil in large nonstick skillet over medium-high heat until hot. Add half of steak to skillet; cook and stir 3 minutes or until meat is barely pink in center. Remove from skillet; set aside. Repeat with remaining steak.

PERFECT PASTA

3. Add vegetable broth, water, soy sauce and remaining ¼ teaspoon red pepper flakes to skillet; bring to a boil over high heat. Add vegetables; return to a boil. Reduce heat to low; simmer, covered, 3 minutes or until vegetables are crisp-tender.

4. Uncover; stir in pasta. Return to a boil over high heat. Reduce heat to medium; simmer, uncovered, 2 minutes, separating pasta with two forks. Return steak and any accumulated juices to skillet; simmer 1 minute or until pasta is tender and steak is hot. Sprinkle with cilantro, if desired.

Makes 4 servings

Nutrients per Serving: Calories: 408 (25% Calories from Fat), Total Fat: 11 g, Saturated Fat: 3 g, Protein: 32 g, Carbohydrate: 44 g, Cholesterol: 137 mg, Sodium: 386 mg, Fiber: 2 g, Sugar: 1 g

Dietary Exchanges: 2 Starch/Bread, 3 Lean Meat, 3 Vegetable, ½ Fat

Szechwan Beef Lo Mein

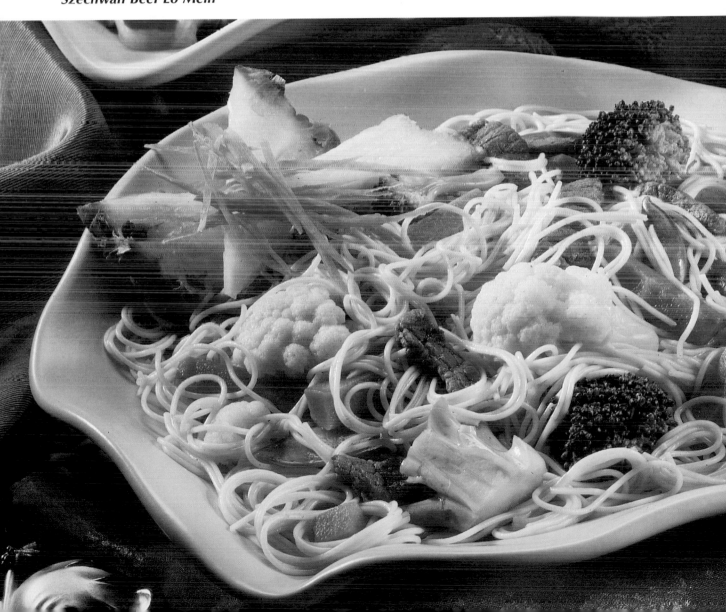

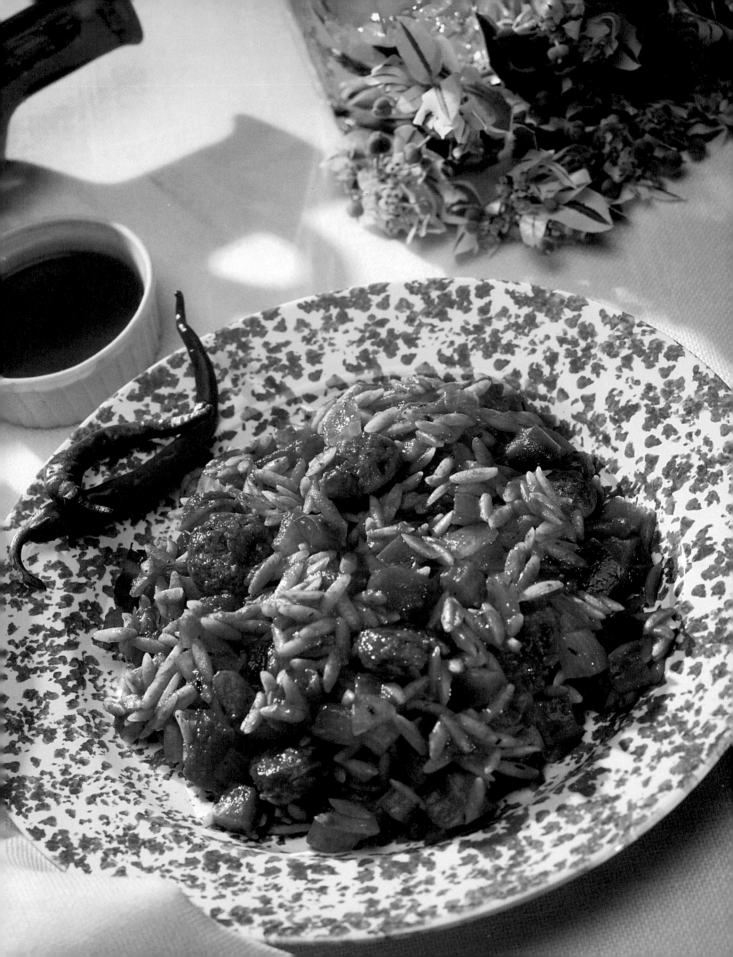

PERFECT PASTA

233 COUNTRY KIELBASA AND VEGETABLES

Nonstick cooking spray
8 ounces turkey kielbasa sausage, cut into $\frac{1}{8}$-inch rounds
1 cup chopped onion
$\frac{3}{4}$ cup chopped green bell pepper
$\frac{1}{2}$ cup finely chopped celery
1 can (16 ounces) diced tomatoes, undrained
$\frac{1}{3}$ cup water
$\frac{1}{2}$ cup orzo pasta
$\frac{1}{2}$ teaspoon dried thyme leaves
2 teaspoons olive oil
Hot pepper sauce

1. Preheat oven to 350°F. Spray large nonstick skillet with cooking spray; heat over high heat until hot. Add sausage; cook and stir 10 to 15 minutes or until sausage is brown. Add onion, pepper and celery; cook an additional 3 minutes.

2. Spoon into 1½-quart casserole. Add tomatoes, water, orzo and thyme. Cover; bake 1 hour, stirring after 30 minutes, or until heated through. Remove from oven. Add olive oil; stir to combine. Let stand, covered, 10 minutes before serving. Serve with pepper sauce. *Makes 4 servings*

Nutrients per Serving: Calories: 260 (24% Calories from Fat), Total Fat: 7 g, Saturated Fat: 2 g, Protein: 16 g, Carbohydrate: 36 g, Cholesterol: 38 mg, Sodium: 691 mg, Fiber: 3 g, Sugar: 7 g

Dietary Exchanges: 1½ Starch/Bread, 1 Lean Meat, 2 Vegetable, 1 Fat

234 STRAW AND HAY

1 cup skim milk
$\frac{1}{2}$ cup nonfat cottage cheese
2 teaspoons cornstarch
$\frac{1}{4}$ teaspoon ground mace
$\frac{1}{8}$ teaspoon black pepper
4 ounces uncooked plain fettuccine
4 ounces uncooked spinach fettuccine
Nonstick cooking spray
4 ounces reduced-fat deli-style ham, diagonally sliced
2 tablespoons snipped chives
1 cup frozen peas, thawed and drained
$\frac{1}{4}$ cup grated Parmesan cheese
$\frac{1}{8}$ teaspoon paprika

1. Combine milk, cottage cheese, cornstarch, mace and pepper in blender or food processor; process until smooth. Set aside.

2. Cook pasta according to package directions, omitting salt. Drain; set aside. Meanwhile, spray large nonstick skillet with cooking spray; heat over medium heat until hot. Add ham and chives; cook and stir until ham is lightly browned. Add milk mixture and peas; cook and stir until thickened.

3. Remove from heat. Add pasta and Parmesan cheese; toss to coat evenly. Sprinkle with paprika; serve immediately. *Makes 4 servings*

Nutrients per Serving: Calories: 348 (11% Calories from Fat), Total Fat: 4 g, Saturated Fat: 2 g, Protein: 25 g, Carbohydrate: 52 g, Cholesterol: 9 mg, Sodium: 592 mg, Fiber: 3 g, Sugar: 5 g

Dietary Exchanges: 3 Starch/Bread, 2 Lean Meat, ½ Fat

Country Kielbasa and Vegetables

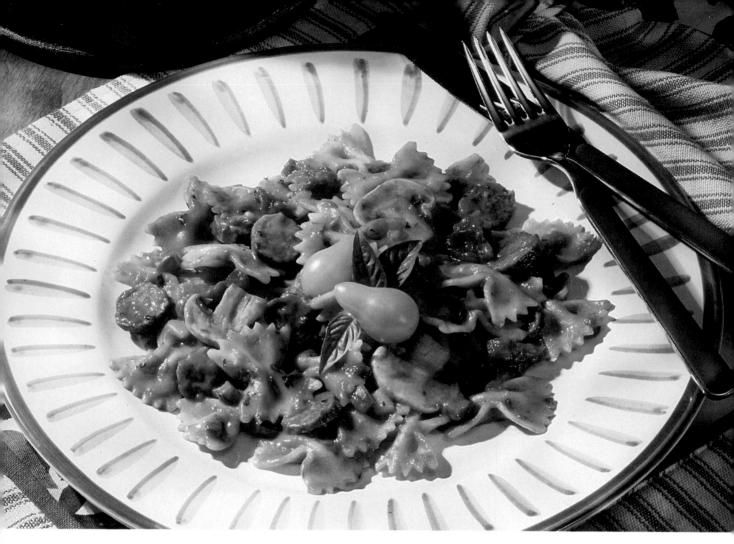

Sausage and Bow Tie Bash

235 SAUSAGE AND BOW TIE BASH

1 can HEALTHY CHOICE® RECIPE
  CREATIONS™ Tomato with Garden
  Herbs Condensed Soup
¼ cup nonfat milk
  Vegetable cooking spray
½ cup *each* diced onion and green bell
  pepper
 2 cloves garlic, minced
½ cup sliced mushrooms
½ teaspoon salt (optional)
 1 (7-ounce package) HEALTHY CHOICE®
  Low Fat Smoked Sausage, cut into
  ⅛-inch slices
 4 cups cooked bow tie pasta

In small bowl, combine soup and milk; mix
well. Set aside. In large nonstick skillet
sprayed with vegetable cooking spray, sauté
onion, pepper and garlic until tender. Add
mushrooms and salt; cook 2 to 3 minutes.
Add sausage and soup mixture; mix well.
Reduce heat; cover and simmer 2 minutes
longer. Add pasta and toss until coated with
sauce.   *Makes 6 servings*

Nutrients per Serving: Calories: 440,
(6% Calories from Fat), Fat: 3 g, Protein: 22 g,
Sodium: 410 mg

Dietary Exchanges: 2½ Starch/Bread,
1 Lean Meat

PERFECT PASTA

236 SWISS CHEESE SAUCED PASTA SHELLS WITH CRUMBLED BACON

1 cup frozen peas
10 ounces uncooked medium shell pasta
2½ cups skim milk
3 tablespoons all-purpose flour
2 teaspoons Dijon mustard
½ teaspoon salt
⅛ teaspoon black pepper
3 ounces sliced reduced-fat Swiss cheese
4 slices reduced-sodium bacon, cooked and crumbled
1 tablespoon grated Parmesan cheese

1. Preheat oven to 325°F. Spray 12×8-inch baking pan with nonstick cooking spray; set aside. Place peas in colander. Cook pasta according to package directions, omitting salt. Drain over peas in colander; set aside.

2. Meanwhile, whisk together milk, flour, mustard, salt and pepper in large skillet. Cook over medium heat, stirring constantly, 5 minutes or until thickened. Remove from heat. Add Swiss cheese; whisk until smooth.

3. Place peas and pasta on bottom of prepared pan. Pour sauce evenly over pasta and peas; top with crumbled bacon. Bake 20 to 25 minutes. Remove from oven. Sprinkle with Parmesan cheese; let stand 5 minutes before serving.

Makes 4 servings

Nutrients per Serving: Calories: 486 (17% Calories from Fat), Total Fat: 9 g, Saturated Fat: 3 g, Protein: 26 g, Carbohydrate: 74 g, Cholesterol: 23 mg, Sodium: 528 mg, Fiber: 2 g, Sugar: 9 g

Dietary Exchanges: 4½ Starch/Bread, 1 Lean Meat, ½ Milk, 1½ Fat

237 STIR–FRIED PORK LO MEIN

Nonstick cooking spray
6 green onions, cut into 1-inch pieces
½ teaspoon garlic powder
½ teaspoon ground ginger
6 ounces pork loin roast, thinly sliced
3 cups shredded green cabbage
½ cup shredded carrot
½ cup snow peas
½ cup fat-free reduced-sodium chicken broth
2 teaspoons cornstarch
2 tablespoons hoisin sauce (optional)
1 tablespoon reduced-sodium soy sauce
8 ounces hot cooked linguine

1. Spray wok with cooking spray; heat over medium heat until hot. Add onions, garlic powder and ginger; stir-fry 30 seconds. Add pork; stir-fry 2 minutes or until pork is no longer pink. Add vegetables; stir-fry 3 minutes or until vegetables are crisp-tender.

2. Blend chicken broth, cornstarch, hoisin sauce and soy sauce in small bowl. Add to wok; cook and stir until mixture boils and thickens. Serve over pasta.

Makes 4 servings

Nutrients per Serving: Calories: 310 (13% Calories from Fat), Total Fat: 4 g, Saturated Fat: 1 g, Protein: 20 g, Carbohydrate: 48 g, Cholesterol: 25 mg, Sodium: 228 mg, Fiber: 4 g, Sugar: 4 g

Dietary Exchanges: 3 Starch/Bread, 1 Lean Meat, 1½ Vegetable

PERFECT PASTA

238 LEMON CHICKEN AND VEGETABLES

8 ounces uncooked spaghetti
1 pound boneless skinless chicken breasts
1 large green bell pepper, cut in half
1 large red bell pepper, cut in half
1 medium yellow squash, cut in half lengthwise
½ cup finely chopped parsley
⅓ cup dry white wine
2 tablespoons lemon juice
2 tablespoons olive oil
3 cloves garlic, minced
2 teaspoons finely grated lemon peel
¼ teaspoon salt
¼ teaspoon black pepper

1. Cook pasta according to package directions, omitting salt. Drain; set aside.

2. To prevent sticking, spray grid with nonstick cooking spray. Prepare coals for grilling. Place chicken, bell peppers and squash on grill 5 to 6 inches from medium-hot coals. Grill 10 to 12 minutes or until chicken is no longer pink in center and vegetables are soft to the touch. Remove from grill; cool slightly. Cut into ½-inch pieces.

3. Combine parsley, wine, lemon juice, oil, garlic, lemon peel, salt and black pepper in medium bowl. Toss cooked chicken and vegetables with ⅓ cup sauce. Toss pasta with remaining sauce. Place chicken and vegetables over pasta; serve immediately.

Makes 8 servings

Nutrients per Serving: Calories: 255 (20% Calories from Fat), Total Fat: 6 g, Saturated Fat: 1 g, Protein: 18 g, Carbohydrate: 31 g, Cholesterol: 34 mg, Sodium: 101 mg, Fiber: 1 g, Sugar: trace

Dietary Exchanges: 1½ Starch/Bread, 2 Lean Meat, 1½ Vegetable

239 SPICY MESQUITE CHICKEN FETTUCCINE

8 ounces uncooked fettuccine
1 tablespoon chili powder
1 teaspoon ground cumin
1 teaspoon paprika
¼ teaspoon ground red pepper
2 teaspoons vegetable oil
1 pound mesquite marinated chicken breasts, cut into bite-size pieces

1. Cook pasta according to package directions, omitting salt. Drain; set aside.

2. Combine chili powder, cumin, paprika and pepper in small bowl; set aside.

3. Heat oil in large nonstick skillet over medium-high heat until hot. Add chili powder mixture; cook 30 seconds, stirring constantly. Add chicken; cook and stir 5 to 6 minutes or until no longer pink in center and lightly browned. Add pasta to skillet; stir. Cook 1 to 2 minutes or until heated through. Sprinkle with additional chili powder, if desired. Garnish with fresh cilantro and red bell pepper, if desired.

Makes 4 servings

Nutrients per Serving: Calories: 520 (14% Calories from Fat), Total Fat: 8 g, Saturated Fat: 2 g, Protein: 44 g, Carbohydrate: 71 g, Cholesterol: 144 mg, Sodium: 699 mg, Fiber: 2 g, Sugar: 6 g

Dietary Exchanges: 4 Starch/Bread, 4 Lean Meat

Spicy Mesquite Chicken Fettuccine

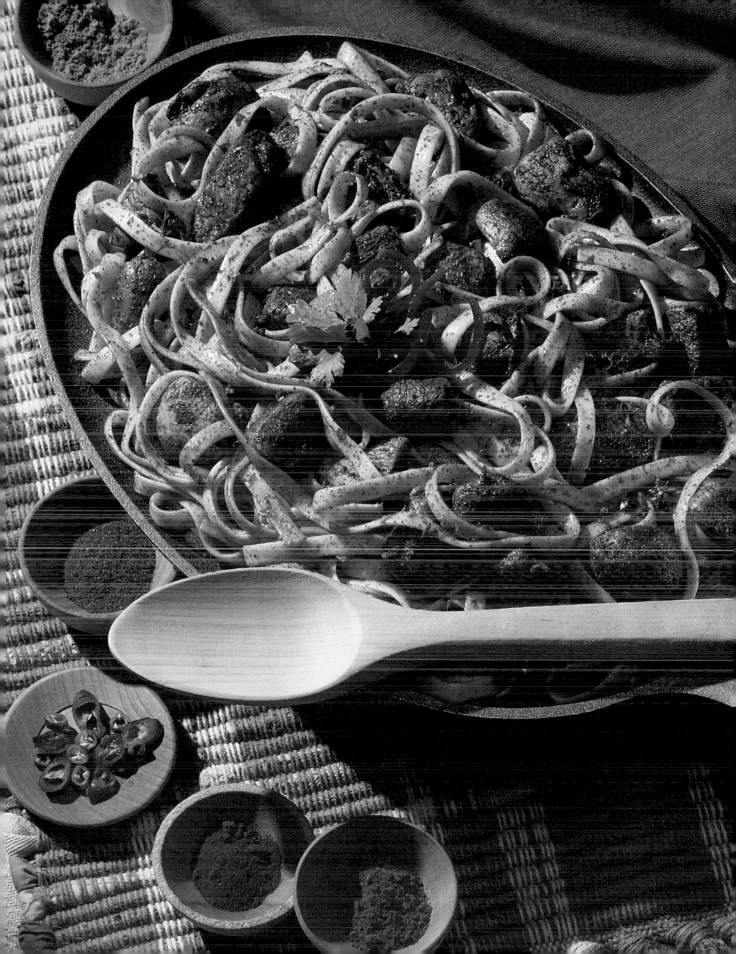

PERFECT PASTA

240 PLUM CHICKEN

6 ounces fresh uncooked Chinese egg
    noodles
¼ cup plum preserves or jam
3 tablespoons rice wine vinegar
3 tablespoons reduced-sodium soy sauce
1 tablespoon cornstarch
3 teaspoons oil, divided
1 small red onion, thinly sliced
2 cups fresh snow peas, diagonally sliced
12 ounces boneless skinless chicken
    breasts, cut into thin strips
4 medium plums or apricots, pitted and
    sliced

1. Cook noodles according to package
directions, omitting salt. Drain; keep warm.

2. Stir together plum preserves, vinegar, soy
sauce and cornstarch; set aside.

3. Heat 2 teaspoons oil in large nonstick
skillet or wok. Add onion; cook and stir
2 minutes or until slightly softened. Add
snow peas; cook and stir 3 minutes. Remove
vegetables to medium bowl.

4. Heat remaining 1 teaspoon oil in same
skillet. Add chicken; cook and stir over
medium-high heat 2 to 3 minutes or until no
longer pink in center. Push chicken to one
side of skillet.

5. Stir sauce; add to skillet. Cook and stir
until thick and bubbly. Stir in vegetables and
plums; coat evenly. Cook 3 minutes or until
heated through. Toss with noodles; serve
immediately.   *Makes 4 servings*

Nutrients per Serving: Calories: 415
(11% Calories from Fat), Total Fat: 5 g,
Saturated Fat: 1 g, Protein: 21 g,
Carbohydrate: 73 g, Cholesterol: 43 mg,
Sodium: 307 mg, Fiber: 3 g, Sugar: 23 g

Dietary Exchanges: 3 Starch/Bread,
1½ Lean Meat, 1½ Fruit, 1 Vegetable

241 CHICKEN TETRAZZINI

Vegetable cooking spray
2 cups sliced mushrooms
½ cup chopped onion
1 can HEALTHY CHOICE® RECIPE
    CREATIONS™ Cream of Roasted
    Chicken with Herbs Condensed Soup
½ cup nonfat milk
1½ tablespoons dry sherry
½ teaspoon salt (optional)
2 cups 1-inch cooked chicken cubes
⅓ cup fat free shredded Parmesan cheese,
    divided
¼ cup chopped fresh parsley
4 cups cooked spaghetti

In large saucepan sprayed with vegetable
cooking spray, sauté mushrooms and onion
until tender. Stir in soup, milk, sherry and
salt; heat through. Add chicken, ¼ cup
Parmesan cheese and parsley; blend well.
Add cooked spaghetti; toss to coat. Top with
remaining Parmesan cheese.

    Makes 4 servings

Nutrients per Serving: Calories: 390
(16% Calories from Fat), Fat: 7 g, Protein: 27 g,
Sodium: 410 mg

Dietary Exchanges: 4 Starch/Bread,
2 Lean Meat

Plum Chicken

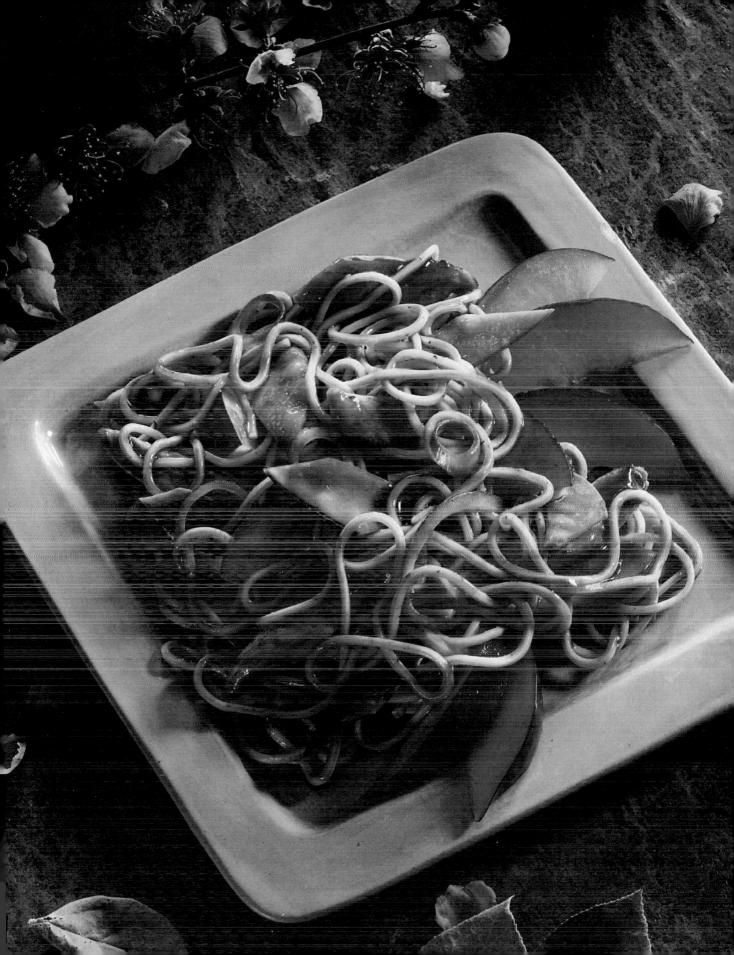

PERFECT PASTA

242 CHICKEN CHOW MEIN

6 ounces uncooked fresh Chinese egg
    noodles
    Nonstick cooking spray
½ cup fat-free reduced-sodium
    chicken broth
2 tablespoons reduced-sodium soy sauce
1½ teaspoons cornstarch
½ teaspoon dark sesame oil
½ teaspoon black pepper
⅛ teaspoon Chinese 5-spice powder
6 ounces boneless skinless chicken
    breasts, coarsely chopped
2 green onions, sliced
2 cups thinly sliced bok choy
1½ cups mixed frozen vegetables, thawed
    and drained
1 can (8 ounces) sliced water chestnuts,
    rinsed and drained
1 cup fresh bean sprouts

1. Preheat oven to 400°F. Cook noodles according to package directions, omitting salt; drain. Rinse under cold running water until cool; drain. Lightly spray 9-inch cake pan with cooking spray. Spread noodles in pan, pressing firmly; lightly spray top of noodles with cooking spray. Bake 10 minutes.

2. Invert noodles onto baking sheet or large plate. Carefully slide noodle cake back into cake pan; bake 10 to 15 minutes or until top is crisp and lightly browned. Transfer to serving platter. Whisk together next 6 ingredients in small bowl until cornstarch is dissolved; set aside.

3. Spray large nonstick skillet with cooking spray. Add chicken and green onions; cook, stirring frequently, until chicken is no longer pink, about 5 minutes. Stir in bok choy, mixed vegetables and water chestnuts; cook 3 minutes or until vegetables are crisp-tender. Push vegetables to one side of

skillet; stir in sauce. Cook and stir until thickened, about 2 minutes. Stir in bean sprouts; spoon over noodle cake.

Makes 4 servings

Nutrients per Serving: Calories: 284 (6% Calories from Fat), Total Fat: 2 g, Saturated Fat: trace, Protein: 16 g, Carbohydrate: 52 g, Cholesterol: 22 mg, Sodium: 322 mg, Fiber: 3 g, Sugar: 5 g

Dietary Exchanges: 2 Starch/Bread, 1 Lean Meat, 3 Vegetable

243 CHICKEN NOODLE ROLL–UPS

9 uncooked lasagna noodles (about
    9 ounces)
8 ounces boneless skinless chicken
    breasts, cut into chunks
    Nonstick cooking spray
2 cups finely chopped broccoli
2 cups 1% low-fat cottage cheese
1 egg
2 teaspoons snipped fresh chives
¼ teaspoon ground nutmeg
¼ teaspoon black pepper
1 tablespoon reduced-calorie margarine
2 tablespoons all-purpose flour
1 cup fat-free reduced-sodium
    chicken broth
½ cup skim milk
½ teaspoon dry mustard
1 medium tomato, seeded and chopped

1. Cook lasagna noodles according to package directions, omitting salt; drain. Rinse under cold running water; drain. Place in single layer on aluminum foil.

2. Preheat oven to 375°F. Place chicken in food processor; process until finely chopped. Spray large nonstick skillet with cooking spray; heat over medium heat until

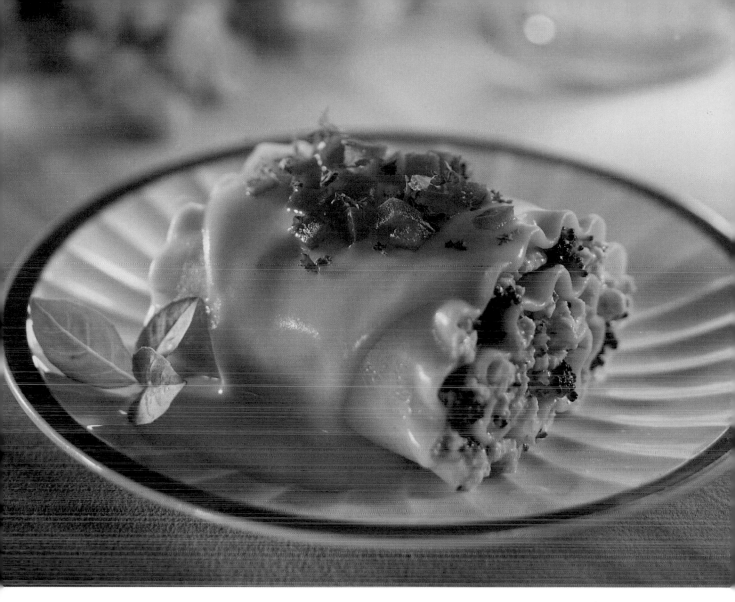

Chicken Noodle Roll-Up

hot. Add chicken; cook 4 minutes or until chicken is no longer pink. Stir in broccoli; cook until broccoli is crisp-tender, about 3 minutes. Cool.

3. Combine cottage cheese, egg, chives, nutmeg and pepper; stir in chicken mixture. Spread a generous ⅓ cup filling over each lasagna noodle. Roll up noodles, starting at short end. Place filled rolls, seam side down, in 10×8-inch baking dish; set aside.

4. Melt margarine in small saucepan. Stir in flour; cook 1 minute. Whisk in chicken broth, milk and mustard; cook, stirring constantly, until thickened. Pour sauce over filled rolls; sprinkle with tomato. Cover dish with foil; bake 30 to 35 minutes or until filling is set. *Makes 9 servings*

Nutrients per Serving: Calories: 179 (22% Calories from Fat), Total Fat: 4 g, Saturated Fat: 1 g, Protein: 18 g, Carbohydrate: 17 g, Cholesterol: 46 mg, Sodium: 291 mg, Fiber: 2 g, Sugar: 3 g

Dietary Exchanges: 1 Starch/Bread, 2 Lean Meat

PERFECT PASTA

244 FAMILY–STYLE CREAMY CHICKEN AND NOODLES

8 ounces uncooked yolk-free wide egg noodles
4 cups water
1 pound boneless skinless chicken breasts
1½ cups chopped onions
¾ cup chopped celery
½ teaspoon salt
½ teaspoon dried thyme leaves
1 bay leaf
⅛ teaspoon white pepper
1 can (10 ounces) reduced-sodium cream of chicken soup
½ cup nonfat buttermilk

1. Cook pasta according to package directions, omitting salt. Drain; set aside.

2. Meanwhile, bring water to a boil in Dutch oven over high heat. Add chicken breasts, onions, celery, salt, thyme, bay leaf and pepper; return to a boil. Reduce heat to low; simmer, uncovered, 35 minutes. Remove chicken; cut into ½-inch pieces. Set aside.

3. Increase heat to high; return liquid in Dutch oven to a boil. Continue cooking until liquid and vegetables have reduced to 1 cup. Remove from heat; remove and discard bay leaf. Whisk in soup and buttermilk until well blended; heat 1 minute or until heated through. Add chicken pieces and pasta; toss to blend. *Makes 4 servings*

Nutrients per Serving: Calories: 411 (16% Calories from Fat), Total Fat: 7 g, Saturated Fat: 2 g, Protein: 34 g, Carbohydrate: 52 g, Cholesterol: 70 mg, Sodium: 741 mg, Fiber: 2 g, Sugar: 3 g

Dietary Exchanges: 3 Starch/Bread, 3 Lean Meat, 1 Vegetable

245 EASY TEX–MEX BAKE

8 ounces uncooked thin mostaccioli
1 pound ground turkey breast
⅔ cup bottled medium or mild salsa
1 package (10 ounces) frozen corn, thawed and drained
1 container (16 ounces) 1% low-fat cottage cheese
1 egg
1 tablespoon minced fresh cilantro
½ teaspoon white pepper
¼ teaspoon ground cumin
½ cup (2 ounces) shredded Monterey Jack cheese

1. Cook pasta according to package directions, omitting salt. Drain; set aside.

2. Spray large nonstick skillet with nonstick cooking spray; heat over medium heat until hot. Add turkey; cook until no longer pink, about 5 minutes. Stir in salsa and corn; remove from heat.

3. Preheat oven to 350°F. Combine cottage cheese, egg, cilantro, pepper and cumin in small bowl.

4. Spoon ½ turkey mixture in bottom of 11½×7½-inch baking dish; top with pasta. Spoon cottage cheese mixture over pasta; top with remaining turkey mixture. Sprinkle cheese over casserole.

5. Bake 25 to 30 minutes or until heated through. *Makes 6 servings*

Nutrients per Serving: Calories: 365 (15% Calories from Fat), Total Fat: 6 g, Saturated Fat: 3 g, Protein: 38 g, Carbohydrate: 39 g, Cholesterol: 99 mg, Sodium: 800 mg, Fiber: 4 g, Sugar: 3 g

Dietary Exchanges: 2 Starch/Bread, 4 Lean Meat

Easy Tex-Mex Bake

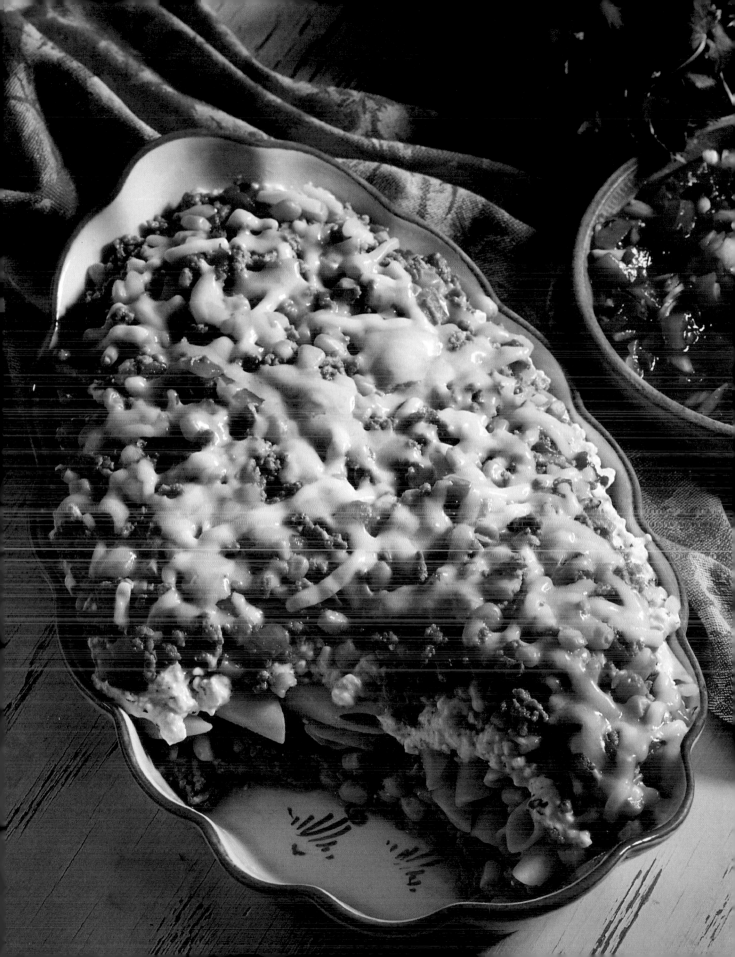

PERFECT PASTA

246 BEEFY TURKEY AND NOODLES

Nonstick cooking spray
8 ounces lean ground turkey
1 package (8 ounces) sliced fresh mushrooms
1 cup chopped onions
1 cup chopped green bell pepper
1½ cups water
1 tablespoon beef bouillon granules
1 can (6 ounces) no-salt-added tomato paste
1 teaspoon dried Italian seasoning
1 teaspoon Worcestershire sauce
¼ teaspoon sugar
5 ounces uncooked yolk-free egg noodles

1. Spray large nonstick skillet with cooking spray; heat over high heat until hot. Add turkey; brown over medium-high heat 6 to 8 minutes or until no longer pink, stirring to separate turkey; drain fat. Remove from skillet; set aside.

2. Add mushrooms to skillet; cook and stir 3 minutes. Add onions and pepper; cook and stir 5 minutes or until onions are tender. Add water, bouillon granules, tomato paste, Italian seasoning, Worcestershire sauce, sugar and turkey; blend well. Bring to a boil. Reduce heat to low; simmer, covered, 20 minutes.

3. Meanwhile, cook noodles according to package directions, omitting salt; drain. Add to skillet; stir to combine. Remove from heat; let stand 5 minutes before serving

Makes 4 servings

Nutrients per Serving: Calories: 272 (20% Calories from Fat), Total Fat: 6 g, Saturated Fat: 1 g, Protein: 17 g, Carbohydrate: 40 g, Cholesterol: 45 mg, Sodium: 721 mg, Fiber: 3 g, Sugar: 4 g

Dietary Exchanges: 2 Starch/Bread, 1½ Lean Meat, 2 Vegetable

247 LASAGNA ROLL–UPS

Vegetable cooking spray
1 pound ground turkey breast or extra-lean ground beef
½ cup chopped onion
2 cloves garlic, minced
1 can HEALTHY CHOICE® RECIPE CREATIONS™ Tomato with Garden Herbs Condensed Soup
1 cup chopped zucchini
¾ cup water
1 (15-ounce) container fat free ricotta cheese
½ cup HEALTHY CHOICE® Fat Free Shredded Mozzarella Cheese
1 egg
4 cooked lasagna noodles

In large nonstick skillet sprayed with vegetable cooking spray, cook turkey, onion and garlic until turkey is no longer pink and onion is tender. Add soup, zucchini and water; simmer 5 minutes. Pour soup mixture into shallow 2-quart baking dish.

In medium bowl, combine ricotta and mozzarella cheeses and egg; mix well. Lay lasagna noodles on flat surface; spread ½ cup cheese mixture on each noodle. Roll up noodles, enclosing filling; place rolls seam sides down over soup mixture.

Cover and bake at 375°F 30 minutes; uncover and continue baking 10 minutes longer or until sauce is bubbly. Place lasagna rolls on serving dish; spoon remaining sauce over rolls. *Makes 4 servings*

Nutrients per Serving: Calories: 404 (14% Calories from Fat), Fat: 6 g, Protein: 52 g, Sodium: 558 mg

Dietary Exchanges: 2 Starch/Bread, 4 Lean Meat, 1 Milk

Lasagna Roll-Ups

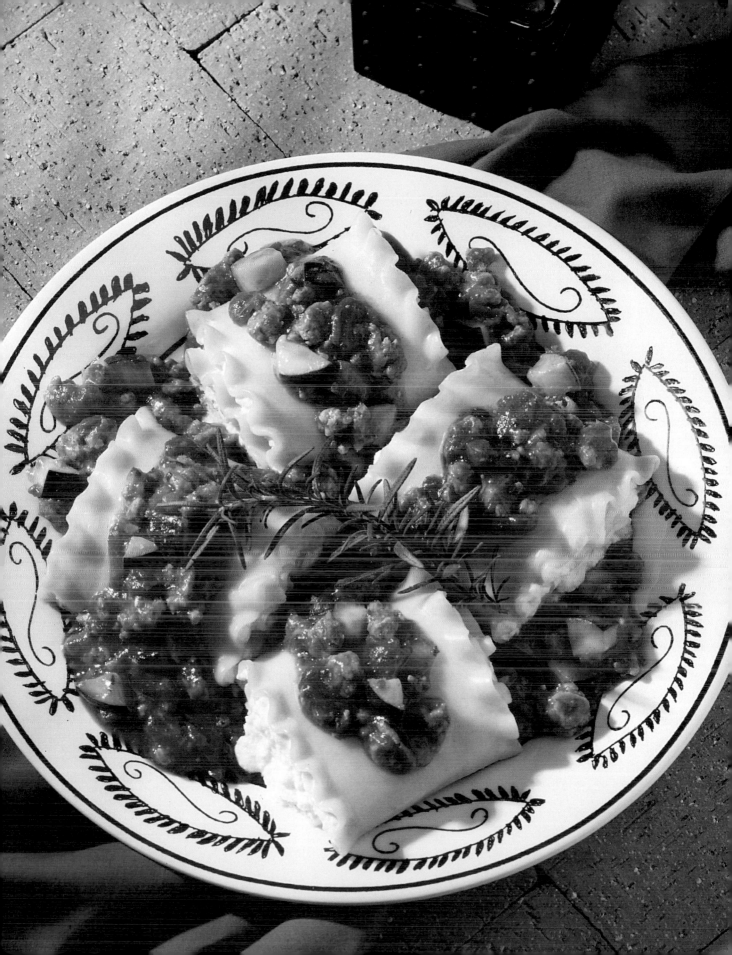

PERFECT PASTA

248 TURKEY & PASTA WITH CILANTRO PESTO

    1 pound turkey tenders, cut into strips
    3 cloves garlic, minced
 ½ teaspoon ground cumin
 ¼ teaspoon ground red pepper
 ¼ teaspoon black pepper
    2 tablespoons olive oil
1½ cups chopped seeded tomatoes
 ½ cup chopped fresh cilantro
 ¼ cup (1 ounce) grated Parmesan cheese
    2 tablespoons orange juice
  12 ounces dry linguine, cooked and
        kept warm

1. Combine turkey, garlic, cumin, red pepper and black pepper in medium bowl; toss to coat. Heat oil in large skillet over medium-high heat until hot. Add turkey mixture; cook and stir 4 to 6 minutes or until turkey is no longer pink in center.

2. Add tomatoes; cook and stir 2 minutes. Stir in cilantro, cheese and orange juice; cook 1 minute.

3. Toss turkey mixture and linguine in large bowl; serve immediately.

Makes 6 servings

Nutrients per Serving: Calories: 365 (22% Calories from Fat), Total Fat: 9 g, Saturated Fat: 2 g, Protein: 23 g, Carbohydrate: 48 g, Cholesterol: 33 mg, Sodium: 112 mg, Fiber: 1 g, Sugar: 2 g

Dietary Exchanges: 3 Starch/Bread, 1½ Lean Meat, 1 Vegetable, 1 Fat

Turkey & Pasta with Cilantro Pesto

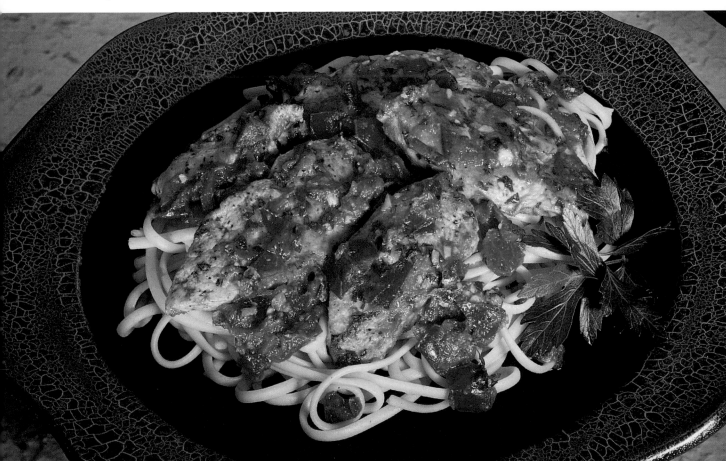

PERFECT PASTA

249 SPICY SHRIMP PUTTANESCA

8 ounces uncooked linguine, capellini or spaghetti
1 tablespoon olive oil
12 ounces medium shrimp, peeled and deveined
4 cloves garlic, minced
3/4 teaspoon red pepper flakes
1 cup finely chopped onion
1 can (14 1/2 ounces) no-salt-added stewed tomatoes, undrained
2 tablespoons tomato paste
2 tablespoons chopped pitted calamata or black olives
1 tablespoon drained capers
1/4 cup chopped fresh basil or parsley

1. Cook linguine according to package directions, omitting salt. Drain; set aside.

2. Meanwhile, heat oil in large nonstick skillet over medium high heat. Add shrimp, garlic and red pepper flakes; cook and stir 3 to 4 minutes or until shrimp are opaque. Transfer shrimp mixture to bowl with slotted spoon; set aside.

3. Add onion to same skillet; cook over medium heat 5 minutes, stirring occasionally. Add tomatoes, tomato paste, olives and capers; simmer, uncovered, 5 minutes.

4. Return shrimp mixture to skillet; simmer 1 minute. Stir in basil; simmer 1 minute. Place linguine in large serving bowl; top with shrimp mixture. *Makes 4 servings*

Nutrients per Serving: Calories: 328 (22% Calories from Fat), Total Fat: 8 g, Saturated Fat: 1 g, Protein: 24 g, Carbohydrate: 42 g, Cholesterol: 131 mg, Sodium: 537 mg, Fiber: 2 g, Sugar: 4 g

Dietary Exchanges: 2 Starch/Bread, 1 1/2 Lean Meat, 2 Vegetable, 1 Fat

250 CHEESE TORTELLINI WITH TUNA

1 tuna steak* (about 6 ounces)
1 package (9 ounces) reduced-fat cheese tortellini
1 cup finely chopped red bell pepper
1 cup finely chopped green bell pepper
1/4 cup finely chopped onion
3/4 teaspoon fennel seeds
1/2 cup evaporated skim milk
2 teaspoons all-purpose flour
1/2 teaspoon dry mustard
1/2 teaspoon black pepper

Or, substitute 1 can (6 ounces) tuna packed in water, drained, for tuna steak.

1. Grill or broil tuna 4 inches from heat source until fish just begins to flake, about 7 to 9 minutes. Remove and discard skin. Cut tuna into chunks; set aside.

2. Cook pasta according to package directions, omitting salt. Drain; set aside.

3. Spray large nonstick skillet with nonstick cooking spray. Add bell peppers, onion and fennel seeds; cook over medium heat until crisp-tender.

4. Whisk together milk, flour, mustard and black pepper in small bowl until smooth; add to skillet. Cook until thickened, stirring constantly. Stir in tuna and pasta; reduce heat and simmer until heated through, about 3 minutes. Serve immediately.
Makes 4 servings

Nutrients per Serving: Calories: 180 (19% Calories from Fat), Total Fat: 4 g, Saturated Fat: 2 g, Protein: 16 g, Carbohydrate: 21 g, Cholesterol: 21 mg, Sodium: 160 mg, Fiber: 3 g, Sugar: trace

Dietary Exchanges: 1/2 Starch/Bread, 1 1/2 Lean Meat, 1/2 Milk, 1 Vegetable

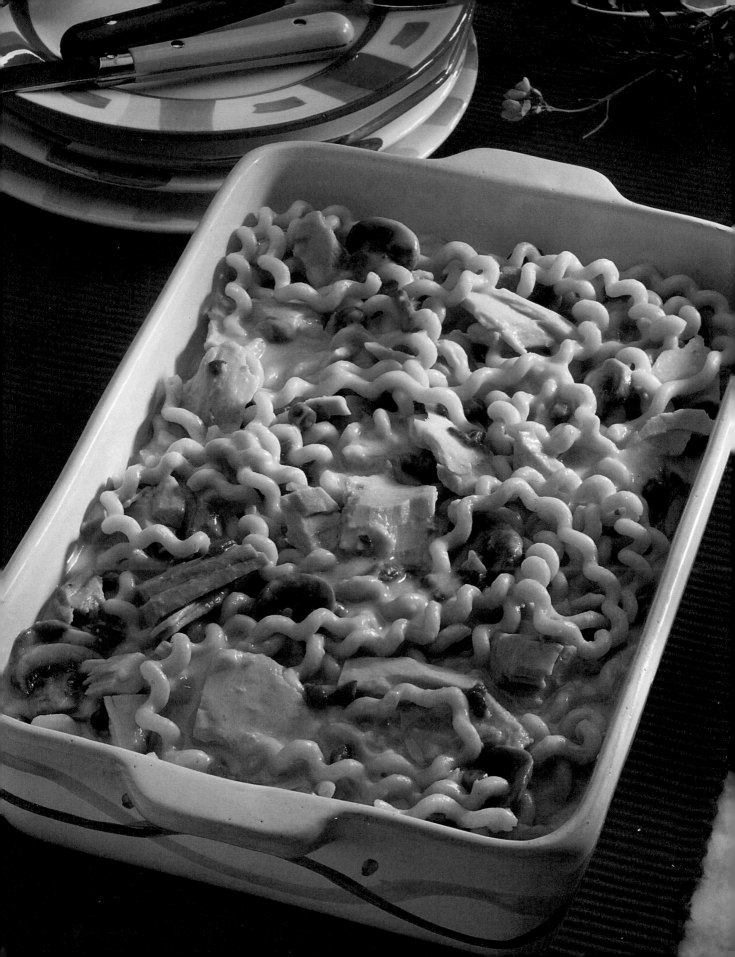

251 CAJUN GRILLED SHRIMP WITH ROTINI AND ROASTED RED PEPPER SAUCE

10 ounces uncooked rotini pasta
2 jars (7 ounces each) roasted peppers packed in water, drained
2 cloves garlic
2 tablespoons olive oil
½ teaspoon salt
¼ cup chicken broth
⅛ teaspoon ground red pepper
   Nonstick cooking spray
12 ounces medium shrimp, peeled and deveined
1½ teaspoons chili powder
1½ teaspoons lemon pepper
¾ teaspoon paprika

1. Cook pasta according to package directions, omitting salt. Drain; set aside.

2. Meanwhile, place peppers, garlic, oil, salt, chicken broth and ground red pepper in food processor or blender; process until smooth. Set aside.

3. Spray large nonstick skillet with cooking spray; heat over medium heat until hot. Add shrimp, chili powder, lemon pepper and paprika; cook and stir 8 minutes or until shrimp are opaque. Add roasted pepper mixture; heat thoroughly. *Do not boil.* Serve over pasta.   *Makes 4 servings*

Nutrients per Serving: Calories: 452 (20% Calories from Fat), Total Fat: 10 g, Saturated Fat: 1 g, Protein: 28 g, Carbohydrate: 62 g, Cholesterol: 130 mg, Sodium: 468 mg, Fiber: 3 g, Sugar: 4 g

Dietary Exchanges: 3 Starch/Bread, 2½ Lean Meat, 3 Vegetable, ½ Fat

Tuna Noodle Casserole

252 TUNA NOODLE CASSEROLE

6 ounces uncooked noodles
1 tablespoon margarine
8 ounces fresh mushrooms, sliced
1 small onion, chopped
1 cup fat-free reduced-sodium chicken broth
1 cup skim milk
¼ cup all-purpose flour
1 can (12 ounces) tuna packed in water, drained
1 cup frozen peas, thawed
1 jar (2 ounces) chopped pimiento, drained
½ teaspoon dried thyme leaves
¼ teaspoon salt
⅛ teaspoon black pepper

1. Cook noodles according to package directions, omitting salt. Drain; set aside.

2. Melt margarine in large nonstick skillet over medium-high heat. Add mushrooms and onion; cook and stir 5 minutes.

3. Whisk together chicken broth, milk and flour in small bowl. Stir into mushroom mixture; bring to a boil. Cook and stir 2 minutes or until thickened. Reduce heat to medium; stir in tuna, peas, pimiento, thyme and salt. Add noodles and pepper; mix well.

4. Preheat oven to 350°F. Spray 2-quart casserole with nonstick cooking spray. Spread noodle mixture in casserole; bake 30 minutes or until bubbly. Let stand 5 minutes before serving.   *Makes 6 servings*

Nutrients per Serving: Calories: 254 (11% Calories from Fat), Total Fat: 3 g, Saturated Fat: 1 g, Protein: 23 g, Carbohydrate: 33 g, Cholesterol: 18 mg, Sodium: 585 mg, Fiber: 2 g, Sugar: 4 g

Dietary Exchanges: 2 Starch/Bread, 2 Lean Meat

PERFECT PASTA

253 CARIBBEAN SHRIMP & PASTA

6 ounces uncooked medium bow tie pasta
1 tablespoon ground allspice
1 tablespoon frozen orange juice
 concentrate, thawed
1 teaspoon ground thyme
1½ teaspoons vegetable oil, divided
 ¼ teaspoon minced scotch bonnet pepper*
12 ounces medium shrimp, peeled and
 deveined
 Nonstick cooking spray
 ½ cup fat-free reduced-sodium chicken
 broth
 ⅓ cup finely chopped green onions, tops
 only
2 tablespoons lemon juice
1 tablespoon dark sesame oil
1 teaspoon Dijon mustard
 ¼ teaspoon salt
1 cup diced papaya
 ¾ cup diced mango

Scotch bonnet peppers can sting and irritate the skin; wear rubber gloves when handling peppers and do not touch eyes. Wash hands after handling.

1. Cook pasta according to package directions, omitting salt. Drain; set aside.

2. Combine allspice, orange juice concentrate, thyme, 1 teaspoon oil and pepper in small bowl. Add shrimp; toss to coat. Spray large nonstick skillet with cooking spray; heat over medium heat until hot. Add shrimp; cook and stir 3 to 5 minutes or until shrimp are opaque. Remove from heat.

3. Combine chicken broth, green onions, lemon juice, sesame oil, mustard, salt and remaining ½ teaspoon oil in large bowl. Add papaya and mango; toss to combine. Add pasta and shrimp; toss again. Serve immediately. *Makes 6 servings*

Nutrients per Serving: Calories: 217 (19% Calories from Fat), Total Fat: 5 g, Saturated Fat: 1 g, Protein: 14 g, Carbohydrate: 30 g, Cholesterol: 87 mg, Sodium: 208 mg, Fiber: 1 g, Sugar: 4 g

Dietary Exchanges: 1½ Starch/Bread, 1½ Lean Meat, ½ Fruit

254 LINGUINE WITH PESTO–MARINARA CLAM SAUCE

1 teaspoon vegetable oil
 ¼ cup chopped shallots
3 cloves garlic, finely chopped
2 cans (6 ounces each) minced clams
1⅓ cups Marinara Sauce (page 237)
2 tablespoons prepared pesto sauce
 ¼ teaspoon red pepper flakes
8 ounces uncooked linguine
 ¼ cup chopped parsley

1. Heat oil in large nonstick saucepan over medium heat until hot. Add shallots and garlic; cook, covered, 2 minutes.

2. Drain clams; reserve ½ cup juice. Add clams, reserved juice, Marinara Sauce, pesto and red pepper flakes to saucepan; cook 10 minutes, stirring occasionally.

3. Prepare linguine according to package directions, omitting salt; drain. Spoon sauce evenly over each serving; top with parsley.
Makes 4 servings

Nutrients per Serving: Calories: 398 (13% Calories from Fat), Total Fat: 6 g, Saturated Fat: 1 g, Protein: 32 g, Carbohydrate: 54 g, Cholesterol: 58 mg, Sodium: 293 mg, Fiber: 4 g, Sugar: 1 g

Dietary Exchanges: 2½ Starch/Bread, 3 Lean Meat, 2½ Vegetable

Linguine with Pesto-Marinara Clam Sauce

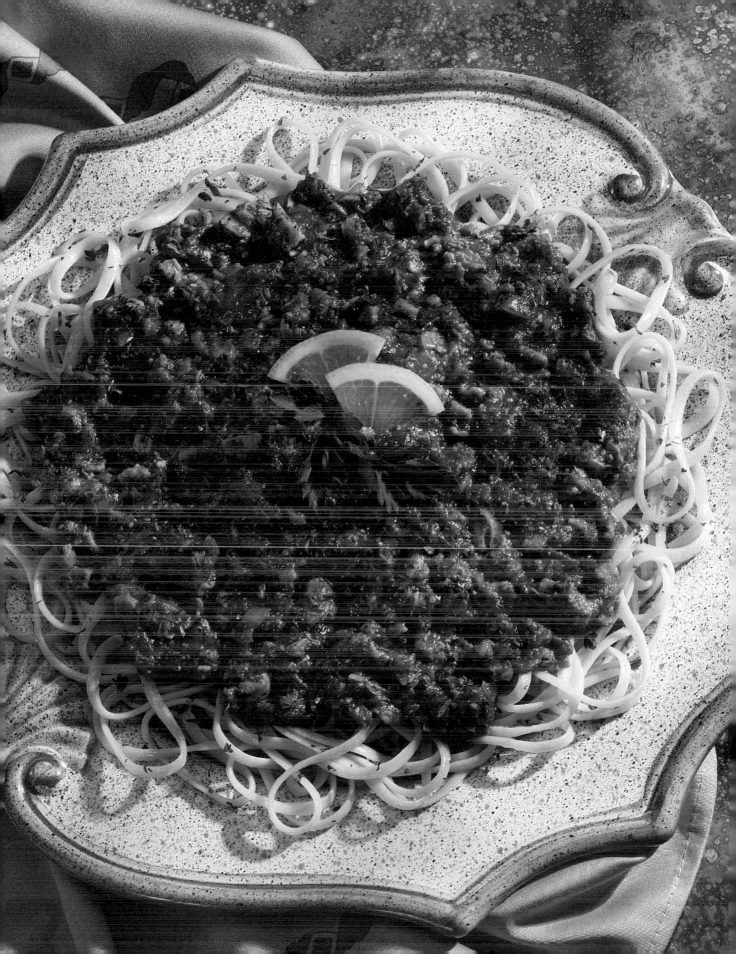

PERFECT PASTA

255 ORANGE GINGER SEAFOOD

     8 ounces uncooked rigatoni
    12 ounces firm, white-fleshed fish
        Salt and black pepper (optional)
        Nonstick cooking spray
     1 cup orange juice, divided
     2 cloves garlic, minced
     2 teaspoons grated fresh ginger
     2 to 3 teaspoons reduced-sodium soy
        sauce
     1 teaspoon cornstarch
     ¾ cup finely chopped seeded fresh plum
        tomatoes
     1 can (11 ounces) mandarin oranges,
        drained

1. Cook pasta according to package directions, omitting salt. Drain; set aside.

2. Season fish with salt and pepper. Spray large nonstick skillet with cooking spray; heat over medium-high heat until hot. Add fish; cook 3 minutes each side, or until fish begins to flake when tested with a fork and is lightly browned. Remove; set aside and keep warm.

3. Heat 1 tablespoon orange juice in same skillet over medium-low heat, scraping browned bits from bottom of skillet. Add garlic and ginger; cook and stir 2 minutes. Reserving ¼ cup juice, add remaining juice and soy sauce to skillet. Bring to a boil over medium-high heat. Stir reserved ¼ cup juice into cornstarch in small bowl until smooth. Add cornstarch mixture to skillet; return to a boil. Stir constantly until slightly thickened. Stir in tomatoes; heat 1 minute. Remove from heat; stir in oranges.

4. Divide pasta among 4 plates; top with fish. Spoon sauce over fish. Garnish with fresh chives and orange peel, if desired.

Makes 4 servings

Nutrients per Serving: Calories: 367 (6% Calories from Fat), Total Fat: 2 g, Saturated Fat: trace, Protein: 25 g, Carbohydrate: 61 g, Cholesterol: 45 mg, Sodium: 167 mg, Fiber: 1 g, Sugar: 8 g

Dietary Exchanges: 3 Starch/Bread, 2 Lean Meat, 1 Fruit

256 SHRIMP & SNOW PEAS WITH FUSILLI

     6 ounces uncooked fusilli
        Nonstick cooking spray
     2 cloves garlic, finely chopped
     ¼ teaspoon red pepper flakes
    12 ounces medium shrimp, peeled and
        deveined
     2 cups snow peas
     1 can (8 ounces) sliced water chestnuts,
        drained
     ⅓ cup sliced green onions
     3 tablespoons lime juice
     2 tablespoons chopped fresh cilantro
     2 tablespoons olive oil
     1 tablespoon reduced-sodium soy sauce
    1½ teaspoons Mexican seasoning

1. Cook pasta according to package directions, omitting salt; drain. Set aside.

2. Spray large nonstick skillet with cooking spray; heat over medium heat until hot. Add garlic and red pepper flakes; stir-fry 1 minute. Add shrimp; stir-fry 5 minutes or until shrimp are opaque. Remove shrimp from skillet.

PERFECT PASTA

3. Add snow peas and 2 tablespoons water to skillet; cook, covered, 1 minute. Uncover; cook and stir 2 minutes or until snow peas are crisp-tender. Remove snow peas from skillet.

4. Combine pasta, shrimp, snow peas, water chestnuts and onions in large bowl. Blend lime juice, cilantro, oil, soy sauce and Mexican seasoning in small bowl. Drizzle over pasta mixture; toss to coat.

Makes 6 servings

Nutrients per Serving: Calories: 228 (24% Calories from Fat), Total Fat: 6 g, Saturated Fat: 1 g, Protein: 15 g, Carbohydrate: 29 g, Cholesterol: 87 mg, Sodium: 202 mg, Fiber: 3 g, Sugar: 9 g

Dietary Exchanges: 1½ Starch/Bread, 1 Lean Meat, 1 Vegetable, 1 Fat

Shrimp & Snow Peas with Fusilli

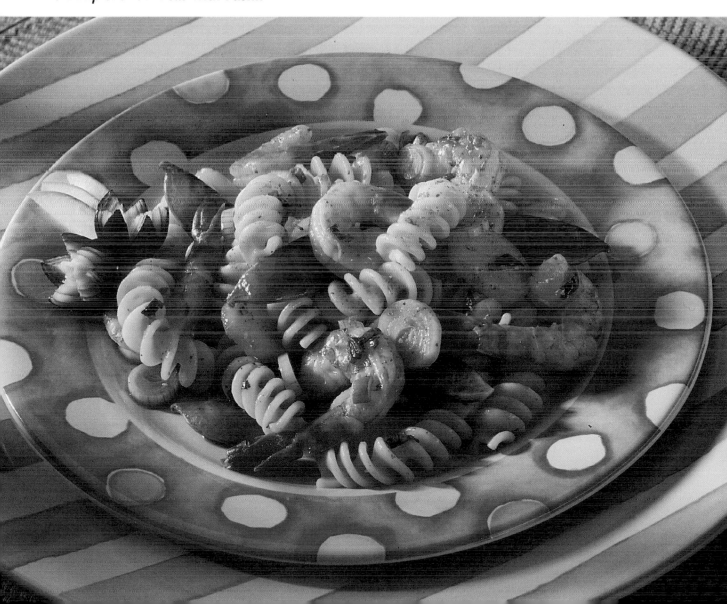

PERFECT PASTA

257 MEDITERRANEAN LINGUINE

8 ounces uncooked linguine
1½ ounces sun-dried tomatoes (not packed in oil)
Nonstick cooking spray
1 package (8 ounces) sliced fresh mushrooms
4 cloves garlic, minced
¾ cup finely chopped onions
½ medium green bell pepper, thinly sliced
1½ teaspoons dried Italian seasoning
½ teaspoon red pepper flakes
2 tablespoons dry red wine
12 ounces medium shrimp, peeled and deveined
12 kalamata olives, pitted and sliced *or*
20 medium pitted black olives, halved
¼ cup chopped parsley
½ teaspoon salt
3 tablespoons grated Parmesan cheese
2 teaspoons olive oil

1. Cook pasta according to package directions, omitting salt. Drain; set aside.

2. Meanwhile, bring 2 cups water to a boil over high heat; add sun-dried tomatoes. Reduce heat to low; simmer, uncovered, 4 minutes. Drain; cool slightly. Cut into thin strips; set aside.

3. Spray large nonstick skillet with cooking spray; heat over medium-high heat until hot. Add mushrooms and garlic; cook 4 minutes. Add onions, bell pepper, Italian seasoning and red pepper flakes; cook 4 minutes. Add wine, tomatoes and shrimp; cook 6 to 8 minutes or until shrimp are opaque.

4. Add olives, parsley, salt, pasta and Parmesan cheese; toss to blend. Remove from heat; drizzle with olive oil. Serve immediately. *Makes 4 servings*

Nutrients per Serving: Calories: 384 (22% Calories from Fat), Total Fat: 10 g, Saturated Fat: 2 g, Protein: 30 g, Carbohydrate: 47 g, Cholesterol: 133 mg, Sodium: 653 mg, Fiber: 2 g, Sugar: 2 g

Dietary Exchanges: 2 Starch/Bread, 3½ Lean Meat, 2 Vegetable

258 CATALAN SPINACH AND PASTA

16 ounces uncooked rotelle pasta
2 cups water
20 ounces fresh spinach, stems removed
⅔ cup raisins, divided
4 teaspoons balsamic vinegar
2 teaspoons olive oil
2 cloves garlic, minced
½ teaspoon salt
¼ teaspoon black pepper
6 tablespoons pine nuts

1. Cook pasta according to package directions, omitting salt. Drain; set aside.

2. Bring water to a boil in large saucepan over high heat. Add spinach; cook, covered, 3 minutes or until spinach leaves start to wilt. Remove from heat; drain. Stir in 5 tablespoons raisins, vinegar, oil, garlic, salt and pepper. Place in food processor or blender; process until smooth. Add spinach mixture and remaining raisins to pasta; sprinkle with pine nuts.

Makes 6 servings

Nutrients per Serving: Calories: 442 (19% Calories from Fat), Total Fat: 10 g, Saturated Fat: 1 g, Protein: 16 g, Carbohydrate: 39 g, Cholesterol: 0 mg, Sodium: 256 mg, Fiber: 3 g, Sugar: 5 g

Dietary Exchanges: 2 Starch/Bread, 1 Vegetable, 1 Fat

259 SANTA FE FUSILLI

1 medium red bell pepper*
2 teaspoons cumin seeds
¾ cup chopped, seeded tomato
¼ cup chopped onion
1 clove garlic, minced
1 tablespoon chili powder
¼ teaspoon red pepper flakes
¼ teaspoon black pepper
1 can (16 ounces) no-salt-added tomato
    purée
⅓ cup water
1 teaspoon sugar
8 ounces uncooked fusilli pasta
1 can (16 ounces) black beans, rinsed and
    drained
1 package (10 ounces) frozen corn,
    thawed and drained
1 can (4 ounces) diced green chilies,
    drained
⅓ cup low-fat sour cream
    Fresh cilantro

Or, substitute 1 jar (7 ounces) roasted peppers.

1. Roast bell pepper over charcoal or gas flame or place under broiler, turning several times, until skin is charred. Cool 10 minutes. Peel and discard charred skin. Cut pepper in half; seed, devein and coarsely chop. Set aside.

2. Place cumin seeds in large nonstick saucepan; cook and stir over medium heat until lightly toasted, about 3 minutes. Stir in tomato, onion, garlic, chili powder, red pepper flakes and black pepper; cook until onion is tender, about 5 minutes. Stir in tomato purée, water and sugar. Reduce heat to low; simmer, covered, 15 minutes.

3. Cook pasta according to package directions, omitting salt. Drain; set aside. Stir in beans, corn, roasted peppers and chilies into vegetable mixture; cook until

heated through, about 8 minutes. Stir in pasta; top with sour cream and cilantro.

Makes 8 servings

Nutrients per Serving: Calories: 228 (9% Calories from Fat), Total Fat: 2 g, Saturated Fat: trace, Protein: 12 g, Carbohydrate: 46 g, Cholesterol: 3 mg, Sodium: 215 mg, Fiber: 8 g, Sugar: 3 g

Dietary Exchanges: 2 Starch/Bread, ½ Lean Meat, 2½ Vegetable

260 CREAMY MACARONI & CHEESE

1 can HEALTHY CHOICE® RECIPE
    CREATIONS™ Cream of Celery with
    Sautéed Onion & Garlic Condensed
    Soup
2 cups HEALTHY CHOICE® Fat Free
    Shredded Cheddar Cheese
½ cup nonfat milk
2 teaspoons *each* minced onion and diced
    red or green bell pepper
2 teaspoons horseradish
½ teaspoon salt (optional)
4 cups cooked small elbow macaroni
    Vegetable cooking spray
3 slices fat free sharp Cheddar cheese

In large bowl, combine soup, shredded cheese, milk, onion, pepper, horseradish and salt; mix well. Add macaroni; mix well.

Place macaroni mixture in 2-quart baking dish sprayed with vegetable cooking spray. Top with cheese slices; cover and bake at 375°F 30 minutes or until hot and bubbly.

Makes 6 servings

Nutrients per Serving: Calories: 247 (6% Calories from Fat), Fat: 2 g, Protein: 20 g, Sodium: 587 mg

Dietary Exchanges: 2 Starch/Bread, 2 Lean Meat

PERFECT PASTA

261 BROCCOLI LASAGNA BIANCA

1 (15- to 16-ounce) container fat-free
    ricotta cheese
1 cup EGG BEATERS® Healthy Real Egg
    Substitute
1 tablespoon minced basil (or 1 teaspoon
    dried basil leaves)
½ cup chopped onion
1 clove garlic, minced
2 tablespoons FLEISCHMANN'S® 70%
    Corn Oil Spread
¼ cup all-purpose flour
2 cups skim milk
2 (10-ounce) packages frozen chopped
    broccoli, thawed and well drained
1 cup (4 ounces) shredded part-skim
    mozzarella cheese
9 lasagna noodles, cooked and drained
1 small tomato, chopped
2 tablespoons grated Parmesan cheese
    Fresh basil leaves, for garnish

In medium bowl, combine ricotta cheese,
Egg Beaters and minced basil; set aside.

In large saucepan, over medium heat, sauté
onion and garlic in spread until tender-crisp.
Stir in flour; cook for 1 minute. Gradually
stir in milk; cook, stirring until mixture
thickens and begins to boil. Remove from
heat; stir in broccoli and mozzarella cheese.

In lightly greased 13×9×2-inch baking dish,
place 3 lasagna noodles; top with ⅓ each
ricotta and broccoli mixtures. Repeat layers
2 more times. Top with tomato; sprinkle with
Parmesan cheese. Bake at 350°F for 1 hour
or until set. Let stand 10 minutes before
serving. Garnish with basil leaves.

Makes 8 servings

Prep Time: 20 minutes
Cook Time: 90 minutes

Nutrients per Serving: Calories: 302,
Total Fat: 7 g, Saturated Fat: 2 g,
Cholesterol: 10 mg, Sodium: 291 mg, Fiber: 2 g

Dietary Exchanges: 2 Starch/Bread,
2 Lean Meat, 2 Vegetable, ½ Milk

262 SPINACH PESTO PASTA

10 ounces uncooked linguine
1 package (10 ounces) frozen chopped
    spinach, thawed and squeezed dry
1 cup water
4 cloves garlic, peeled
2 tablespoons olive oil
2 tablespoons lemon juice
2 tablespoons dried basil leaves
1 teaspoon chicken bouillon granules
¼ to ½ teaspoon black pepper
¼ cup grated Parmesan cheese
½ teaspoon salt, divided
4 plum tomatoes, seeded and chopped

1. Cook pasta according to package
directions, omitting salt. Drain; set aside.

2. Meanwhile, place spinach, water, garlic,
olive oil, lemon juice, basil, bouillon
granules and pepper in food processor or
blender; process until smooth.

3. Place pasta in large bowl. Add spinach
mixture, Parmesan cheese and ¼ teaspoon
salt; toss to coat. Top with tomatoes and
remaining ¼ teaspoon salt.

Makes 4 servings

Nutrients per Serving: Calories: 352
(29% Calories from Fat), Total Fat: 12 g,
Saturated Fat: 2 g, Protein: 15 g,
Carbohydrate: 50 g, Cholesterol: 5 mg,
Sodium: 783 mg, Fiber: 2 g, Sugar: 4 g

Dietary Exchanges: 2½ Starch/Bread,
½ Lean Meat, 2 Vegetable, 2 Fat

Broccoli Lasagna Bianca

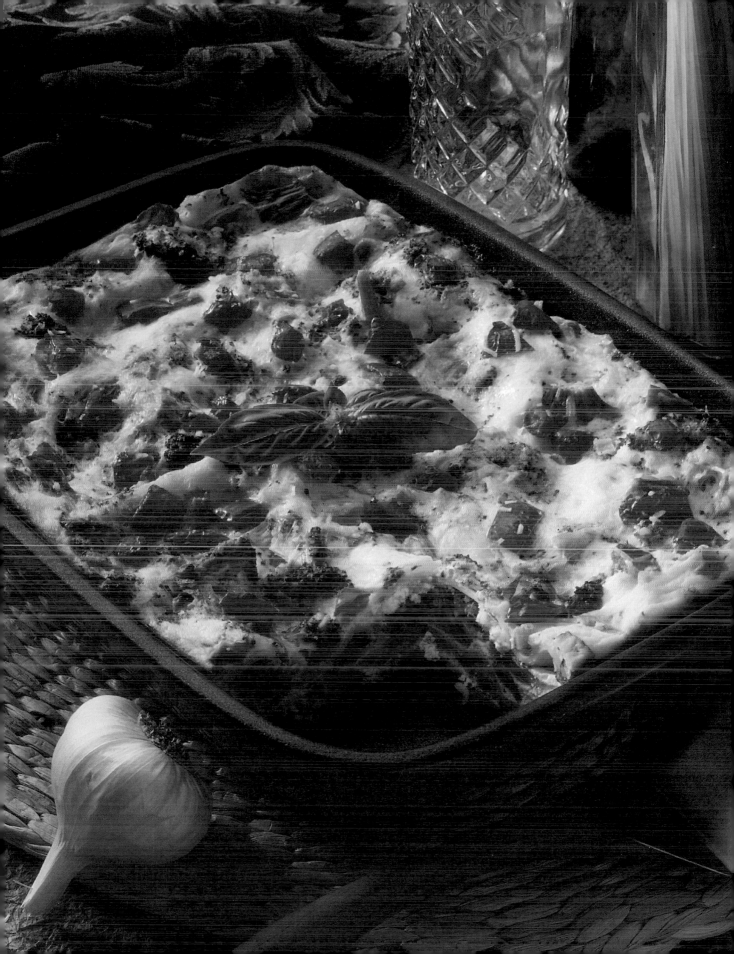

PERFECT PASTA

263 GINGER NOODLES WITH SESAME EGG STRIPS

5 egg whites
6 teaspoons teriyaki sauce, divided
3 teaspoons toasted sesame seeds,* divided
1 teaspoon dark sesame oil
½ cup fat-free reduced-sodium chicken broth
1 tablespoon minced fresh ginger
6 ounces uncooked Chinese rice noodles or vermicelli, cooked and drained
⅓ cup sliced green onions

To toast sesame seeds, spread seeds in small skillet. Shake skillet over medium heat 2 minutes or until seeds begin to pop and turn golden.

1. Beat together egg whites, 2 teaspoons teriyaki sauce and 1 teaspoon sesame seeds.

2. Heat oil in large nonstick skillet over medium heat until hot. Pour egg mixture into skillet; cook 1½ to 2 minutes or until bottom of omelet is set. Turn omelet over; cook 30 seconds to 1 minute. Slide out onto plate; cool and cut into ½-inch strips.

3. Add broth, ginger and remaining 4 teaspoons teriyaki sauce to skillet; bring to a boil over high heat. Reduce heat to medium. Add noodles; heat through. Add omelet strips and onions; heat through. Sprinkle with remaining 2 teaspoons sesame seeds. *Makes 4 side-dish servings*

Nutrients per Serving: Calories: 111 (19% Calories from Fat), Total Fat: 2 g, Saturated Fat: 1 g, Protein: 7 g, Carbohydrate: 16 g, Cholesterol: 0 mg, Sodium: 226 mg, Fiber: trace, Sugar: trace

Dietary Exchanges: 1 Starch/Bread, ½ Lean Meat, ½ Fat

264 BEAN THREADS WITH TOFU AND VEGETABLES

8 ounces firm tofu, drained and cubed
1 tablespoon dark sesame oil
3 teaspoons reduced-sodium soy sauce, divided
1 can (about 14 ounces) fat-free reduced-sodium chicken broth
1 package (3¾ ounces) bean threads
1 package (16 ounces) frozen mixed vegetable medley such as broccoli, carrots and red pepper, thawed
¼ cup rice wine vinegar
½ teaspoon red pepper flakes

1. Place tofu on shallow plate; drizzle with oil and 1½ teaspoons soy sauce.

2. Combine broth and remaining 1½ teaspoons soy sauce in deep skillet or large saucepan. Bring to a boil over high heat; reduce heat. Add bean threads; simmer, uncovered, 7 minutes or until noodles absorb liquid, stirring occasionally to separate noodles.

3. Stir in vegetables and vinegar; heat through. Stir in tofu and red pepper flakes; heat through about 1 minute. *Makes 6 side-dish servings*

Nutrients per Serving: Calories: 167 (30% Calories from Fat), Total Fat: 6 g, Saturated Fat: 1 g, Protein: 8 g, Carbohydrate: 23 g, Cholesterol: 0 mg, Sodium: 130 mg, Fiber: 3 g, Sugar: 2 g

Dietary Exchanges: 1 Starch/Bread, ½ Lean Meat, 1 Vegetable, 1 Fat

Bean Threads with Tofu and Vegetables

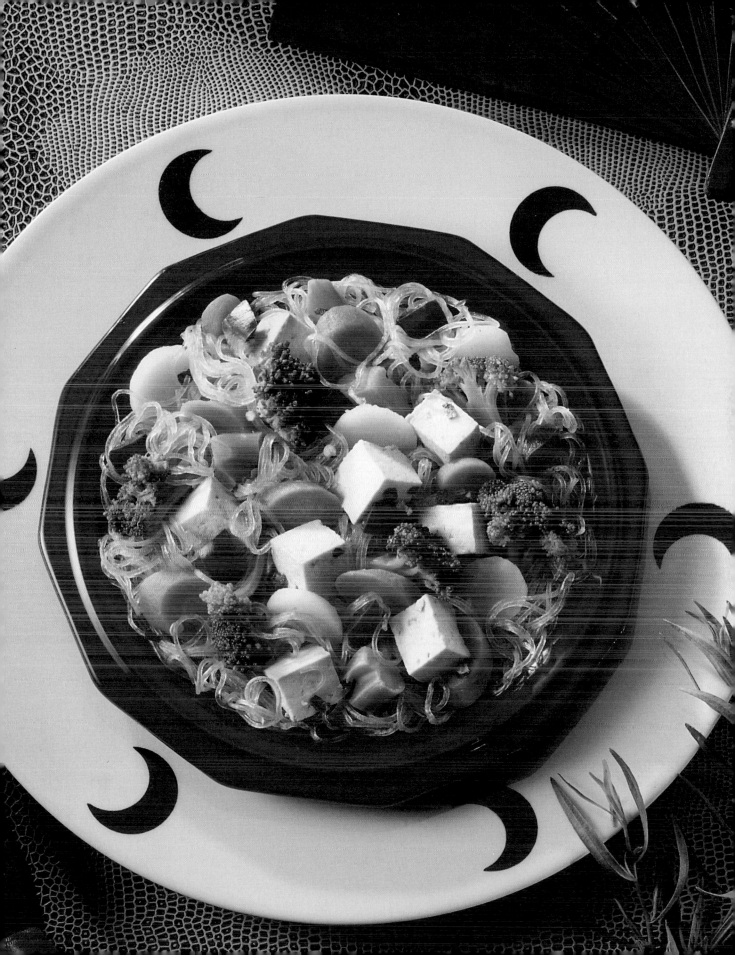

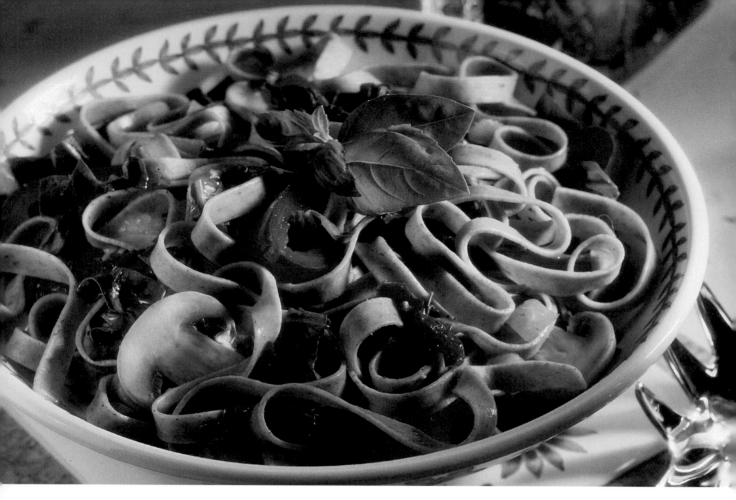

Vegetables with Spinach Fettuccine

265 VEGETABLES WITH SPINACH FETTUCCINE

6 sun-dried tomatoes (not packed in oil)
3 ounces uncooked spinach fettuccine
1 tablespoon olive oil
¼ cup chopped onion
¼ cup sliced red bell pepper
1 clove garlic, minced
½ cup sliced mushrooms
½ cup coarsely chopped fresh spinach
¼ teaspoon salt
¼ teaspoon ground nutmeg
⅛ teaspoon black pepper

1. Place sun-dried tomatoes in small bowl; pour boiling water over tomatoes to cover. Let stand 10 to 15 minutes or until tomatoes are tender. Drain tomatoes; discard liquid. Cut tomatoes into strips.

2. Cook pasta according to package directions, omitting salt. Drain; set aside.

3. Heat oil in large nonstick skillet over medium heat until hot. Add onion, bell pepper and garlic; cook and stir 3 minutes or until vegetables are crisp-tender. Add mushrooms and spinach; cook and stir 1 minute. Add sun-dried tomatoes, pasta, salt, nutmeg and black pepper; cook and stir 1 to 2 minutes or until heated through.

Makes 6 servings

Nutrients per Serving: Calories: 82 (30% Calories from Fat), Total Fat: 3 g, Saturated Fat: trace, Protein: 3 g, Carbohydrate: 13 g, Cholesterol: 3 mg, Sodium: 101 mg, Fiber: 1 g, Sugar: 1 g

Dietary Exchanges: ½ Starch/Bread, 1 Vegetable, ½ Fat

PERFECT PASTA

266 FRESH ASPARAGUS FETTUCCINE PARMESAN

8 ounces uncooked fettuccine
1 pound fresh asparagus *or* 1 package
   (10 ounces) frozen cut asparagus
3 ounces Neufchâtel cheese, softened
½ cup plus 2 tablespoons skim milk
1 tablespoon lemon juice
¼ cup (1 ounce) grated Parmesan cheese,
   divided
¼ teaspoon salt
   Black pepper

1. Cook noodles according to package directions, omitting salt. Drain; set aside.

2. Meanwhile, bring ½ cup water to a boil over high heat in large nonstick skillet. Add asparagus; return to a boil. Reduce heat to low; simmer, covered, 4 minutes or until crisp-tender. Drain; rinse under cold running water. Drain.

3. Place Neufchâtel cheese, milk and lemon juice in food processor or blender; process until smooth.

4. Combine pasta, asparagus and Neufchâtel cheese mixture; return to skillet. Add 3 tablespoons Parmesan cheese and salt; blend. Place in serving dishes; sprinkle with remaining Parmesan cheese and pepper. Serve immediately.   *Makes 4 servings*

Nutrients per Serving: Calories: 287 (26% Calories from Fat), Total Fat: 9 g, Saturated Fat: 4 g, Protein: 16 g, Carbohydrate: 40 g, Cholesterol: 76 mg, Sodium: 421 mg, Fiber: 1 g, Sugar: 2 g

Dietary Exchanges: 2 Starch/Bread, ½ Lean Meat, 2 Vegetable, 1½ Fat

267 SPAGHETTI WITH MARINARA SAUCE

MARINARA SAUCE
1 teaspoon olive oil
¾ cup chopped onion
3 cloves garlic, finely chopped
1 can (16 ounces) no-salt-added tomato
   sauce
1 can (6 ounces) tomato paste
2 bay leaves
1 teaspoon dried oregano leaves
1 teaspoon dried basil leaves
½ teaspoon dried marjoram leaves
½ teaspoon honey
¼ teaspoon black pepper

8 ounces uncooked spaghetti, cooked and
   drained

1. Heat oil in large saucepan over medium-high heat until hot. Add onion and garlic; cook and stir 5 minutes or until onion is tender. Add 2 cups water, tomato sauce, tomato paste, bay leaves, oregano, basil, marjoram, honey and pepper; bring to a boil, stirring occasionally. Reduce heat; simmer 1 hour, stirring occasionally.

2. Remove and discard bay leaves. Measure 2 cups sauce; reserve remaining sauce for another use. Spoon sauce over pasta.
Makes 4 servings

Nutrients per Serving: Calories: 289 (trace Calories from Fat), Total Fat: 2 g, Saturated Fat: trace, Protein: 10 g, Carbohydrate: 58 g, Cholesterol: 0 mg, Sodium: 213 mg, Fiber: 3 g, Sugar: 2 g

Dietary Exchanges: 3 Starch/Bread, 2½ Vegetable

PERFECT PASTA

268 PASTA PRIMAVERA

8 ounces uncooked linguine or medium
    pasta shells
1 tablespoon reduced-calorie margarine
2 green onions, diagonally sliced
1 clove garlic, minced
1 cup fresh sliced mushrooms
1 cup broccoli florets
2½ cups fresh snow peas
4 to 8 asparagus spears, cut into 2-inch
    pieces
1 medium red bell pepper, cut into thin
    strips
½ cup evaporated skim milk
½ teaspoon dried tarragon leaves
½ teaspoon black pepper
⅓ cup grated Parmesan cheese

1. Cook pasta according to package
directions, omitting salt. Drain; set aside.

2. Melt margarine in large nonstick skillet.
Add green onions and garlic; cook and stir
over medium heat until softened. Add
mushrooms and broccoli; cook, covered,
3 minutes or until mushrooms are tender.
Add snow peas, asparagus, bell pepper, milk,
tarragon and black pepper; cook and stir
until vegetables are crisp-tender and lightly
coated.

3. Add pasta and cheese; toss to coat evenly.
Serve immediately.   *Makes 4 servings*

Nutrients per Serving: Calories: 329
(16% Calories from Fat), Total Fat: 6 g,
Saturated Fat: 2 g, Protein: 18 g,
Carbohydrate: 51 g, Cholesterol: 8 mg,
Sodium: 243 mg, Fiber: 6 g, Sugar: 3 g

Dietary Exchanges: 2½ Starch/Bread,
½ Lean Meat, ½ Milk, 1½ Vegetable

269 SPINACH–STUFFED SHELLS

1 package (10 ounces) chopped frozen
    spinach, thawed and drained
1½ cups nonfat ricotta cheese
½ cup grated Parmesan cheese
½ cup cholesterol-free egg substitute
3 cloves garlic, finely chopped
1 teaspoon dried oregano leaves
½ teaspoon salt
½ teaspoon dried basil leaves
½ teaspoon dried marjoram leaves
¼ teaspoon black pepper
24 cooked large pasta shells
2 cans (14½ ounces each) crushed
    tomatoes
1 cup (4 ounces) shredded reduced-fat
    mozzarella cheese

1. Preheat oven to 350°F. Spray 13×9-inch
baking pan with nonstick cooking spray.

2. Combine spinach, ricotta and Parmesan
cheeses, egg substitute and seasonings in
large bowl; spoon into shells. Place shells in
prepared pan; top with tomatoes with liquid
and mozzarella cheese. Bake 20 minutes or
until cheese melts.   *Makes 4 servings*

Nutrients per Serving: Calories: 456
(20% Calories from Fat), Total Fat: 11 g,
Saturate Fat: 6 g, Protein: 38 g,
Carbohydrate: 57 g, Cholesterol: 35 mg,
Sodium: 803 mg, Fiber: 6 g, Sugar: 5 g

Dietary Exchanges: 3 Starch/Bread,
3 Lean Meat, 2 Vegetable

Spinach-Stuffed Shells

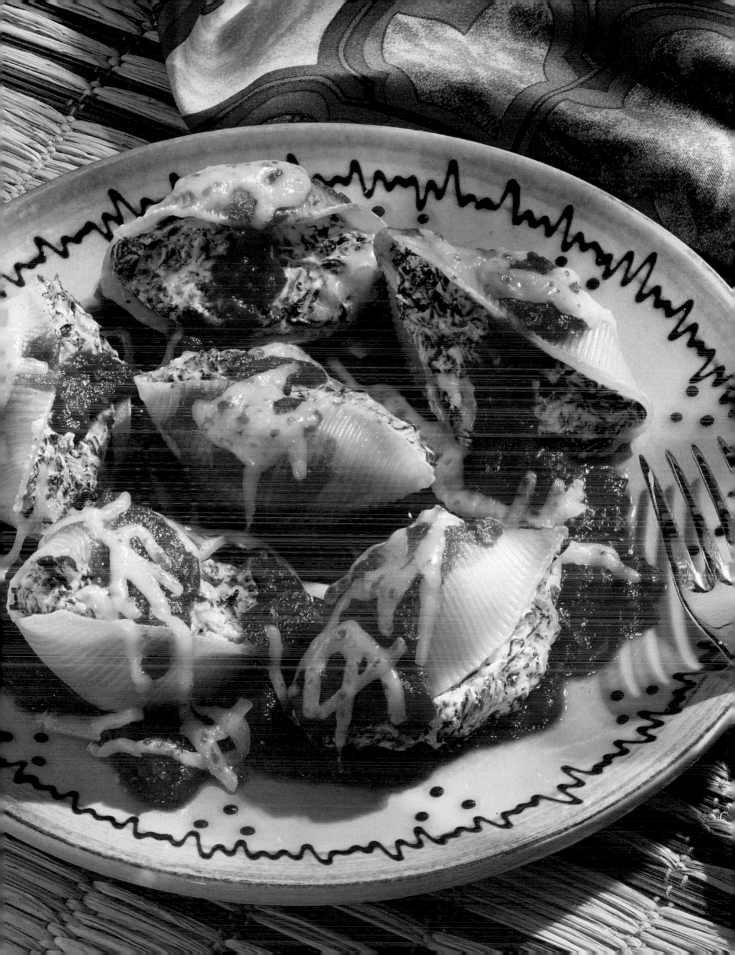

PERFECT PASTA

270 TUSCANY CAVATELLI

16 ounces uncooked cavatelli, penne or ziti pasta
1½ cups diced and seeded plum tomatoes
⅔ cup sliced pimiento-stuffed green olives
¼ cup capers, drained
2 tablespoons olive oil
2 tablespoons grated Parmesan cheese
2 tablespoons balsamic vinegar
2 cloves garlic, minced
½ teaspoon black pepper

1. Cook pasta according to package directions, omitting salt. Drain; set aside.

2. Combine tomatoes, olives, capers, oil, cheese, vinegar, garlic and pepper in a medium bowl. Stir in pasta until thoroughly coated. Serve warm or at room temperature.

Makes 5 servings

Nutrients per serving: Calories: 452 (21% Calories from Fat), Total Fat: 11 g, Saturated Fat: 2 g, Protein: 14 g, Carbohydrate: 75 g, Cholesterol: 2 mg, Sodium: 777 mg, Fiber: 2 g, Sugar: 2 g

Dietary Exchanges: 5 Starch/Bread, 2 Fat

271 LATIN–STYLE PASTA & BEANS

8 ounces uncooked mostaccioli, penne or bow tie pasta
1 tablespoon olive oil
1 medium onion, chopped
1 yellow or red bell pepper, diced
4 cloves garlic, minced
1 can (15 ounces) red or black beans, rinsed and drained
¾ cup canned vegetable broth
¾ cup medium-hot salsa or picante sauce
2 teaspoons ground cumin
⅓ cup coarsely chopped fresh cilantro

1. Cook pasta according to package directions, omitting salt. Drain; set aside.

2. Meanwhile, heat oil in a large skillet over medium heat until hot. Add onion; cook 5 minutes, stirring occasionally. Add bell pepper and garlic; cook 3 minutes, stirring occasionally. Add beans, vegetable broth, salsa and cumin; simmer, uncovered, 5 minutes.

3. Add pasta to skillet; cook 1 minute, tossing frequently. Stir in cilantro.

Makes 4 servings

Nutrients per serving: Calories: 390 (12% Calories from Fat), Total Fat: 6 g, Saturated Fat: 1 g, Protein: 18 g, Carbohydrate: 74 g, Cholesterol: 0 mg, Sodium: 557 mg, Fiber: 8 g, Sugar: 1 g

Dietary Exchanges: 4 Starch/Bread, 1 Lean Meat, 1 Vegetable, ½ Fat

272 FRESH VEGETABLE LASAGNA

8 ounces uncooked lasagna noodles
1 package (10 ounces) frozen chopped spinach, thawed and squeezed dry
1 cup shredded carrots
½ cup sliced green onions
½ cup sliced red bell pepper
¼ cup chopped parsley
½ teaspoon black pepper
1½ cups 1% low-fat cottage cheese
1 cup buttermilk
½ cup plain nonfat yogurt
2 egg whites
1 cup sliced mushrooms
1 can (14 ounces) artichoke hearts, drained and chopped
2 cups (8 ounces) shredded part-skim mozzarella cheese
¼ cup grated Parmesan cheese

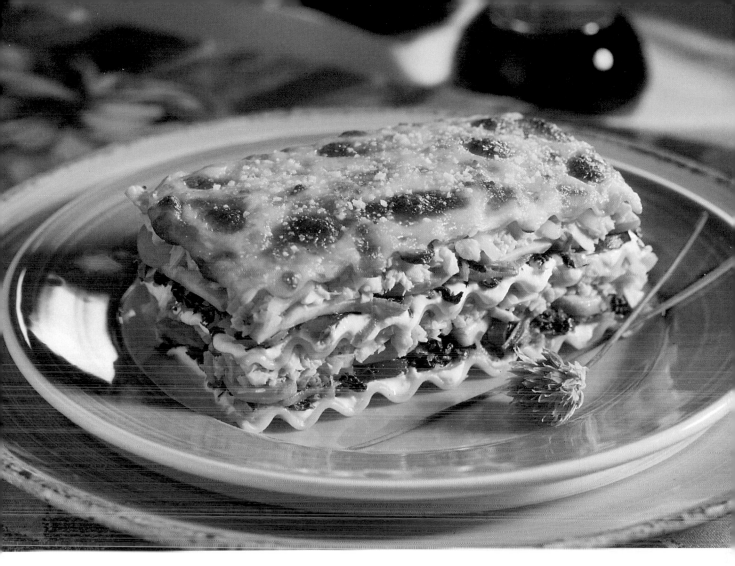

Fresh Vegetable Lasagna

1. Cook pasta according to package directions, omitting salt; drain. Rinse under cold running water until cool; drain. Set aside.

2. Preheat oven to 375°F. Combine spinach, carrots, green onions, bell pepper, parsley and black pepper in large bowl; set aside.

3. Combine cottage cheese, buttermilk, yogurt and egg whites in food processor or blender; process until smooth.

4. Spray 13×9-inch baking pan with nonstick cooking spray. Arrange ⅓ of lasagna noodles in bottom of pan. Spread with half *each* of cottage cheese mixture,

spinach mixture, mushrooms, artichokes and mozzarella. Repeat layers, ending with noodles. Sprinkle with Parmesan cheese.

5. Cover and bake 30 minutes. Uncover; continue baking 20 minutes or until bubbling and heated through. Let stand 10 minutes before serving.   *Makes 8 servings*

Nutrients per Serving: Calories: 250 (26% Calories from Fat), Total Fat: 8 g, Saturated Fat: 4 g, Protein: 22 g, Carbohydrate: 26 g, Cholesterol: 22 mg, Sodium: 508 mg, Fiber: 5 g, Sugar: 6 g

Dietary Exchanges: 1 Starch/Bread, 2 Lean Meat, 2 Vegetable, ½ Fat

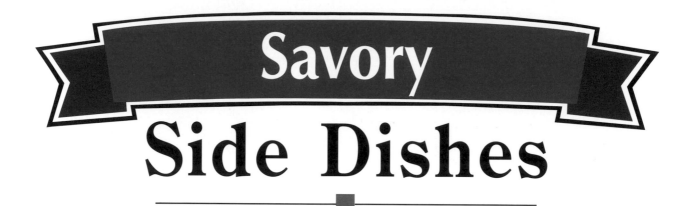

Savory Side Dishes

273 MEDITERRANEAN–STYLE ROASTED VEGETABLES

1½ **pounds red potatoes**
1 **tablespoon plus 1½ teaspoons olive oil, divided**
1 **red bell pepper**
1 **yellow or orange bell pepper**
1 **small red onion**
2 **cloves garlic, minced**
½ **teaspoon salt**
¼ **teaspoon black pepper**
1 **tablespoon balsamic vinegar**
¼ **cup chopped fresh basil leaves**

1. Preheat oven to 425°F. Spray large shallow metal roasting pan with nonstick cooking spray. Cut potatoes into 1½-inch chunks; place in pan. Drizzle 1 tablespoon oil over potatoes; toss to coat. Bake 10 minutes.

2. Cut bell peppers into 1½-inch chunks. Cut onion through the core into ½-inch wedges. Add bell peppers and onion to pan. Drizzle remaining 1½ teaspoons oil over vegetables; sprinkle with garlic, salt and black pepper. Toss well to coat. Return to oven; bake 18 to 20 minutes or until vegetables are brown and tender, stirring once.

3. Transfer to large serving bowl. Drizzle vinegar over vegetables; toss to coat. Add basil; toss again. Serve warm or at room temperature with additional black pepper, if desired. *Makes 6 servings*

Nutrients per Serving: Calories: 170 (19% Calories from Fat), Total Fat: 4 g, Saturated Fat: trace, Protein: 3 g, Carbohydrate: 33 g, Cholesterol: 0 mg, Sodium: 185 mg, Fiber: 1 g, Sugar: trace

Dietary Exchanges: 2 Starch/Bread, ½ Fat

Mediterranean-Style Roasted Vegetables

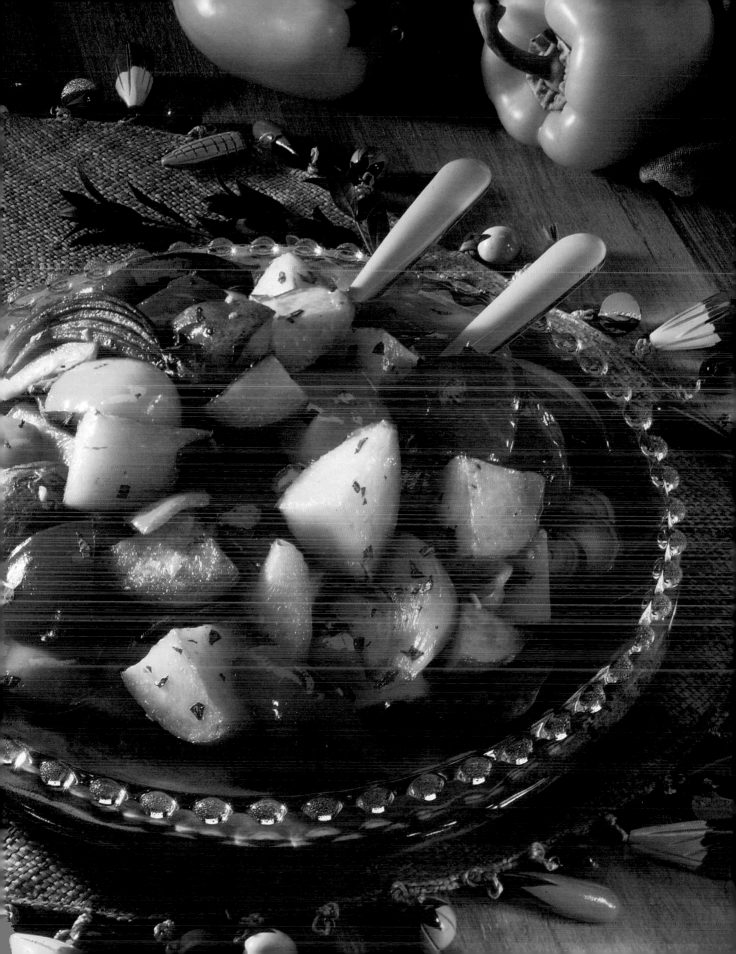

SAVORY SIDE DISHES

274 BROCCOLI AND CHEESE TOPPED POTATOES

4 large baking potatoes
2 cups broccoli florets
1 cup skim milk
½ cup nonfat cottage cheese
1 teaspoon dry mustard
½ teaspoon red pepper flakes
1 cup (4 ounces) shredded reduced-fat sharp Cheddar cheese, divided
1 cup (4 ounces) shredded part-skim mozzarella cheese
2 tablespoons all-purpose flour

1. Pierce potatoes several times with fork. Place in microwave oven on paper towel; microwave at HIGH 15 minutes or just until softened. Let stand 5 minutes.

2. Bring water to a boil in medium saucepan over medium heat. Add broccoli; cook 5 minutes or until broccoli is crisp-tender. Drain. Add milk, cottage cheese, mustard and red pepper flakes to broccoli in saucepan; bring to boil. Remove from heat.

3. Combine ¾ cup Cheddar, mozzarella and flour in medium bowl. Toss to coat cheese with flour; add to broccoli mixture. Cook and stir over medium-low heat until cheese is melted and mixture is thickened.

4. Cut potatoes open. Divide broccoli mixture evenly among potatoes; sprinkle with remaining ¼ cup Cheddar cheese.

Makes 4 servings

Nutrients per Serving: Calories: 381 (22% Calories from Fat), Total Fat: 9 g, Saturated Fat: 5 g, Protein: 24 g, Carbohydrate: 51 g, Cholesterol: 33 mg, Sodium: 647 mg, Fiber: 2 g, Sugar: 4 g

Dietary Exchanges: 3 Starch/Bread, 2 Lean Meat, 1 Vegetable, ½ Fat

275 SCALLOPED POTATOES

2 tablespoons margarine
3 tablespoons all-purpose flour
2½ cups skim milk
3 tablespoons grated Parmesan cheese
Black pepper
2 pounds baking potatoes, peeled and thinly sliced
Ground nutmeg
Salt
½ cup (2 ounces) shredded reduced-fat Swiss cheese, divided
3 tablespoons thinly sliced chives, divided

1. Preheat oven to 350°F. Spray 2-quart glass casserole with nonstick cooking spray.

2. Melt margarine in medium saucepan. Add flour; cook over medium-low heat 1 to 2 minutes, stirring constantly. Gradually whisk in milk; bring to a boil. Cook, whisking constantly, 1 to 2 minutes or until mixture thickens. Stir in Parmesan cheese; season to taste with pepper.

3. Layer ⅓ potatoes in bottom of prepared casserole. Sprinkle potatoes with nutmeg, salt, ⅓ Swiss cheese and 1 tablespoon chives. Spoon ⅓ margarine mixture over chives. Repeat layers, ending with margarine mixture.

4. Bake 1 hour and 15 minutes or until potatoes are fork-tender. Cool slightly before serving; garnish with additional fresh chives, if desired.

Makes 8 servings

Nutrients per Serving: Calories: 185 (24% Calories from Fat), Total Fat: 5 g, Saturated Fat: 2 g, Protein: 8 g, Carbohydrate: 27 g, Cholesterol: 8 mg, Sodium: 140 mg, Fiber: 0 g, Sugar: 3 g

Dietary Exchanges: 1½ Starch/Bread, ½ Lean Meat, ½ Fat

Broccoli and Cheese Topped Potatoes

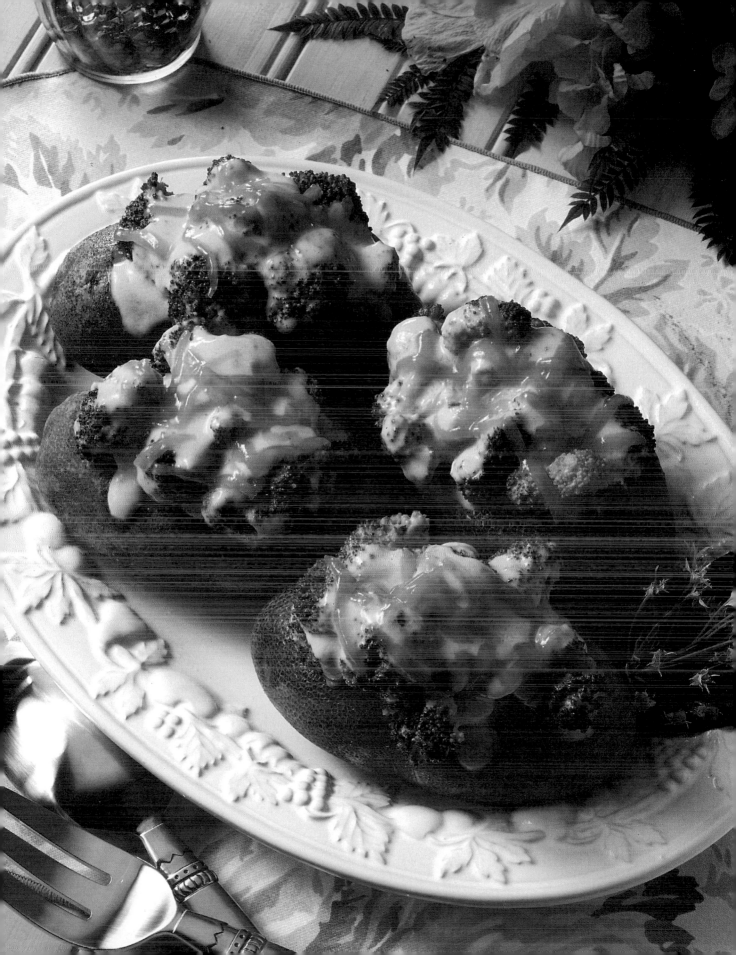

SAVORY SIDE DISHES

276 POTATO PANCAKES WITH APPLE–CHERRY CHUTNEY

Apple-Cherry Chutney (recipe follows)
1 pound baking potatoes, about 2 medium
½ small onion
3 egg whites
2 tablespoons all-purpose flour
½ teaspoon salt
¼ teaspoon black pepper
4 teaspoons vegetable oil, divided

1. Prepare Apple-Cherry Chutney; set aside.

2. Peel potatoes; cut into chunks. Combine potatoes, onion, egg whites, flour, salt and pepper in food processor or blender; process until almost smooth (mixture will appear grainy).

3. Heat large nonstick skillet 1 minute over medium heat. Add 1 teaspoon oil. Spoon 2 tablespoons batter per pancake into skillet. Cook 3 pancakes at a time, 3 minutes per side or until golden brown. Repeat with remaining batter, adding 1 teaspoon oil with each batch. Serve with Apple-Cherry Chutney.
Makes 1 dozen pancakes (2 pancakes per serving)

APPLE–CHERRY CHUTNEY
1 cup chunky applesauce
½ cup canned tart cherries, drained
2 tablespoons brown sugar
1 teaspoon lemon juice
½ teaspoon ground cinnamon
⅛ teaspoon ground nutmeg

1. Combine all ingredients in small saucepan; bring to a boil. Reduce heat; simmer 5 minutes. Serve warm.
Makes 1½ cups

Nutrients per Serving: Calories: 164 (17% Calories from Fat), Total Fat: 3 g, Saturated Fat: trace, Protein: 4 g, Carbohydrate: 31 g, Cholesterol: 0 mg, Sodium: 214 mg, Fiber: 1 g, Sugar: 2 g

Dietary Exchanges: 1½ Starch/Bread, ½ Fruit, ½ Fat

277 ZUCCHINI CAKES

3 teaspoons reduced-calorie margarine, divided
2 tablespoons finely chopped red onion
1 zucchini
½ baking potato, peeled
¼ cup cholesterol-free egg substitute
4½ teaspoons bread crumbs
1 teaspoon chopped dill
Pinch white pepper

1. Melt 1½ teaspoons margarine in large skillet. Add onion; cook and stir 5 minutes or until tender.

2. Shred zucchini and potato with grater; drain. Combine onion, zucchini, potato, egg substitute, bread crumbs, dill and pepper in medium bowl.

3. Melt remaining 1½ teaspoons margarine in large skillet. Drop 4 heaping ¼-cupfuls mixture into skillet; flatten. Cook 10 minutes or until golden brown, turning once.
Makes 2 servings

Nutrients per Serving: Calories: 111 (24% Calories from Fat), Total Fat: 3 g, Saturated Fat: 1 g, Protein: 5 g, Carbohydrate: 17 g, Cholesterol: 0 mg, Sodium: 123 mg, Fiber: 1 g, Sugar: 2 g

Dietary Exchanges: 1 Starch/Bread, ½ Vegetable, ½ Fat

Potato Pancakes with Apple-Cherry Chutney

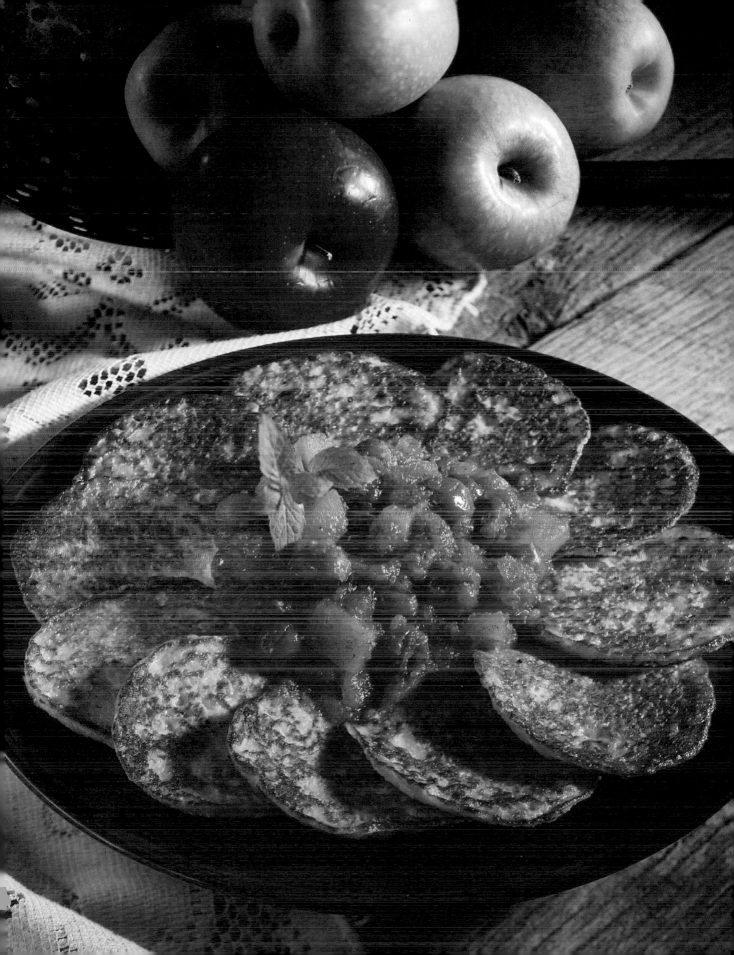

SAVORY SIDE DISHES

278 GRATIN OF TWO POTATOES

2 large baking potatoes (about 1¼ pounds)
2 large sweet potatoes (about 1¼ pounds)
1 tablespoon unsalted butter
1 large sweet or yellow onion, thinly sliced, separated into rings
2 teaspoons all-purpose flour
1 cup canned fat-free reduced-sodium chicken broth
½ teaspoon salt
¼ teaspoon white pepper *or* ⅛ teaspoon ground red pepper
¾ cup freshly grated Parmesan cheese

1. Cook baking potatoes in large pot of boiling water 10 minutes. Add sweet potatoes; return to a boil. Simmer, uncovered, 25 minutes or until tender. Drain; cool under cold running water. Drain.

2. Meanwhile, melt butter in large nonstick skillet over medium-high heat. Add onion; cover and cook 3 minutes or until wilted. Uncover; cook over medium-low heat 10 to 12 minutes or until tender, stirring occasionally. Sprinkle with flour; cook 1 minute, stirring frequently. Add chicken broth, salt and pepper; bring to a boil over high heat. Reduce heat to medium; simmer, uncovered, 2 minutes or until sauce thickens, stirring occasionally.

3. Preheat oven to 375°F. Spray 13×9-inch baking dish with nonstick cooking spray. Peel potatoes; cut crosswise into ¼-inch slices. Layer half of baking and sweet potato slices in prepared dish. Spoon half of onion mixture evenly over potatoes. Repeat layering with remaining potatoes and onion mixture. Cover with foil. Bake 25 minutes or until heated through.

4. Preheat broiler. Uncover potatoes; sprinkle evenly with cheese. Broil, 5 inches from heat, 3 to 4 minutes or until cheese is bubbly and light golden brown.

Makes 6 servings

Nutrients per Serving: Calories: 261 (21% Calories from Fat), Total Fat: 6 g, Saturated Fat: 4 g, Protein: 9 g, Carbohydrate: 43 g, Cholesterol: 15 mg, Sodium: 437 mg, Fiber: 1 g, Sugar: 1 g

Dietary Exchanges: 3 Starch/Bread, ½ Lean Meat, ½ Fat

279 SWEET POTATO PUFFS

2 pounds sweet potatoes
⅓ cup orange juice
1 egg, beaten
1 tablespoon grated orange peel
½ teaspoon ground nutmeg
¼ cup chopped pecans

1. Peel sweet potatoes; cut into 1-inch pieces. Place potatoes in medium saucepan. Add enough water to cover; bring to a boil over medium-high heat. Cook 10 to 15 minutes or until tender. Drain potatoes and place in large bowl; mash until smooth. Add orange juice, egg, orange peel and nutmeg; mix well.

2. Preheat oven to 375°F. Spray baking sheet with nonstick cooking spray. Spoon potato mixture into 10 mounds on prepared baking sheet. Sprinkle pecans on tops of mounds.

3. Bake 30 minutes or until centers are hot.

Makes 10 servings

Nutrients per Serving: Calories: 105 (22% Calories from Fat), Total Fat: 3 g, Saturated Fat: trace, Protein: 2 g, Carbohydrate: 19 g, Cholesterol: 21 mg, Sodium: 15 mg, Fiber: trace, Sugar: 1 g

Dietary Exchanges: 1 Starch/Bread, ½ Fat

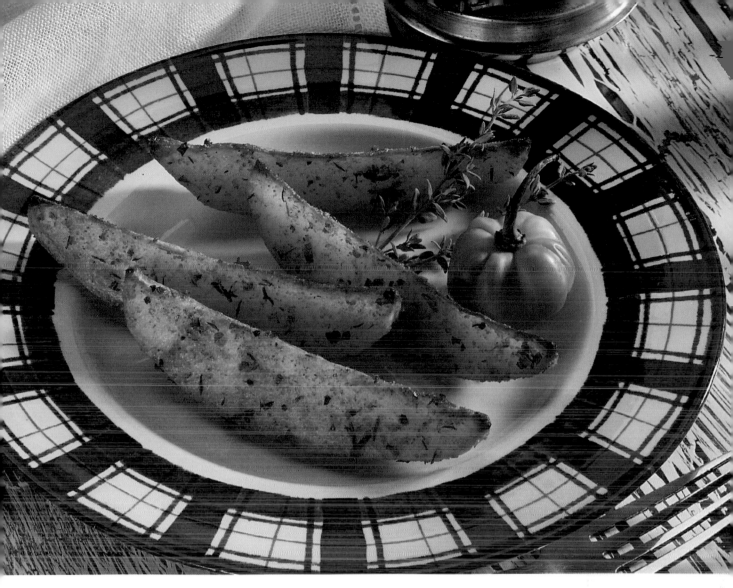

Roast Cajun Potatoes

280 ROAST CAJUN POTATOES

1 pound baking potatoes
2 tablespoons finely chopped parsley
2 teaspoons canola oil
½ teaspoon garlic powder
½ teaspoon onion powder
½ teaspoon ground red pepper
½ teaspoon dried thyme leaves
¼ teaspoon black pepper

1. Preheat oven to 400°F. Peel potatoes; cut each potato lengthwise into 8 wedges. Place on ungreased jelly-roll pan.

2. Toss potatoes with parsley, oil, garlic powder, onion powder, red pepper, thyme and black pepper until evenly coated.

3. Bake 50 minutes, turning wedges halfway through cooking time. Serve immediately.
Makes 4 servings

Nutrients per Serving: Calories: 120 (18% Calories from Fat), Total Fat: 2 g, Saturated Fat: trace, Protein: 2 g, Carbohydrate: 23 g, Cholesterol: 0 mg, Sodium: 7 mg, Fiber: 2 g, Sugar: 0 g

Dietary Exchanges: 1½ Starch/Bread, ½ Fat

SAVORY SIDE DISHES

281 COUNTRY–STYLE MASHED POTATOES

4 pounds Yukon gold or baking potatoes, unpeeled and cut into 1-inch pieces
6 large cloves garlic, peeled
½ cup nonfat sour cream
½ cup skim milk, warmed
2 tablespoons margarine
2 tablespoons finely chopped fresh rosemary *or* 1 teaspoon dried rosemary
2 tablespoons finely chopped fresh thyme *or* ½ teaspoon dried thyme leaves
2 tablespoons finely chopped parsley

1. Place potatoes and garlic in medium saucepan; cover with water. Bring to a boil. Reduce heat; simmer, covered, about 15 minutes or until potatoes are fork-tender. Drain.

2. Place potatoes and garlic in large bowl; beat with electric mixer just until mashed. Beat in sour cream, milk and margarine until almost smooth. Mix in rosemary, thyme and parsley. *Makes 8 servings*

Nutrients per Serving: Calories: 191 (8% Calories from Fat), Total Fat: 2 g, Saturated Fat: 0 g, Protein: 4 g, Carbohydrate: 40 g, Cholesterol: 0 mg, Sodium: 38 mg, Fiber: 0 g, Sugar: trace

Dietary Exchanges: 2½ Starch/Bread

282 ROASTED POTATOES AND PEARL ONIONS

3 pounds red potatoes, well-scrubbed and cut into 1½-inch cubes
1 package (10 ounces) pearl onions, peeled
2 tablespoons olive oil
2 teaspoons dried basil or thyme leaves
1 teaspoon paprika
¾ teaspoon dried rosemary
¾ teaspoon salt
¾ teaspoon black pepper

1. Preheat oven to 400°F. Spray large shallow roasting pan (do not use glass or potatoes will not brown) with nonstick cooking spray.

2. Add potatoes and onions to pan; drizzle with oil. Combine basil, paprika, rosemary, salt and pepper in small bowl; mix well. Sprinkle over potatoes and onions; toss well to coat.

3. Bake 20 minutes; toss well. Continue baking 15 to 20 minutes or until potatoes are browned and tender. *Makes 10 servings*

Nutrients per Serving: Calories: 236 (11% Calories from Fat), Total Fat: 3 g, Saturated Fat: trace, Protein: 4 g, Carbohydrate: 49 g, Cholesterol: 0 mg, Sodium: 278 mg, Fiber: trace, Sugar: 1 g

Dietary Exchanges: 3 Starch/Bread, ½ Fat

Country-Style Mashed Potatoes

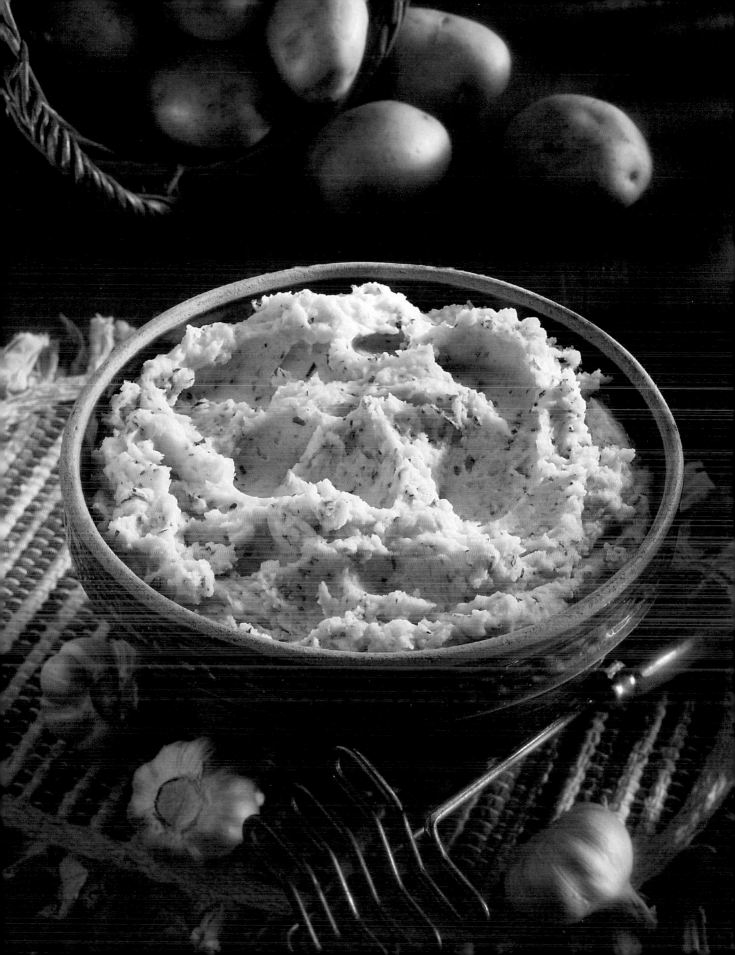

SAVORY SIDE DISHES

283 SPIRITED SWEET POTATO CASSEROLE

2½ pounds sweet potatoes
2 tablespoons reduced-calorie margarine
⅓ cup 1% low-fat or skim milk
¼ cup packed brown sugar
2 tablespoons bourbon or apple juice
1 teaspoon ground cinnamon
1 teaspoon vanilla
2 egg whites
½ teaspoon salt
⅓ cup chopped pecans

1. Preheat oven to 375°F. Bake potatoes 50 to 60 minutes or until very tender. Cool 10 minutes; leave oven on. Scoop pulp from warm potatoes into large bowl; discard potato skins. Add margarine to bowl; mash with potato masher until potatoes are fairly smooth and margarine has melted. Stir in milk, brown sugar, bourbon, cinnamon and vanilla; mix well.

2. Beat egg whites with electric mixer at high speed until soft peaks form. Add salt; beat until stiff peaks form. Fold egg whites into sweet potato mixture.

3. Spray 1½-quart souffle dish with nonstick cooking spray. Spoon sweet potato mixture into dish; top with pecans.

4. Bake 30 to 35 minutes or until casserole is puffed and pecans are toasted. Serve immediately.   *Makes 8 servings*

Nutrients per Serving: Calories: 203 (21% Calories from Fat), Total Fat: 5 g, Saturated Fat: 1 g, Protein: 3 g, Carbohydrate: 35 g, Cholesterol: trace, Sodium: 202 mg, Fiber: trace, Sugar: 1 g

Dietary Exchanges: 2 Starch/Bread, 1½ Fat

284 POTATOES AU GRATIN

1 pound baking potatoes
4 teaspoons reduced-calorie margarine
4 teaspoons all-purpose flour
1¼ cups skim milk
¼ teaspoon ground nutmeg
¼ teaspoon paprika
   Pinch white pepper
½ cup thinly sliced red onion, divided
⅓ cup whole wheat bread crumbs
1 tablespoon finely chopped red onion
1 tablespoon grated Parmesan cheese

1. Spray 4- or 6-cup casserole with nonstick cooking spray; set aside.

2. Place potatoes in large saucepan; add water to cover. Bring to a boil over high heat. Boil 12 minutes or until potatoes are tender. Drain; let potatoes stand 10 minutes or until cool enough to handle.

3. Melt margarine in small saucepan over medium heat. Add flour; cook and stir 3 minutes. Gradually whisk in milk; cook and stir 8 minutes or until sauce thickens. Remove saucepan from heat; stir in nutmeg, paprika and pepper.

4. Preheat oven to 350°F. Cut potatoes into thin slices. Arrange half of potato slices in prepared casserole; sprinkle with half of onion slices. Repeat layers. Spoon sauce over potato mixture. Combine bread crumbs, finely chopped red onion and cheese in small bowl; sprinkle mixture evenly over sauce. Bake 20 minutes. Let stand 5 minutes before serving.
                    Makes 4 servings

Nutrients per Serving: Calories: 178 (14% Calories from Fat), Total Fat: 3 g, Saturated Fat: 1 g, Protein: 6 g, Carbohydrate: 33 g, Cholesterol: 2 mg, Sodium: 144 mg, Fiber: 2 g, Sugar: 4 g

Dietary Exchanges: 2 Starch/Bread, ½ Vegetable, ½ Fat

SAVORY SIDE DISHES

285 SPINACH PARMESAN RISOTTO

3⅔ cups fat-free reduced-sodium
    chicken broth
½ teaspoon white pepper
    Nonstick cooking spray
1 cup uncooked arborio rice
1½ cups chopped fresh spinach
½ cup frozen green peas
1 tablespoon minced fresh dill *or*
    1 teaspoon dried dill weed
½ cup grated Parmesan cheese
1 teaspoon grated lemon peel

1. Combine chicken broth and pepper in medium saucepan; cover. Bring to a simmer over medium-low heat; maintain simmer by adjusting heat.

2. Spray large saucepan with cooking spray; heat over medium-low heat until hot. Add rice; cook and stir 1 minute. Stir in ⅔ cup hot chicken broth; cook, stirring constantly until chicken broth is absorbed.

3. Stir remaining hot chicken broth into rice mixture, ½ cup at a time, stirring constantly until all chicken broth is absorbed before adding next ½ cup. When adding last ½ cup chicken broth, stir in spinach, peas and dill. Cook, stirring gently until all chicken broth is absorbed and rice is just tender but still firm to the bite. (Total cooking time for chicken broth absorption is 35 to 40 minutes.)

4. Remove saucepan from heat; stir in cheese and lemon peel.

Makes 6 servings

Nutrients per Serving: Calories: 179 (15% Calories from Fat), Total Fat: 3 g, Saturated Fat: 2 g, Protein: 7 g, Carbohydrate: 30 g, Cholesterol: 7 mg, Sodium: 198 mg, Fiber: 1 g, Sugar: 1 g

Dietary Exchanges: 2 Starch/Bread, ½ Lean Meat

Spinach Parmesan Risotto

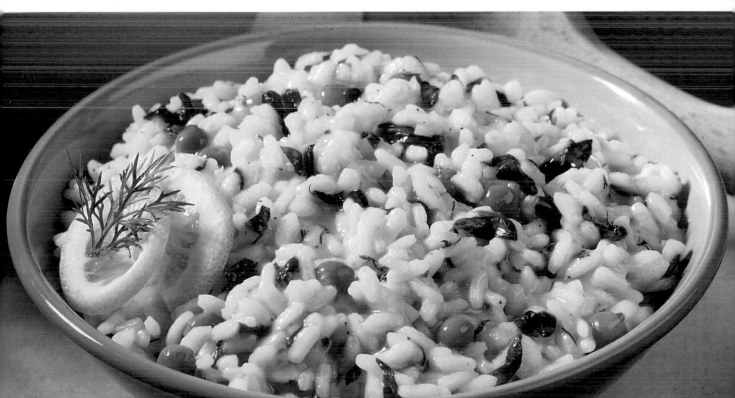

SAVORY SIDE DISHES

286 WILD & BROWN RICE WITH EXOTIC MUSHROOMS

1²/₃ cups packaged unseasoned wild & brown rice blend
  6 cups water
  ½ ounce dried porcini or morel mushrooms
  ¾ cup boiling water
  2 tablespoons margarine
  8 ounces cremini or button mushrooms, sliced
  2 cloves garlic, minced
  2 tablespoons chopped fresh thyme *or* 2 teaspoons dried thyme leaves
  1 teaspoon salt
  ¼ teaspoon black pepper
  ½ cup sliced green onions

1. Combine rice and water in large saucepan; bring to a boil over high heat. Cover; simmer over low heat until rice is tender (check package for cooking time). Drain, but do not rinse.

2. Meanwhile, combine porcini mushrooms and boiling water in small bowl; let stand 30 minutes or until mushrooms are tender. Drain mushrooms, reserving liquid. Chop mushrooms; set aside.

3. Melt margarine in large, deep skillet over medium heat. Add cremini mushrooms and garlic; cook and stir 5 minutes. Sprinkle thyme, salt and pepper over mushrooms; cook and stir 1 minute or until mushrooms are tender.

4. Stir rice, porcini mushrooms and reserved mushroom liquid into skillet; cook and stir over medium-low heat 5 minutes or until hot. Stir in green onions.

Makes 8 servings

Nutrients per Serving: Calories: 175 (21% Calories from Fat), Total Fat: 4 g, Saturated Fat: 1 g, Protein: 5 g, Carbohydrate: 30 g, Cholesterol: 0 mg, Sodium: 304 mg, Fiber: 2 g, Sugar: 1 g

Dietary Exchanges: 2 Starch/Bread, 1 Fat

287 RICE PILAF WITH DRIED CHERRIES AND ALMONDS

  ½ cup slivered almonds
  2 tablespoons margarine
  2 cups uncooked rice
  ½ cup chopped onion
  1 can (about 14 ounces) vegetable broth
1½ cups water
  ½ cup dried cherries

1. To toast almonds, cook and stir in large nonstick skillet over medium heat until lightly browned. Remove from skillet; cool.

2. Melt margarine in skillet over low heat. Add rice and onion; cook and stir until rice is lightly browned. Add broth and water; bring to a boil over high heat. Reduce heat to low; simmer, covered, 15 minutes.

3. Stir in almonds and cherries. Simmer 5 minutes or until liquid is absorbed and rice is tender. *Makes 12 servings*

Nutrients per Serving: Calories: 174 (24% Calories from Fat), Total Fat: 5 g, Saturated Fat: 1 g, Protein: 3 g, Carbohydrate: 29 g, Cholesterol: 0 mg, Sodium: 37 mg, Fiber: 1 g, Sugar: 2 g

Dietary Exchanges: 2 Starch/Bread, 1 Fat

Wild & Brown Rice with Exotic Mushrooms

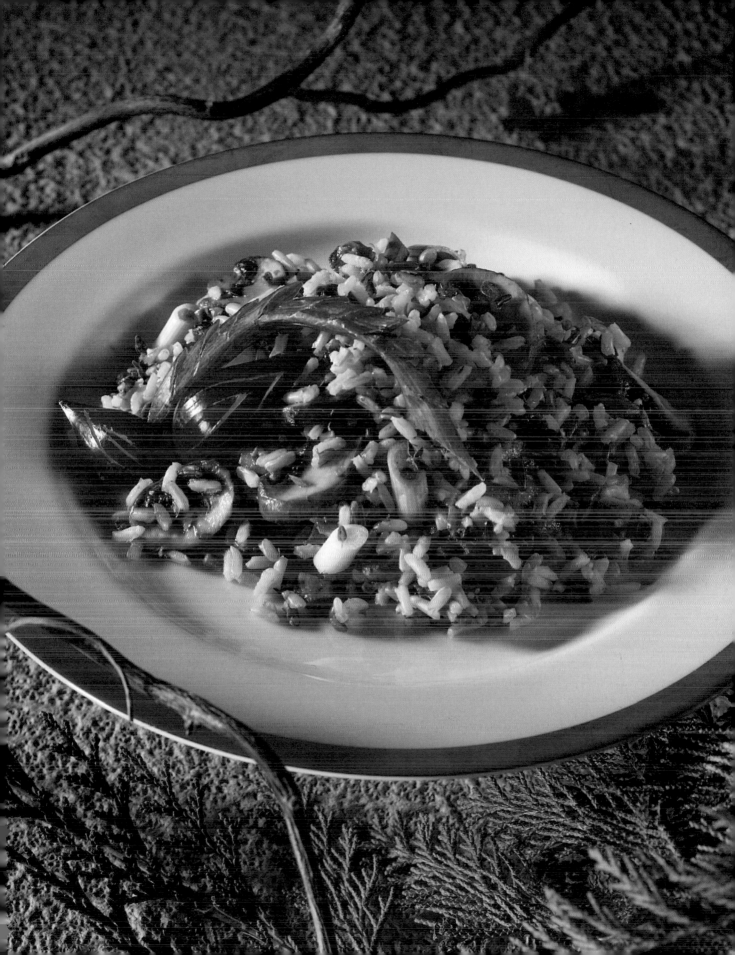

SAVORY SIDE DISHES

288 PESTO–PASTA STUFFED TOMATOES

3 ounces uncooked star or other small
  pasta
4 large tomatoes
1 cup loosely packed fresh basil
1 clove garlic, minced
3 tablespoons reduced-calorie mayonnaise
1 tablespoon skim milk
¼ teaspoon black pepper
1 cup shredded zucchini
4 teaspoons grated Parmesan cheese

1. Cook pasta according to package directions, omitting salt. Drain and rinse; set aside.

2. Cut tops from tomatoes; scoop out and discard all but ½ cup tomato pulp. Chop tomato pulp; add to pasta. Place tomatoes, cut side down, on paper towels; let drain 5 minutes.

3. Preheat oven to 350°F. Place basil and garlic in blender or food processor; process until finely chopped. Add mayonnaise, milk and black pepper; process until smooth.

4. Combine pasta mixture, zucchini and basil mixture; toss to coat evenly. Place tomatoes, cut side up, in 8-inch baking dish. Divide pasta mixture evenly among tomatoes, mounding filling slightly; sprinkle with cheese.

5. Bake 10 to 15 minutes or until heated through. *Makes 4 servings*

Nutrients per Serving: Calories: 155 (33% Calories from Fat), Total Fat: 6 g, Saturated Fat: 1 g, Protein: 6 g, Carbohydrate: 22 g, Cholesterol: 2 mg, Sodium: 154 mg, Fiber: 3 g, Sugar: 4 g

Dietary Exchanges: 1 Starch/Bread, 1½ Vegetable, 1 Fat

289 SPICY CHICK–PEAS & COUSCOUS

1 can (about 14 ounces) vegetable broth
1 teaspoon ground coriander
½ teaspoon ground cardamom
½ teaspoon turmeric
½ teaspoon hot pepper sauce
¼ teaspoon salt
⅛ teaspoon cinnamon
1 cup julienned carrots
1 can (15 ounces) chick-peas, rinsed and
  drained
1 cup frozen peas
1 cup quick-cooking couscous
2 tablespoons chopped fresh mint or
  parsley

1. Combine vegetable broth, coriander, cardamom, turmeric, pepper sauce, salt and cinnamon in large saucepan; bring to a boil over high heat. Add carrots; reduce heat and simmer 5 minutes. Add chick-peas and peas; return to a simmer. Simmer, uncovered, 2 minutes.

2. Stir in couscous. Cover; remove from heat. Let stand 5 minutes or until liquid is absorbed. Sprinkle with mint.

Makes 6 servings

Nutrients per Serving: Calories: 226 (6% Calories from Fat), Total Fat: 2 g, Saturated Fat: trace, Protein: 9 g, Carbohydrate: 44 g, Cholesterol: 0 mg, Sodium: 431 mg, Fiber: 10 g, Sugar: 3 g

Dietary Exchanges: 3 Starch/Bread

Spicy Chick-peas & Couscous

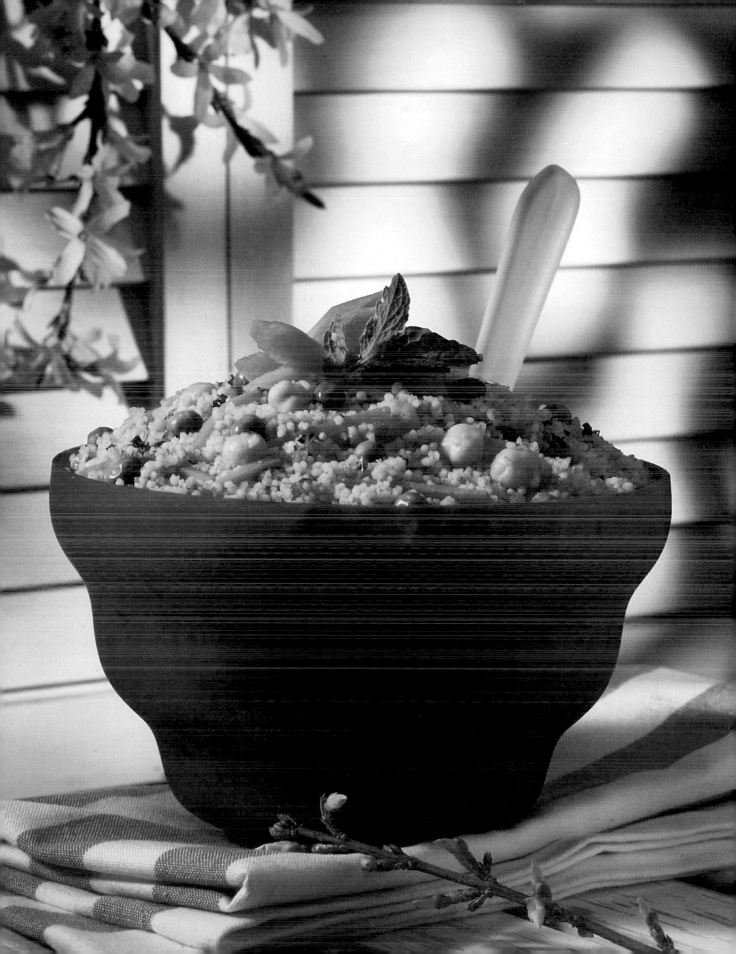

SAVORY SIDE DISHES

290 GREEN PEA & RICE ALMONDINE

2 teaspoons reduced-calorie margarine
1 cup frozen baby green peas
¼ teaspoon ground cardamom
¼ teaspoon ground cinnamon
   Pinch ground cloves
   Pinch white pepper
¾ cup cooked white rice
2 teaspoons slivered almonds

Melt margarine in medium nonstick skillet over medium heat. Add peas, cardamom, cinnamon, cloves and pepper; cook and stir 10 minutes or until peas are tender. Add rice; cook until heated through, stirring occasionally. Sprinkle almonds evenly over servings.   *Makes 4 servings*

Nutrients per Serving: Calories: 100 (16% Calories from Fat), Total Fat: 2 g, Saturated Fat: trace, Protein: 3 g, Carbohydrate: 18 g, Cholesterol: 0 mg, Sodium: 57 mg, Fiber: 2 g, Sugar: 2 g

Dietary Exchanges: 1 Starch/Bread, ½ Fat

Spaghetti Squash Primavera

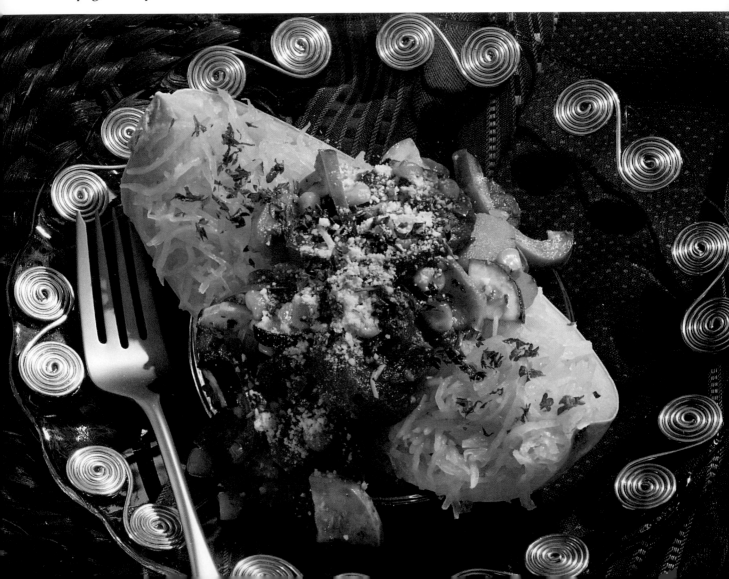

SAVORY SIDE DISHES

291 SPAGHETTI SQUASH PRIMAVERA

2 teaspoons vegetable oil
½ teaspoon finely chopped garlic
¼ cup finely chopped red onion
¼ cup thinly sliced carrot
¼ cup thinly sliced red bell pepper
¼ cup thinly sliced green bell pepper
1 can (14½ ounces) Italian-style stewed tomatoes
½ cup thinly sliced yellow squash
½ cup thinly sliced zucchini
½ cup frozen corn, thawed
½ teaspoon dried oregano leaves
⅛ teaspoon dried thyme leaves
1 spaghetti squash (about 2 pounds)
4 teaspoons grated Parmesan cheese (optional)
2 tablespoons finely chopped parsley

1. Heat oil in large skillet over medium-high heat until hot. Add garlic; cook and stir 3 minutes. Add onion, carrot and peppers; cook and stir 3 minutes. Add tomatoes, squash, zucchini, corn, oregano and thyme; cook 5 minutes or until heated through, stirring occasionally.

2. Cut squash lengthwise in half; remove seeds. Cover with plastic wrap; microwave at HIGH 9 minutes or until squash separates easily into strands when tested with fork.

3. Cut each squash half lengthwise in half; separate strands with fork. Spoon vegetables evenly over squash. Top servings evenly with cheese, if desired and parsley.

Makes 4 servings

Nutrients per Serving: Calories: 101 (25% Calories from Fat), Total Fat: 3 g, Saturated Fat: trace, Protein: 3 g, Carbohydrate: 18 g, Cholesterol: 0 mg, Sodium: 11 mg, Fiber: 5 g, Sugar: 3 g

Dietary Exchanges: 1 Starch/Bread, 1 Vegetable, ½ Fat

292 SPICY SPANISH RICE

1 teaspoon canola oil
1 cup uncooked white rice
1 medium onion, chopped
2 cups chicken stock or canned low sodium chicken broth, defatted
1 cup GUILTLESS GOURMET® Salsa (medium)
Green chili pepper strips (optional)

Heat large skillet over medium-high heat until hot. Add oil; swirl to coat skillet. Add rice; cook and stir until lightly browned. Remove rice to small bowl. Add onion to same skillet; cook and stir until onion is translucent. Add stock and salsa to skillet; return rice to skillet. Bring to a boil. Reduce heat to low; cover and simmer until liquid is absorbed and rice is tender. Serve hot. Garnish with pepper, if desired.

Makes 4 servings

Nutrients per Serving: Calories: 293 (8% Calories from Fat), Total Fat: 2 g, Saturated Fat: 0 g, Protein: 7 g, Carbohydrate: 58 g, Cholesterol: 0 mg, Sodium: 353 mg, Fiber: 1 g

Dietary Exchanges: 3 Starch/Bread, 1 Vegetable

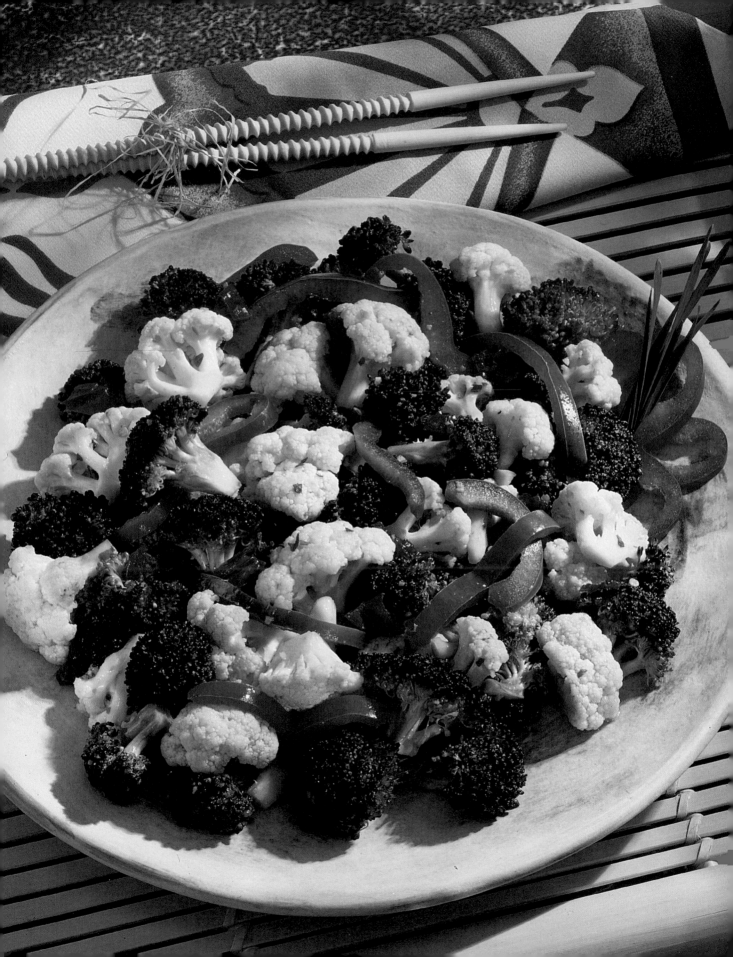

SAVORY SIDE DISHES

293 SPICY SESAME NOODLES

6 ounces uncooked dry soba (buckwheat) noodles
2 teaspoons dark sesame oil
1 tablespoon sesame seeds
½ cup fat-free reduced-sodium chicken broth
1 tablespoon creamy peanut butter
4 teaspoons reduced-sodium soy sauce
½ cup thinly sliced green onions
½ cup minced red bell pepper
1½ teaspoons finely chopped, seeded jalapeño pepper*
1 clove garlic, minced
¼ teaspoon red pepper flakes

*Jalapeño peppers can sting and irritate the skin; wear rubber gloves when handling peppers and do not touch eyes. Wash hands after handling.

1. Cook noodles according to package directions. (Do not overcook.) Rinse noodles thoroughly with cold water to stop cooking and remove salty residue; drain. Place noodles in large bowl; toss with oil.

2. Place sesame seeds in small skillet. Cook over medium heat about 3 minutes or until seeds begin to pop and turn golden brown, stirring frequently. Remove from heat; set aside.

3. Combine chicken broth and peanut butter in small bowl with wire whisk until blended. (Mixture may look curdled.) Stir in soy sauce, green onions, bell pepper, jalapeño pepper, garlic and red pepper flakes.

4. Pour mixture over noodles; toss to coat. Cover and let stand 30 minutes at room temperature or refrigerate up to 24 hours. Sprinkle with toasted sesame seeds before serving. *Makes 6 servings*

Broccoli & Cauliflower Stir-Fry

Nutrients per Serving: Calories: 145 (23% Calories from Fat), Total Fat: 4 g, Saturated Fat: 1 g, Protein: 6 g, Carbohydrate: 24 g, Cholesterol: 0 mg, Sodium: 358 mg, Fiber: 1 g, Sugar: 1 g

Dietary Exchanges: 1½ Starch/Bread, ½ Vegetable, ½ Fat

294 BROCCOLI & CAULIFLOWER STIR–FRY

2 sun-dried tomatoes (not packed in oil)
4 teaspoons reduced-sodium soy sauce
1 tablespoon rice wine vinegar
1 teaspoon brown sugar
1 teaspoon dark sesame oil
⅛ teaspoon red pepper flakes
2¼ teaspoons vegetable oil
2 cups cauliflower florets
2 cups broccoli florets
1 clove garlic, finely chopped
⅓ cup thinly sliced red or green bell pepper

1. Place tomatoes in small bowl; cover with boiling water. Let stand 5 minutes. Drain; coarsely chop. Meanwhile, blend soy sauce, vinegar, sugar, sesame oil and red pepper flakes in small bowl.

2. Heat vegetable oil in wok or large nonstick skillet over medium-high heat until hot. Add cauliflower, broccoli and garlic; stir-fry 4 minutes. Add tomatoes and bell pepper; stir-fry 1 minute. Add soy sauce mixture; cook and stir until heated through. Serve immediately. *Makes 2 servings*

Nutrients per Serving: Calories: 214 (30% Calories from Fat), Total Fat: 8 g, Saturated Fat: 1 g, Protein: 9 g, Carbohydrate: 32 g, Cholesterol: 0 mg, Sodium: 443 mg, Fiber: 5 g, Sugar: 2 g

Dietary Exchanges: 6 Vegetable, 1½ Fat

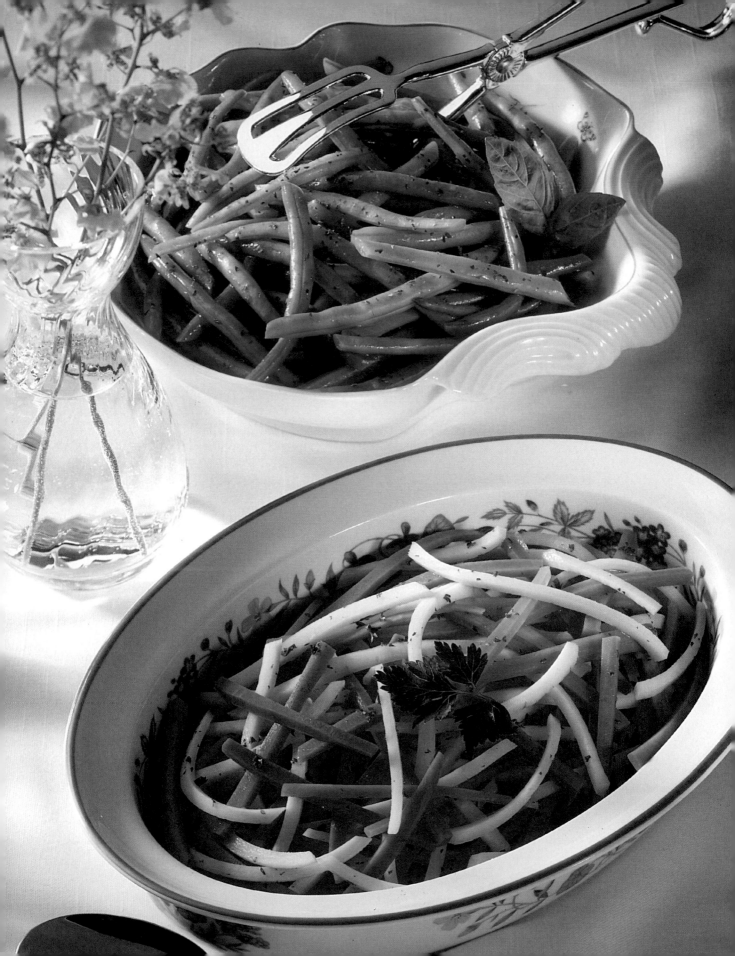

SAVORY SIDE DISHES

295 HERBED GREEN BEANS

1 pound fresh green beans, stem ends
  removed
1 teaspoon olive oil
2 tablespoons chopped fresh basil *or*
  2 teaspoons dried basil leaves

1. Steam green beans 5 minutes or until crisp-tender. Rinse under cold running water; drain. Set aside.

2. Just before serving, heat oil over medium-low heat in large nonstick skillet. Add basil; cook and stir 1 minute, then add green beans. Cook until heated through. Garnish with additional fresh basil, if desired. Serve immediately.   *Makes 6 servings*

Nutrients per Serving: Calories: 26 (26% Calories from Fat), Total Fat: 1 g, Saturated Fat: trace, Protein: 1 g, Carbohydrate: 5 g, Cholesterol: 0 mg, Sodium: 10 mg, Fiber: 0 g, Sugar: 0 g

Dietary Exchanges: 1 Vegetable

296 HONEY GLAZED CARROTS AND PARSNIPS

½ pound carrots, peeled and cut into
  julienned strips
½ pound parsnips, peeled and cut into
  julienned strips
¼ cup chopped fresh parsley
2 tablespoons honey

1. Steam carrots and parsnips 3 to 4 minutes until crisp-tender. Rinse under cold running water; drain and set aside.

Top to bottom: *Herbed Green Beans and Honey Glazed Carrots and Parsnips*

2. Just before serving, combine carrots, parsnips, parsley and honey in large saucepan or skillet. Cook over medium heat just until heated through. Garnish with fresh Italian parsley, if desired. Serve immediately.   *Makes 6 servings*

Nutrients per Serving: Calories: 69 (2% Calories from Fat), Total Fat: trace, Saturated Fat: trace, Protein: 1 g, Carbohydrate: 17 g, Cholesterol: 0 mg, Sodium: 19 mg, Fiber: 3 g, Sugar: 8 g

Dietary Exchanges: 2½ Vegetable

297 BOSTON BAKED BEANS

2 cans (15 ounces each) navy or Great
  Northern beans, rinsed and drained
½ cup beer (not dark beer)
⅓ cup minced red or yellow onion
⅓ cup ketchup
3 tablespoons light molasses
2 teaspoons Worcestershire sauce
1 teaspoon dry mustard
½ teaspoon ground ginger
4 slices turkey bacon

1. Preheat oven to 350°F. Arrange beans in 11×7-inch glass baking dish. Combine remaining ingredients, except bacon, in medium bowl. Pour over beans; toss to coat.

2. Cut bacon into 1-inch pieces; arrange in single layer over beans. Bake, uncovered, 40 to 45 minutes or until most of liquid is absorbed and bacon is browned.
          Makes 8 servings

Nutrients per Serving: Calories: 179 (10% Calories from Fat), Total Fat: 2 g, Saturated Fat: 1 g, Protein: 10 g, Carbohydrate: 31 g, Cholesterol: 5 mg, Sodium: 728 mg, Fiber: trace, Sugar: 6 g

Dietary Exchanges: 2 Starch/Bread, ½ Fat

SAVORY SIDE DISHES

298 INDIAN–STYLE VEGETABLE STIR–FRY

1 teaspoon canola oil
1 teaspoon curry powder
1 teaspoon ground cumin
⅛ teaspoon red pepper flakes
1½ teaspoons finely chopped, seeded
    jalapeño pepper*
2 cloves garlic, minced
¾ cup chopped red bell pepper
¾ cup thinly sliced carrots
3 cups cauliflower florets
½ cup water, divided
½ teaspoon salt
2 teaspoons finely chopped cilantro
    (optional)

Jalapeño peppers can sting and irritate the skin; wear rubber gloves when handling peppers and do not touch eyes. Wash hands after handling.

1. Heat oil in large nonstick skillet over medium-high heat. Add curry powder, cumin and red pepper flakes; cook and stir about 30 seconds.

2. Stir in jalapeño and garlic. Add bell pepper and carrots; mix well to coat with spices. Add cauliflower; reduce heat to medium.

3. Stir in ¼ cup water; cook and stir until water evaporates. Add remaining ¼ cup water; cover and cook about 8 to 10 minutes or until vegetables are crisp-tender, stirring occasionally.

4. Add salt; mix well. Sprinkle with cilantro; serve immediately.   *Makes 6 servings*

Nutrients per Serving: Calories: 40 (22% Calories from Fat), Total Fat: 1 g, Saturated Fat: trace, Protein: 2 g, Carbohydrate: 7 g, Cholesterol: 0 mg, Sodium: 198 mg, Fiber: 1 g, Sugar: 1 g

Dietary Exchanges: 1½ Vegetable

299 HAWAIIAN STIR–FRY

1 can (8 ounces) pineapple chunks in juice
2 teaspoons cornstarch
1 tablespoon vegetable oil
1 red bell pepper, cut into strips
1 teaspoon curry powder
8 ounces (about 3 cups) snow peas, ends
    trimmed
⅓ cup diagonally sliced green onions
2 teaspoons reduced-sodium soy sauce

1. Drain pineapple; reserve juice. Combine juice and cornstarch in small bowl; stir to blend. Set aside.

2. Heat large skillet or wok 1 minute over medium-high heat. Add oil, pepper and curry powder; stir-fry 1 minute. Add pineapple chunks; stir-fry 1 minute. Add snow peas; stir-fry 1 minute. Add pineapple juice mixture; bring sauce to a boil. Boil 1 minute to thicken sauce.

3. Stir in green onions and soy sauce.
    Makes 6 servings

Nutrients per Serving: Calories: 77 (28% Calories from Fat), Total Fat: 3 g, Saturated Fat: trace, Protein: 2 g, Carbohydrate: 13 g, Cholesterol: 0 mg, Sodium: 61 mg, Fiber: 1 g, Sugar: 6 g

Dietary Exchanges: ½ Fruit, 1 Vegetable, ½ Fat

Hawaiian Stir-Fry

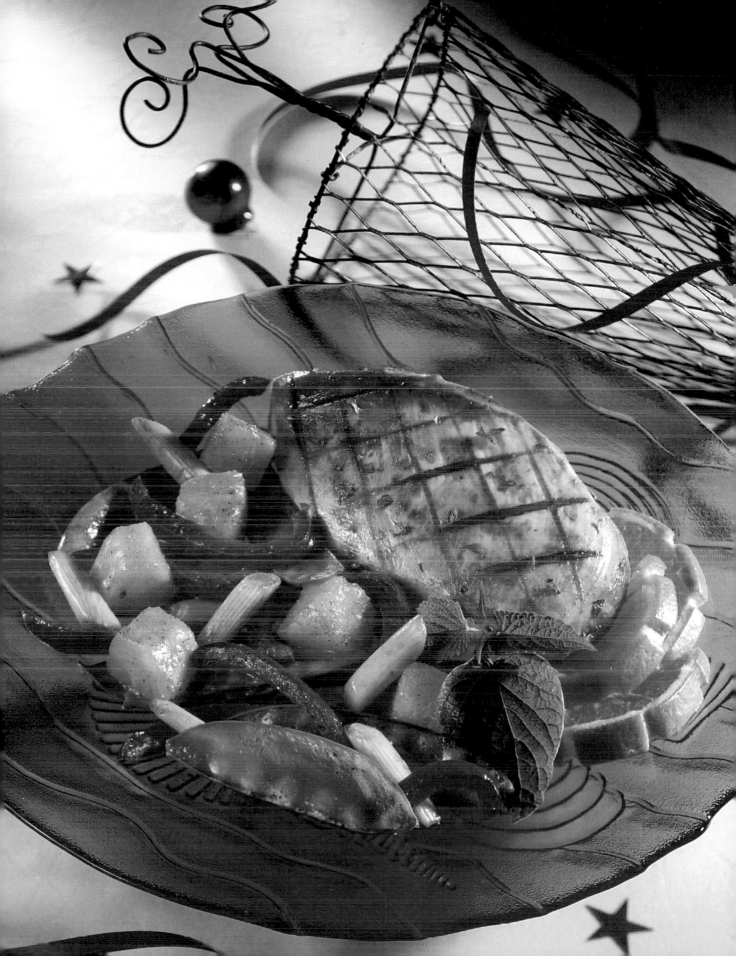

SAVORY SIDE DISHES

300 MOO SHU VEGETABLES

6 dried Chinese black mushrooms
2 tablespoons vegetable oil
2 cloves garlic, minced
2 cups shredded napa or green cabbage
1 red bell pepper, cut into short, thin strips
1 cup fresh bean sprouts or canned bean sprouts, rinsed and drained
2 large green onions, cut into short, thin strips
1 tablespoon teriyaki sauce
⅓ cup plum sauce
8 (6-inch) flour tortillas, warmed

1. Soak mushrooms in warm water 20 minutes. Drain; squeeze out excess water. Discard stems; slice caps.

2. Heat oil in wok or large nonstick skillet over medium heat until hot. Add garlic; stir-fry 30 seconds.

3. Add cabbage, mushrooms and bell pepper; stir-fry 3 minutes. Add bean sprouts and green onions; cook and stir 2 minutes. Add teriyaki sauce; stir-fry 30 seconds or until mixture is hot.

4. Spread about 2 teaspoons plum sauce on each tortilla. Spoon heaping ¼ cupful of vegetable mixture over sauce. Fold bottom of each tortilla up over filling, then fold sides over filling.   *Makes 8 servings*

Nutrients per Serving: Calories: 147 (22% Calories from Fat), Total Fat: 4 g, Saturated Fat: 1 g, Protein: 4 g, Carbohydrate: 26 g, Cholesterol: 0 mg, Sodium: 207 mg, Fiber: 2 g, Sugar: 2 g

Dietary Exchanges: 1½ Starch/Bread, 1 Vegetable, ½ Fat

301 SPICY SOUTHWESTERN VEGETABLE SAUTÉ

1 bag (16 ounces) frozen green beans
2 tablespoons water
1 tablespoon olive oil
1 red bell pepper, chopped
1 medium yellow summer squash or zucchini, chopped
1 jalapeño pepper,* seeded and chopped
½ teaspoon garlic powder
½ teaspoon ground cumin
½ teaspoon chili powder
¼ cup sliced green onions
2 tablespoons chopped fresh cilantro (optional)
1 tablespoon brown sugar

Jalapeños can sting and irritate the skin; wear rubber gloves when handling peppers and do not touch eyes. Wash hands after handling.

1. Heat large skillet over medium heat until hot; add green beans, water and oil. Cover; cook 4 minutes, stirring occasionally.

2. Add bell pepper, squash, jalapeño, garlic powder, cumin and chili powder; cook uncovered, stirring occasionally, 4 minutes or until vegetables are crisp-tender. Stir in green onions, cilantro, if desired, and brown sugar.   *Makes 6 servings*

Nutrients per Serving: Calories: 67 (30% Calories from Fat), Total Fat: 3 g, Saturated Fat: trace, Cholesterol: 0 mg, Sodium: 110 mg, Carbohydrate: 11 g, Fiber: 2 g, Protein: 2 g, Sugar: trace

Dietary Exchanges: 2 Vegetable, ½ Fat

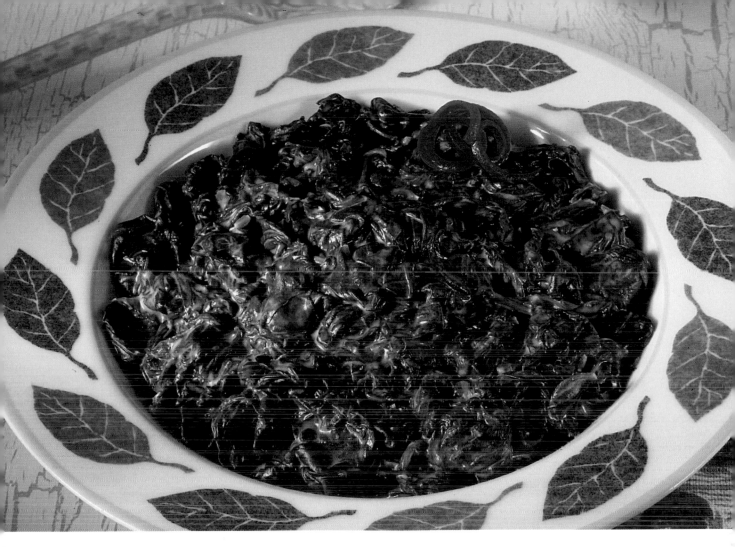

Creamed Spinach

302 CREAMED SPINACH

3 cups water
2 bags (10 ounces each) fresh spinach, washed, stemmed and chopped
2 teaspoons margarine
2 tablespoons all-purpose flour
1 cup skim milk
2 tablespoons grated Parmesan cheese
⅛ teaspoon white pepper
Ground nutmeg

1. Bring water to a boil; add spinach. Reduce heat; simmer, covered, about 5 minutes or until spinach is wilted. Drain; set aside.

2. Melt margarine in small saucepan; stir in flour and cook over medium-low heat 1 minute, stirring constantly. Gradually whisk in milk; bring to a boil. Cook, whisking constantly, 1 to 2 minutes or until mixture thickens. Stir in cheese and pepper.

3. Stir spinach into sauce; heat thoroughly. Spoon into serving bowl; sprinkle lightly with nutmeg. *Makes 4 servings*

Nutrients per Serving: Calories: 91 (30% Calories from Fat), Total Fat: 3 g, Saturated Fat: 1 g, Protein: 7 g, Carbohydrate: 10 g, Cholesterol: 3 mg, Sodium: 188 mg, Fiber: 0 g, Sugar: 3 g

Dietary Exchanges: ½ Starch/Bread, 1 Vegetable, ½ Fat

SAVORY SIDE DISHES

303 ZUCCHINI SHANGHAI STYLE

4 dried Chinese black mushrooms
½ cup fat-free reduced-sodium chicken broth
2 tablespoons ketchup
2 teaspoons dry sherry
1 teaspoon reduced-sodium soy sauce
1 teaspoon red wine vinegar
¼ teaspoon sugar
1½ teaspoons vegetable oil, divided
1 teaspoon minced fresh ginger
1 clove garlic, minced
1 large tomato, peeled, seeded and chopped
1 green onion, finely chopped
4 tablespoons water, divided
1 teaspoon cornstarch
1 pound zucchini (about 3 medium), diagonally cut into 1-inch pieces
½ small yellow onion, cut into wedges and separated

1. Soak mushrooms in warm water 20 minutes. Drain, reserving ¼ cup liquid. Squeeze out excess water. Discard stems; slice caps. Combine reserved ¼ cup mushroom liquid, chicken broth, ketchup, sherry, soy sauce, vinegar and sugar in small bowl. Set aside.

2. Heat 1 teaspoon oil in large saucepan over medium heat. Add ginger and garlic; stir-fry 10 seconds. Add mushrooms, tomato and green onion; stir-fry 1 minute. Add chicken broth mixture; bring to a boil over high heat. Reduce heat to medium; simmer 10 minutes.

3. Combine 1 tablespoon water and cornstarch in small bowl; set aside. Heat remaining ½ teaspoon oil in large nonstick skillet over medium heat. Add zucchini and yellow onion; stir-fry 30 seconds. Add remaining 3 tablespoons water. Cover and cook 3 to 4 minutes or until vegetables are

crisp-tender, stirring occasionally. Add tomato mixture to skillet. Stir cornstarch mixture and add to skillet. Cook until sauce boils and thickens.   *Makes 4 servings*

Nutrients per Serving: Calories: 72 (23% Calories from Fat), Total Fat: 2 g, Saturated Fat: trace, Protein: 3 g, Carbohydrate: 12 g, Cholesterol: 0 mg, Sodium: 156 mg, Fiber: 3 g, Sugar: 3 g

Dietary Exchanges: 2 Vegetable, 1 Fat

304 CARROT AND PARSNIP PURÉE

1 pound carrots, peeled
1 pound parsnips, peeled
1 cup chopped onion
1 cup vegetable broth
1 tablespoon margarine
⅛ teaspoon ground nutmeg

1. Cut carrots and parsnips crosswise into ½-inch pieces.

2. Combine carrots, parsnips, onion and vegetable broth in medium saucepan. Cover; bring to a boil over high heat. Reduce heat; simmer, covered, 20 to 22 minutes or until vegetables are very tender.

3. Drain vegetables, reserving broth. Combine vegetables, margarine, nutmeg and ¼ cup reserved broth in food processor; process until smooth. Serve immediately.
        Makes 10 servings

Nutrients per Serving: Calories: 78 (15% Calories from Fat), Total Fat: 1 g, Saturated Fat: trace, Protein: 1 g, Carbohydrate: 16 g, Cholesterol: 0 mg, Sodium: 56 mg, Fiber: 3 g, Sugar: trace

Dietary Exchanges: 3 Vegetable

Carrot and Parsnip Purée

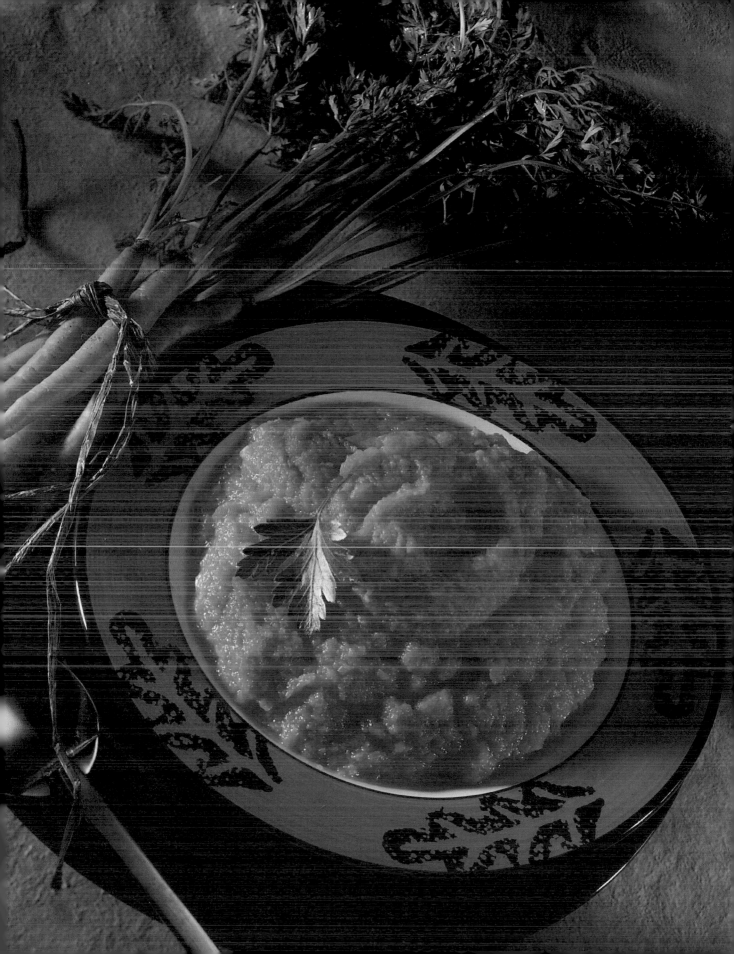

SAVORY SIDE DISHES

305 GREEN BEAN CASSEROLE

Ranch-Style White Sauce (recipe
  follows)
1 cup chopped onion
2 cloves garlic, minced
1½ cups sliced fresh mushrooms
1¼ pounds fresh green beans, cooked until
  crisp-tender
1 cup fresh bread crumbs
  Nonstick cooking spray
2 tablespoons minced parsley

1. Preheat oven to 350°F. Prepare Ranch-Style White Sauce; set aside. Spray medium skillet with nonstick cooking spray; heat over medium-high heat until hot. Add onion and garlic; cook 2 to 3 minutes or until tender. Remove half of onion mixture; set aside.

2. Add mushrooms to skillet; cook about 5 minutes or until tender. Combine mushroom mixture, beans and sauce in 1½-quart casserole.

3. Spray medium skillet with nonstick cooking spray; heat over medium heat until hot. Add bread crumbs; spray top of crumbs lightly with nonstick cooking spray. Cook 3 to 4 minutes or until crumbs are golden. Stir in reserved onion mixture and parsley. Sprinkle bread crumb mixture over casserole. Bake, uncovered, 20 to 30 minutes or until heated through.

Makes 6 servings

RANCH–STYLE WHITE SAUCE
1½ tablespoons margarine
3 tablespoons all-purpose flour
1½ cups skim milk
3 to 4 teaspoons ranch salad dressing mix
¼ to ½ teaspoon white pepper

1. Melt margarine in small saucepan over low heat. Stir in flour; cook 1 to 2 minutes, stirring constantly. Gradually whisk in milk; bring to a boil. Cook, whisking constantly, 1 to 2 minutes or until thickened. Stir in dressing mix and pepper.

Makes 1½ cups

Nutrients per Serving: Calories: 123 (24% Calories from Fat), Total Fat: 3 g, Saturated Fat: 1 g, Protein: 5 g, Carbohydrate: 19 g, Cholesterol: 1 mg, Sodium: 200 mg, Fiber: 1 g, Sugar: 4 g

Dietary Exchanges: 1 Starch/Bread, 1½ Vegetable, ½ Fat

306 BROCCOLI WITH CREAMY LEMON SAUCE

2 tablespoons fat-free mayonnaise
4½ teaspoons low-fat sour cream
1 tablespoon skim milk
1 to 1½ teaspoons lemon juice
⅛ teaspoon ground turmeric
1¼ cups hot cooked broccoli florets

Combine all ingredients except broccoli in top of double boiler. Cook over simmering water 5 minutes or until heated through, stirring constantly. Serve over hot cooked broccoli. *Makes 2 servings*

Nutrients per Serving: Calories: 44 (18% Calories from Fat), Total Fat: 1 g, Saturated Fat: trace, Protein: 2 g, Carbohydrate: 7 g, Cholesterol: 4 mg, Sodium: 216 mg, Fiber: 2 g, Sugar: 2 g

Dietary Exchanges: 2 Vegetable

Green Bean Casserole

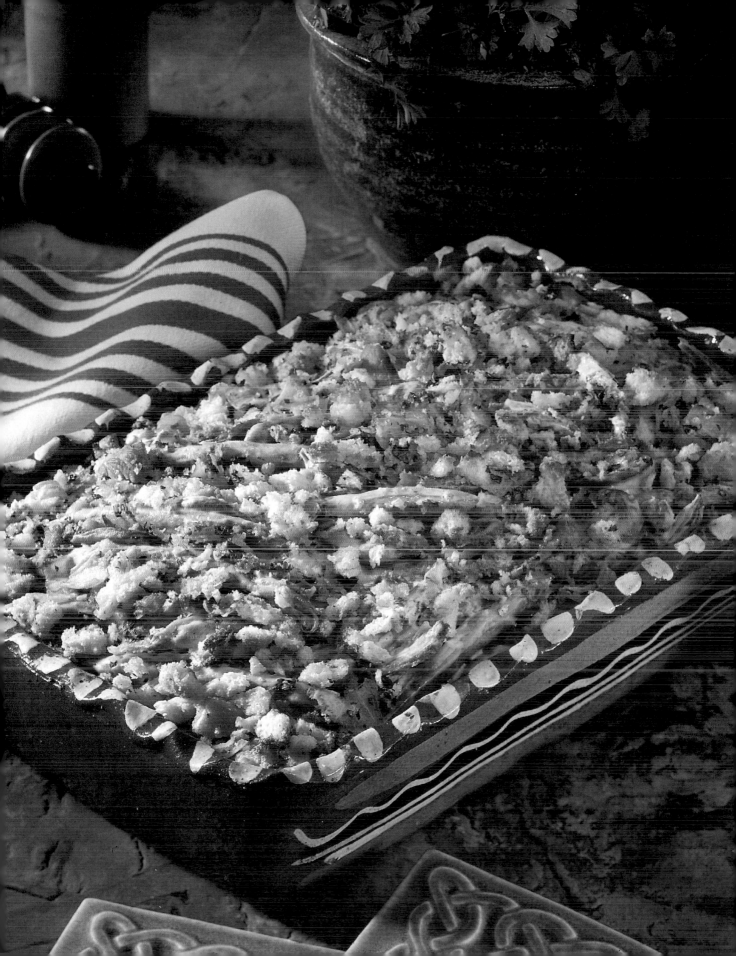

SAVORY SIDE DISHES

307 BAKED CORN TIMBALES

6 sun-dried tomatoes (not packed in oil)
2 whole eggs
2 egg whites
2 cups frozen corn, thawed
¾ cup evaporated skimmed milk
1 teaspoon salt
1 teaspoon dry mustard
1 teaspoon hot pepper sauce

1. Preheat oven to 350°F. Spray 6 (6-ounce) ramekins or small ovenproof dishes with nonstick cooking spray.

2. Place sun-dried tomatoes in small bowl; cover with hot water. Let stand 15 minutes. Drain; finely chop.

3. Beat whole eggs and egg whites in medium bowl with wire whisk until frothy. Fold in tomatoes, corn, milk, salt, mustard and hot pepper sauce until well combined. Fill ramekins ¾ full with mixture.

4. Place ramekins in large roasting pan; pour hot water around ramekins to depth of about ½ inch. Bake 35 minutes or until set and lightly browned. Invert ramekins onto serving plate to release timbales. Serve immediately. *Makes 6 servings*

Nutrients per Serving: Calories: 128 (13% Calories from Fat), Total Fat: 2 g, Saturated Fat: 1 g, Protein: 9 g, Carbohydrate: 22 g, Cholesterol: 72 mg, Sodium: 449 mg, Fiber: 2 g, Sugar: 1 g

Dietary Exchanges: 1 Starch/Bread, ½ Lean Meat, 1 Vegetable

308 SOUTHERN–STYLE SUCCOTASH

2 tablespoons margarine
1 cup chopped onion
1 package (10 ounces) frozen lima beans, thawed
1 cup frozen corn, thawed
½ cup chopped red bell pepper
1 can (15 to 16 ounces) hominy, drained
⅓ cup fat-free reduced-sodium chicken broth
½ teaspoon salt
¼ teaspoon hot pepper sauce
¼ cup chopped green onion tops or chives

1. Melt margarine in large nonstick skillet over medium heat. Add onion; cook and stir 5 minutes. Add lima beans, corn and bell pepper; cook and stir 5 minutes.

2. Add hominy, chicken broth, salt and pepper sauce; simmer 5 minutes or until most of liquid has evaporated. Remove from heat; stir in green onions.

Makes 6 servings

Nutrients per Serving: Calories: 175 (23% Calories from Fat), Total Fat: 5 g, Saturated Fat: 1 g, Protein: 6 g, Carbohydrate: 29 g, Cholesterol: 0 mg, Sodium: 406 mg, Fiber: 5 g, Sugar: 3 g

Dietary Exchanges: 2 Starch/Bread, 1 Fat

Baked Corn Timbale

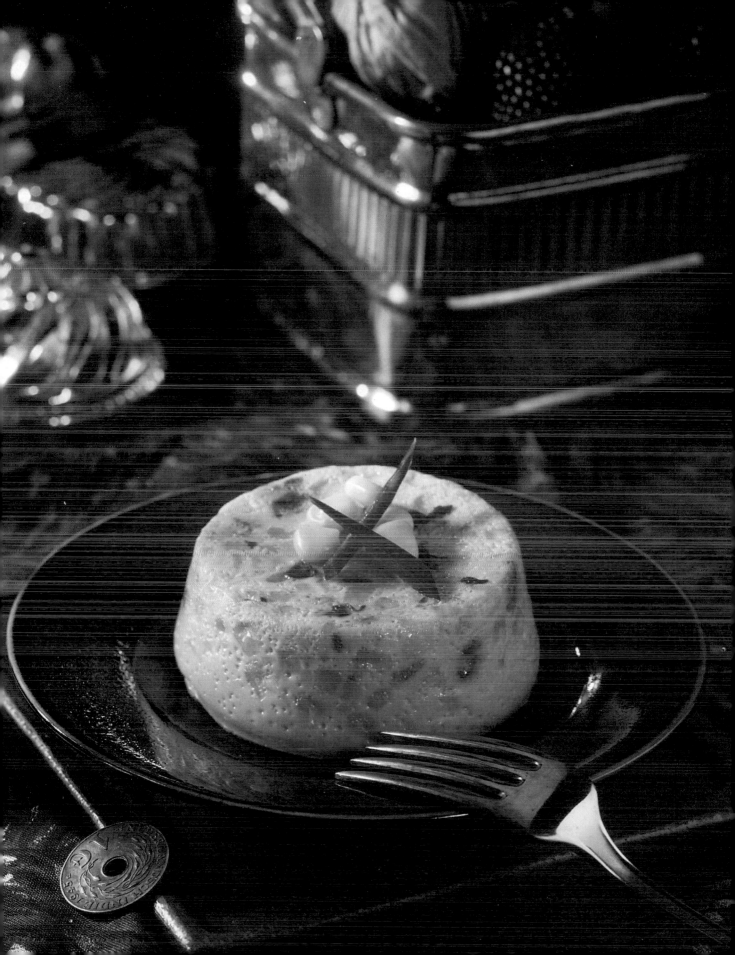

309 GLAZED MAPLE ACORN SQUASH

 1 large acorn or golden acorn squash
¼ cup water
 2 tablespoons pure maple syrup
 1 tablespoon margarine or butter, melted
¼ teaspoon cinnamon

1. Preheat oven to 375°F.

2. Cut stem and blossom ends from squash. Cut squash crosswise into four equal slices. Discard seeds and membrane. Place water in 13×9-inch baking dish. Arrange squash in dish; cover with foil. Bake 30 minutes or until tender.

3. Combine syrup, margarine and cinnamon in small bowl; mix well. Uncover squash; pour off water. Brush squash with syrup mixture, letting excess pool in center of squash.

4. Return to oven; bake 10 minutes or until syrup mixture is bubbly.

Makes 4 servings

Nutrients per Serving: Calories: 161 (16% Calories from Fat), Total Fat: 3 g, Saturated Fat: 2 g, Protein: 2 g, Carbohydrates: 35 g, Cholesterol: 8 mg, Sodium: 39 mg, Fiber: 4 g, Sugar 14 g

Dietary Exchanges: 2 Starch/Bread, ½ Fat

310 CHUNKY SPICED APPLESAUCE

3½ pounds tart cooking apples (about 8 large), peeled and chopped
½ cup water
7¼ teaspoons EQUAL® MEASURE™ or 24 packets EQUAL® sweetener or 1 cup EQUAL® SPOONFUL™
½ teaspoon ground cinnamon
¼ teaspoon ground nutmeg
 1 to 2 dashes salt

• Combine apples and water in large saucepan; heat to boiling. Reduce heat and simmer, covered, until apples are tender, 20 to 25 minutes.

• Mash apples coarsely with fork; stir in Equal®, cinnamon, nutmeg and salt. Serve warm, or refrigerate and serve chilled.

Makes 10 (½-cup) servings

NOTE: Amount of Equal® may vary depending on the tartness of the apples.

Nutrients per Serving: Calories: 104, Fat: 1 g, Protein: 0 g, Carbohydrates: 27 g, Cholesterol: 0 mg, Sodium: 14 mg

Dietary Exchanges: 1½ Fruit

Glazed Maple Acorn Squash

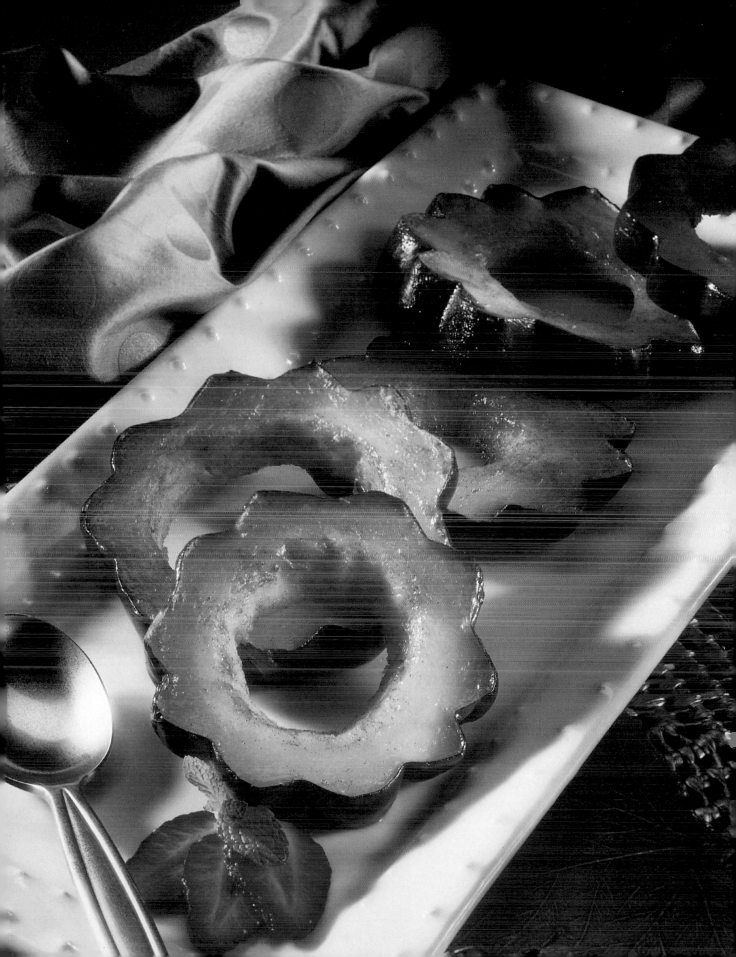

SAVORY SIDE DISHES

311 REFRIGERATOR CORN RELISH

2 cups cut fresh corn (4 ears) *or*
    1 (10-ounce) package frozen corn
½ cup vinegar
⅓ cup cold water
1 tablespoon cornstarch
¼ cup chopped onion
¼ cup chopped celery
¼ cup chopped green or red bell pepper
2 tablespoons chopped pimiento
1 teaspoon ground turmeric
½ teaspoon salt
½ teaspoon dry mustard
1¾ teaspoons EQUAL® MEASURE™ or
    6 packets EQUAL® sweetener or
    ¼ cup EQUAL® SPOONFUL™

• Cook corn in boiling water until crisp-tender, 5 to 7 minutes; drain and set aside. Combine vinegar, water and cornstarch in large saucepan; stir until cornstarch is dissolved. Add corn, onion, celery, pepper, pimiento, turmeric, salt and mustard. Cook and stir until thickened and bubbly. Cook and stir 2 minutes more. Remove from heat; stir in Equal®. Cool. Cover and store in refrigerator up to 2 weeks. Serve with beef, pork or poultry. *Makes 2½ cups*

Nutrition information per serving:
(2 tablespoons), Calories: 22, Fat: 0 g, Protein: 1 g, Carbohydrates: 5 g, Cholesterol: 0 mg, Sodium: 57 mg

Dietary Exchanges: ½ Starch/Bread

312 QUICK REFRIGERATOR SWEET PICKLES

5 cups thinly sliced cucumbers
2 cloves garlic, halved
2 cups water
1 teaspoon mustard seed
1 teaspoon celery seed
1 teaspoon ground turmeric
2 cups sliced onions
1 cup julienne carrot strips
2 cups vinegar
3 tablespoons plus 1¾ teaspoons EQUAL®
    MEASURE™ or 36 packets EQUAL®
    sweetener or 1½ cups EQUAL®
    SPOONFUL™

• Place cucumbers and garlic in glass bowl. Combine water, mustard seed, celery seed and turmeric in medium saucepan. Bring to boiling. Add onion and carrots; cook 2 minutes. Add vinegar; bring just to boiling. Remove from heat; stir in Equal®. Pour over cucumbers and garlic. Cool. Cover and chill at least 24 hours before serving. Store in refrigerator up to 2 weeks.

Makes about 6 cups

Nutrition information per serving: (¼ cup), Calories: 8, Fat: 0 g, Protein: 0 g, Carbohydrates: 3 g, Cholesterol: 0 mg, Sodium: 3 mg

Dietary Exchanges: Free Food

Left to right: *Refrigerator Corn Relish and Quick Refrigerator Sweet Pickles*

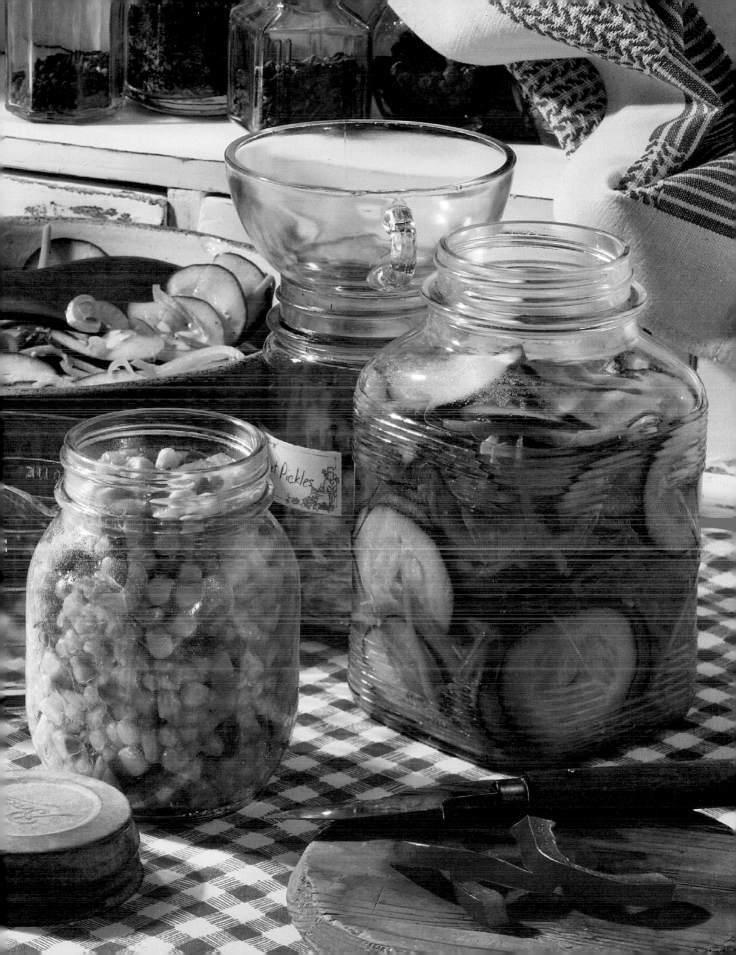

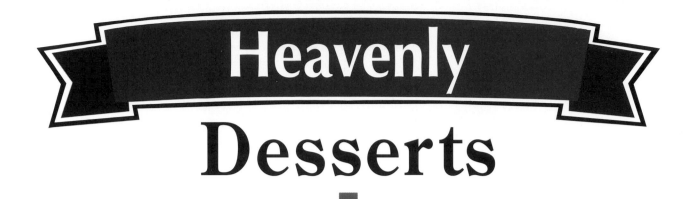

Heavenly
Desserts

313 MIXED BERRY CHEESECAKE

CRUST
1½ **cups fruit-juice-sweetened breakfast cereal flakes***
15 **dietetic butter-flavored cookies***
1 **tablespoon vegetable oil**

CHEESECAKE
2 **packages (8 ounces each) fat-free cream cheese, softened**
2 **cartons (8 ounces each) nonfat raspberry yogurt**
1 **package (8 ounces) Neufchâtel cheese, softened**
½ **cup all-fruit seedless blackberry preserves**
½ **cup all-fruit blueberry preserves**
6 **packages artificial sweetener *or* equivalent of ¼ cup sugar**
1 **tablespoon vanilla**
¼ **cup water**
1 **package (0.3 ounce) sugar-free strawberry-flavored gelatin**

TOPPING
3 **cups fresh or frozen unsweetened mixed berries, thawed**

*Available in the health food section of supermarkets.

1. Preheat oven to 400°F. Spray 10-inch springform pan with nonstick cooking spray.

2. To prepare crust, combine cereal, cookies and oil in food processor; process with on/off pulses until finely crushed. Press firmly onto bottom and ½ inch up side of pan. Bake 5 to 8 minutes or until crust is golden brown.

3. To prepare cheesecake, combine cream cheese, yogurt, Neufchatel cheese, preserves, artificial sweetener and vanilla in large bowl. Beat at high speed until smooth.

4. Combine water and gelatin in small microwavable bowl; microwave at HIGH for 30 seconds to 1 minute or until water is boiling and gelatin is dissolved. Cool slightly. Add to cheese mixture; beat 2 to 3 minutes or until well blended. Pour into springform pan; cover and refrigerate at least 24 hours. Top cheesecake with berries before serving.
Makes 12 servings

Nutrients per Serving: Calories: 248 (25% Calories from Fat), Total Fat: 7 g, Saturated Fat: 3 g, Protein: 10 g, Carbohydrate: 35 g, Cholesterol: 15 mg, Sodium: 386 mg, Fiber: 2 g, Sugar: 6 g

Dietary Exchanges: ½ Starch/Bread, 1 Lean Meat, 2 Fruit, ½ Fat

Mixed Berry Cheesecake

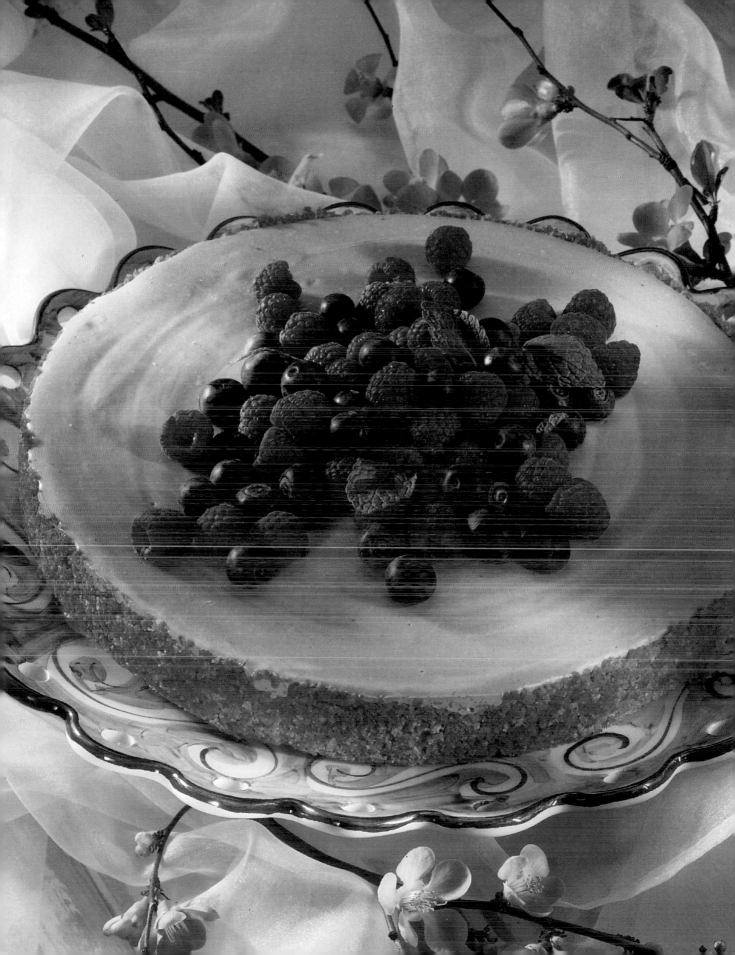

HEAVENLY DESSERTS

314 ORANGE CHIFFON CHEESECAKE

2 cups graham cracker crumbs
8 tablespoons light margarine, melted
1 teaspoon EQUAL® MEASURE™ or
    3 packets EQUAL® sweetener or
    2 tablespoons EQUAL® SPOONFUL™
1 cup orange juice
1 envelope (¼ ounce) unflavored gelatin
12 ounces reduced-fat cream cheese,
    softened
1 cup part-skim ricotta cheese
3½ teaspoons EQUAL® MEASURE™ or
    12 packets EQUAL® sweetener or
    ½ cup EQUAL® SPOONFUL™
2 cups light whipped topping
2 medium oranges, peeled, seeded and
    chopped
    Orange sections (optional)

• Spray 9-inch springform pan with nonstick cooking spray. Mix graham cracker crumbs, margarine and 1 teaspoon Equal® Measure™ or 3 packets Equal® sweetener or 2 tablespoons Equal® Spoonful™. Pat mixture evenly on bottom and halfway up side of pan. Bake in preheated 350°F oven 8 to 10 minutes or until set. Cool.

• Pour orange juice into small saucepan. Sprinkle gelatin over orange juice and let soften 1 minute. Heat, stirring constantly, until gelatin dissolves, about 3 minutes. Blend cream cheese and ricotta cheese in large bowl until smooth; stir in 3½ teaspoons Equal® Measure™ or 12 packets Equal® sweetener or ½ cup Equal® Spoonful™. Add gelatin mixture to cheese mixture; blend until smooth. Fold whipped topping into cheese mixture. Stir in chopped oranges. Spoon into prepared crust and spread evenly.

• Chill 6 hours or overnight. Remove side of pan; place cheesecake on serving plate. Garnish with orange sections, if desired.

Makes 16 servings

Nutrients per Serving: Calories: 204, Fat: 11 g, Protein: 6 g, Carbohydrates: 20 g, Cholesterol: 17 mg, Sodium: 209 mg

Dietary Exchanges: 1 Starch/Bread, ½ Milk, 2 Fat

315 TURTLE CHEESECAKE

6 tablespoons reduced-calorie margarine
1½ cups graham cracker crumbs
2 envelopes unflavored gelatin
2 packages (8 ounces each) fat-free cream
    cheese
2 cups 1% low-fat cottage cheese
1 cup sugar
1½ teaspoons vanilla
1 container (8 ounces) thawed reduced-fat
    nondairy whipped topping
¼ cup prepared fat-free caramel topping
¼ cup prepared fat-free hot fudge topping
¼ cup chopped pecans

1. Preheat oven to 350°F. Spray bottom and side of 9-inch springform pan with nonstick cooking spray. Melt margarine in small saucepan over medium heat; stir in graham cracker crumbs. Press crumb mixture firmly onto bottom and side of prepared pan; bake 10 minutes. Cool.

2. Place ½ cup cold water in small saucepan; sprinkle gelatin over water. Let stand 3 minutes to soften. Heat gelatin mixture over low heat until completely dissolved, stirring constantly.

HEAVENLY DESSERTS

3. Combine cream cheese, cottage cheese, sugar and vanilla in food processor or blender; process until smooth. Add gelatin mixture; process until well blended. Fold in whipped topping; pour into prepared crust. Refrigerate 4 hours or until set.

4. Loosen cake from side of pan. Remove side of pan from cake. Drizzle caramel and hot fudge toppings over cake; sprinkle pecans evenly over top of cake before serving.   *Makes 16 servings*

Nutrients per Serving: Calories: 231 (26% Calories from Fat), Total Fat: 7 g, Saturated Fat: 3 g, Protein: 9 g, Carbohydrate: 33 g, Cholesterol: 1 mg, Sodium: 419 mg, Fiber: trace, Sugar: 18 g

Dietary Exchanges: 2 Starch/Bread, ½ Lean Meat, 1 Fat

Turtle Cheesecake

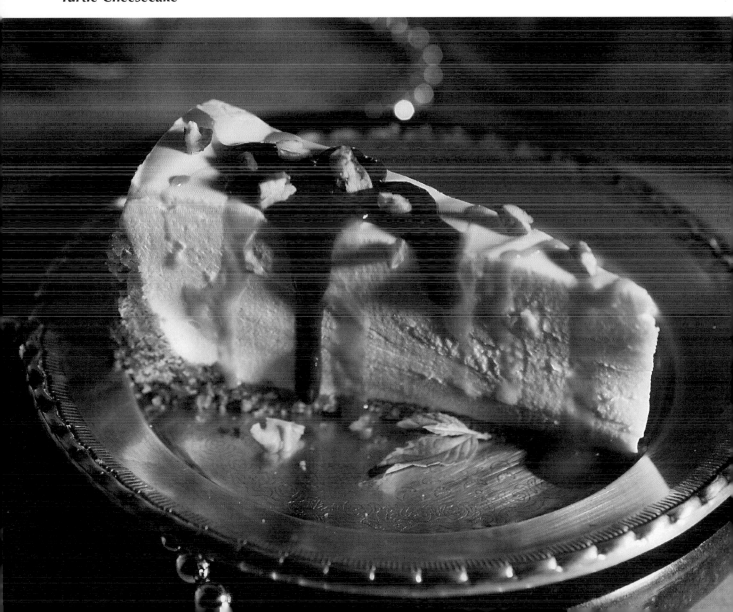

HEAVENLY DESSERTS

316 CHOCOLATE–BERRY CHEESECAKE

1 cup chocolate wafer crumbs
1 container (12 ounces) fat-free cream cheese
1 package (8 ounces) Neufchâtel cheese
²⁄₃ cup sugar
½ cup cholesterol-free egg substitute
3 tablespoons skim milk
1¼ teaspoons vanilla
1 cup mini semisweet chocolate chips
2 tablespoons all-fruit raspberry preserves
2½ cups fresh strawberries, hulled and halved

1. Preheat oven to 350°F. Spray bottom of 9-inch springform pan with nonstick cooking spray.

2. Press chocolate wafer crumbs firmly onto bottom and side of prepared pan. Bake 10 minutes. Remove from oven; cool. *Reduce oven temperature to 325°F.*

3. Combine cheeses in large bowl with electric mixer; beat at medium speed until well blended. Beat in sugar until well blended. Beat in egg substitute, milk and vanilla until well blended. Stir in mini chips with spoon; pour batter into pan.

4. Bake 40 minutes or until center is set. Remove from oven; cool 10 minutes in pan on wire rack. Carefully loosen cheesecake from edge of pan. Cool completely.

5. Remove side of pan from cake. Blend preserves and 2 tablespoons water in medium bowl until smooth. Add strawberries; toss to coat. Arrange strawberries on top of cake. Refrigerate 1 hour before serving.

Makes 16 servings

Nutrients per Serving: Calories: 197, (29% Calories from Fat), Total Fat: 7 g, Saturated Fat: 2 g, Protein: 7 g, Carbohydrate: 29 g, Cholesterol: 7 mg, Sodium: 290 mg, Fiber: trace, Sugar: 20 g

Dietary Exchanges: 1 Starch/Bread, ½ Lean Meat, 1 Fruit, 1 Fat

317 RICH CHOCOLATE CHEESECAKE

1¼ cups graham cracker crumbs
4 tablespoons margarine, melted
1 teaspoon EQUAL® MEASURE™ or
    3 packets EQUAL® sweetener or
    2 tablespoons EQUAL® SPOONFUL™
2 packages (8 ounces each) reduced-fat cream cheese, softened
1 package (8 ounces) fat-free cream cheese, softened
5½ teaspoons EQUAL® MEASURE™ or
    18 packets EQUAL® sweetener or
    ¾ cup EQUAL® SPOONFUL™
2 eggs
2 egg whites
2 tablespoons cornstarch
1 cup reduced-fat sour cream
⅓ cup European or Dutch-process cocoa
1 teaspoon vanilla
    Fresh mint sprigs, raspberries, nonfat whipped topping and orange peel (optional)

• Mix graham cracker crumbs, margarine and 1 teaspoon Equal® Measure™ *or* 3 packets Equal® sweetener *or* 2 tablespoons Equal® Spoonful™ in bottom of 9-inch springform pan. Pat mixture evenly on bottom and ½ inch up side of pan.

• Beat cream cheese and 5½ teaspoons Equal® Measure™ *or* 18 packets Equal® sweetener *or* ¾ cup Equal® Spoonful™ in

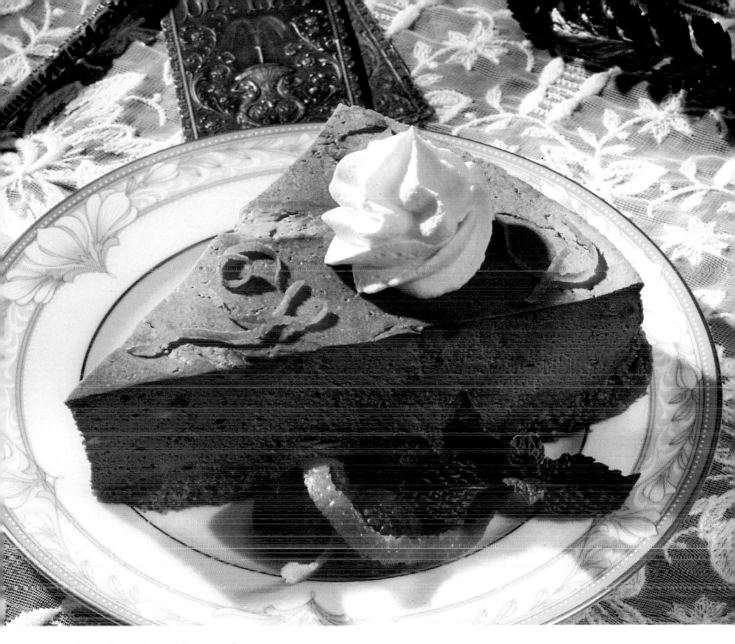

Rich Chocolate Cheesecake

large bowl until fluffy; beat in eggs, egg whites and cornstarch. Mix in sour cream, cocoa and vanilla until well blended. Pour mixture into crust.

• Place cheesecake in roasting pan on oven rack; add 1 inch hot water to roasting pan. Bake cheesecake in preheated 300°F oven just until set in the center, 45 to 50 minutes. Remove cheesecake from roasting pan; return cheesecake to oven. Turn oven off

and let cheesecake cool 3 hours in oven with door ajar. Refrigerate 8 hours or overnight. Remove side of pan; place cheesecake on serving plate. Garnish, if desired.

Makes 16 servings

Nutrients per Serving: Calories: 189, Fat: 11 g, Protein: 8 g, Carbohydrates: 14 g, Cholesterol: 51 mg, Sodium: 280 mg

Dietary Exchanges: 1 Milk, 2 Fat

HEAVENLY DESSERTS

318 BLUEBERRY CHIFFON CAKE

3 tablespoons reduced-calorie margarine
¾ cup graham cracker crumbs
2 cups fresh or thawed frozen blueberries
2 envelopes unflavored gelatin
2 containers (8 ounces each) fat-free cream cheese
1 container (8 ounces) Neufchâtel cheese
¾ cup sugar, divided
⅔ cup nonfat sour cream
½ cup lemon juice
1 tablespoon grated lemon peel
6 egg whites*

Use only grade A clean, uncracked eggs.

1. Preheat oven to 350°F.

2. Melt margarine in small saucepan over medium heat; stir in graham cracker crumbs. Press crumb mixture firmly onto bottom and 1 inch up side of 9-inch springform pan; bake 10 minutes. Remove from oven; cool 10 minutes. Arrange blueberries in a single layer on top of crust; refrigerate.

3. Place ½ cup cold water in small saucepan; sprinkle gelatin over water. Let stand 3 minutes to soften; heat over low heat until completely dissolved, stirring constantly.

4. Beat cheeses and ½ cup sugar in large bowl at medium speed until well blended. Beat in sour cream, lemon juice and lemon peel. Beat in gelatin mixture.

5. With clean, dry beaters, beat egg whites in medium bowl at medium speed until soft peaks form. Gradually add remaining ¼ cup sugar; beat at high speed until stiff peaks form. Fold egg whites into cream cheese mixture; spoon mixture into prepared crust. Cover; refrigerate 6 hours or until firm.

Makes 16 servings

Nutrients per Serving: Calories: 165 (28% Calories from Fat), Total Fat: 5 g, Saturated Fat: 2 g, Protein: 10 g, Carbohydrate: 20 g, Cholesterol: 14 mg, Sodium: 342 mg, Fiber: 1 g, Sugar: 10 g

Dietary Exchanges: ½ Starch/Bread, 1 Lean Meat, 1 Fruit, ½ Fat

319 BROWNIE CAKE DELIGHT

1 package reduced-fat fudge brownie mix
⅓ cup all-fruit strawberry preserves
2 cups thawed reduced-fat nondairy whipped topping
¼ teaspoon almond extract
2 cups strawberries, hulled and halved
¼ cup chocolate sauce

1. Prepare brownies according to package directions, substituting 11×7-inch baking pan. Cool completely in pan.

2. Whisk preserves in small bowl until smooth. Combine whipped topping and almond extract in medium bowl.

3. Cut brownie crosswise in half. Place half of brownie, flat-side down, on serving dish; spread with preserves and 1 cup whipped topping. Place second half of brownie, flat-side down, over bottom layer; spread with remaining whipped topping. Arrange strawberries on whipped topping. Drizzle chocolate sauce onto cake before serving.

Makes 16 servings

Nutrients per Serving: Calories: 193 (14% Calories from Fat), Total Fat: 3 g, Saturated Fat: trace, Protein: 2 g, Carbohydrate: 41 g, Cholesterol: trace, Sodium: 140 mg, Fiber: trace, Sugar: 9 g

Dietary Exchanges: 2 Starch/Bread, ½ Fruit, ½ Fat

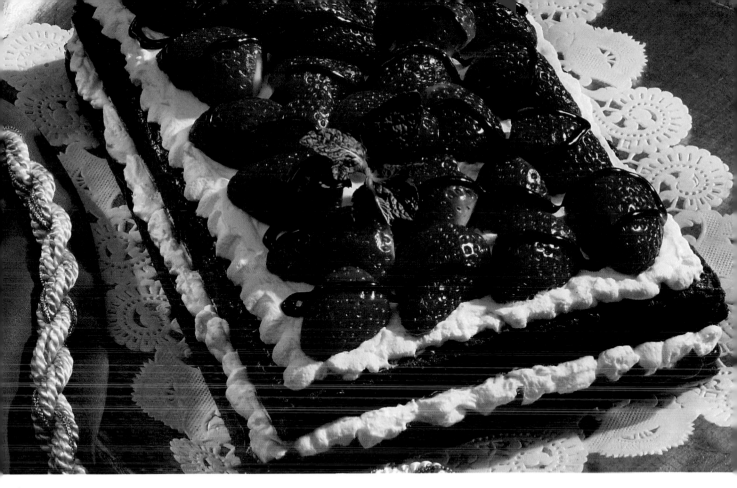

Brownie Cake Delight

320 DATE CAKE SQUARES

1¼ cups water
 1 cup chopped dates
 ¾ cup chopped pitted prunes
 ½ cup dark raisins
 8 tablespoons margarine, cut into pieces
 2 eggs
 1 teaspoon vanilla
 1 cup all-purpose flour
5½ teaspoons EQUAL® MEASURE™ or
   18 packets EQUAL® sweetener or
   ¾ cup EQUAL® SPOONFUL™
 1 teaspoon baking soda
 ½ teaspoon ground cinnamon
 ¼ teaspoon ground nutmeg
 ¼ teaspoon salt
 ¼ cup chopped walnuts

• Combine water, dates, prunes, and raisins in medium saucepan; heat to boiling. Reduce heat and simmer, uncovered, until fruit is tender and water is absorbed, about 10 minutes. Remove from heat and add margarine, stirring until melted; cool to room temperature.

• Mix eggs and vanilla into fruit mixture; mix in combined flour, Equal®, baking soda, cinnamon, nutmeg and salt. Spread batter evenly in greased 11×7×2-inch baking dish; sprinkle with walnuts.

• Bake in preheated 350°F oven until cake springs back when touched lightly, 30 to 35 minutes. Cool on wire rack; cut into squares.   *Makes 2 dozen squares*

Nutrients per Serving: (1 square),
Calories: 117, Fat: 5 g, Protein: 2 g,
Carbohydrate: 17 g, Cholesterol: 18 mg,
Sodium: 126 mg

Dietary Exchanges: ½ Bread, ½ Fruit, 1 Fat

HEAVENLY DESSERTS

321 MAPLE PUMPKIN PIE

1⅓ cups all-purpose flour
⅓ cup plus 1 tablespoon sugar, divided
¾ teaspoon salt, divided
2 tablespoons vegetable shortening
2 tablespoons margarine
4 to 5 tablespoons ice water
1 can (15 ounces) solid-pack pumpkin
2 egg whites
1 cup evaporated skimmed milk
⅓ cup maple syrup
1 teaspoon ground cinnamon
½ teaspoon ground ginger

1. Combine flour, 1 tablespoon sugar and ¼ teaspoon salt in medium bowl; cut in shortening and margarine with pastry blender or two knives until mixture forms coarse crumbs. Mix in ice water, 1 tablespoon at a time, until mixture comes together and forms a soft dough. Wrap in plastic wrap; refrigerate 30 minutes.

2. Preheat oven to 425°F. Roll out pastry on floured surface to ⅛-inch thickness; cut into 12-inch circle. Ease pastry into 9-inch pie plate; turn edge under and flute edge.

3. Combine pumpkin, remaining ⅓ cup sugar, egg whites, milk, syrup, cinnamon, ginger and remaining ½ teaspoon salt in large bowl; mix well. Pour into unbaked pie shell. Bake 15 minutes; *reduce oven temperature to 350°F.* Continue baking 45 to 50 minutes or until center is set. Transfer to wire cooling rack; let stand at least 30 minutes before serving.

Makes 10 servings

Nutrients per Serving: Calories: 198 (22% Calories from Fat), Total Fat: 5 g, Saturated Fat: 1 g, Protein: 5 g, Carbohydrate: 34 g, Cholesterol: 1 mg, Sodium: 231 mg, Fiber: 2 g, Sugar: 14 g

Dietary Exchanges: 2 Starch/Bread, 1 Fat

322 CHERRY LATTICE PIE

2 packages (16 ounces each) frozen no-sugar-added pitted cherries
12¾ teaspoons EQUAL® MEASURE™ or
    42 packets EQUAL® sweetener or
    1¾ cups EQUAL® SPOONFUL™
4 teaspoons all-purpose flour
4 teaspoons cornstarch
¼ teaspoon ground nutmeg
5 to 7 drops red food color
    Reduced-Fat Pie Pastry (2 recipes for double crust) (page 289) or favorite pastry for double crust 9-inch pie

• Thaw cherries completely in strainer set in bowl; reserve ¾ cup cherry juice. Mix Equal®, flour, cornstarch and nutmeg in small saucepan; stir in cherry juice and heat to boiling. Boil, stirring constantly, 1 minute. Remove from heat and stir in cherries; stir in food color.

• Roll half of pastry on floured surface into circle 1 inch larger than inverted 9-inch pie pan; ease pastry into pan. Pour cherry mixture into pastry. Roll remaining pastry on floured surface to ⅛-inch thickness; cut into 10 to 12 strips, ½ inch wide. Arrange pastry strips over filling and weave into lattice design. Trim ends of lattice strips; fold edge of lower crust over ends of lattice strips. Seal and flute edge.

• Bake in preheated 425°F oven until pastry is browned, 35 to 40 minutes. Cool on wire rack. *Makes 8 servings*

Nutrients per Serving: Calories: 330, Fat: 12 g, Protein: 5 g, Carbohydrate: 51 g, Cholesterol: 0 mg, Sodium: 269 mg

Dietary Exchanges: 2 Starch/Bread, 1½ Fruit, 2½ Fat

Cherry Lattice Pie

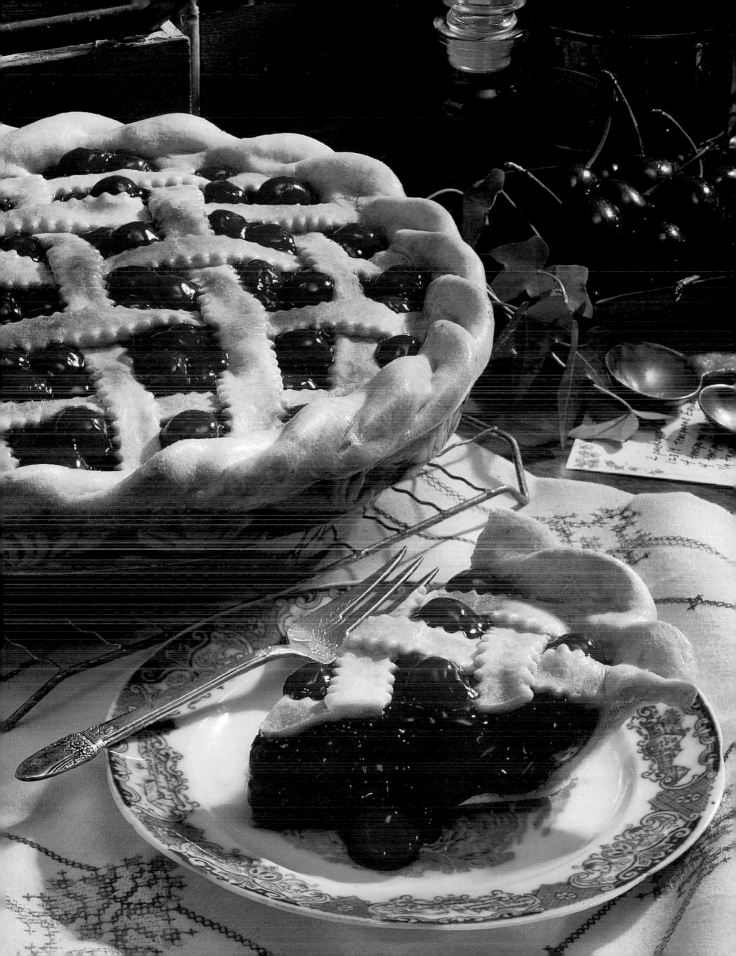

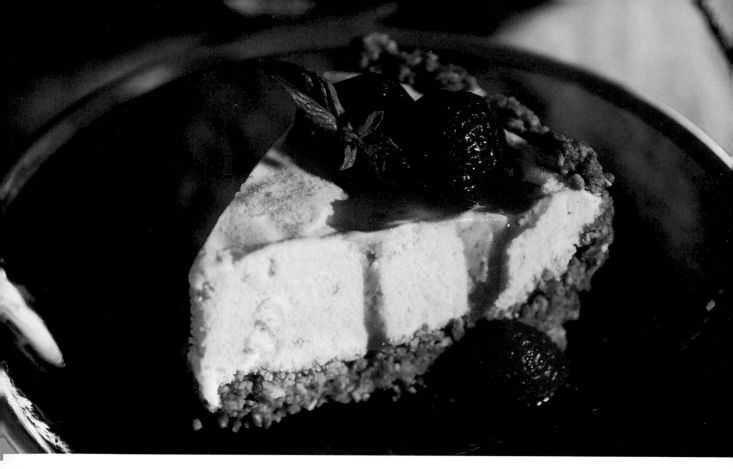

Strawberry Margarita Pie

323 STRAWBERRY MARGARITA PIE

3 tablespoons margarine
2 tablespoons honey
1½ cups crushed pretzels
3 cups low-fat sugar-free strawberry
frozen yogurt, softened
1½ cups thawed reduced-fat nondairy
whipped topping
2 teaspoons grated lime peel, divided
1 package (16 ounces) strawberries in
syrup, thawed
1 tablespoon lime juice
1 tablespoon tequila (optional)

1. Combine margarine and honey in medium microwavable bowl; microwave on HIGH 30 seconds or until smooth when stirred. Add pretzels; stir until evenly coated. Press onto bottom and side of 9-inch pie plate; freeze 30 minutes or until firm.

2. Combine frozen yogurt, whipped topping and 1 teaspoon lime peel in medium bowl; fold with rubber spatula. Spoon into crust; freeze 2 hours or until firm.

3. Combine strawberries, lime juice and remaining 1 teaspoon lime peel in small bowl; stir to blend.

4. Cut pie into 8 slices; serve with strawberry mixture. Add tequila to strawberry mixture just before serving, if desired. *Makes 8 servings*

Nutrients per Serving: Calories: 306 (23% Calories from Fat), Total Fat: 8 g, Saturated Fat: 3 g, Protein: 5 g, Carbohydrate: 56 g, Cholesterol: 19 mg, Sodium: 390 mg, Fiber: 3 g, Sugar: 26 g

Dietary Exchanges: 2½ Starch/Bread, 1 Fruit, 1½ Fat

HEAVENLY DESSERTS

324 BLUEBERRY LATTICE PIE

6 cups fresh blueberries or 2 packages
    (16 ounces each) frozen unsweetened
    blueberries
3 tablespoons lemon juice
6 tablespoons cornstarch
8 teaspoons EQUAL® MEASURE™ or
    27 packets EQUAL® sweetener or
    1 cup plus 2 tablespoons EQUAL®
    SPOONFUL™
Reduced-Fat Pie Pastry (recipe follows),
    (2 recipes for double crust) or favorite
    pastry for double crust 9-inch pie

• Toss blueberries and lemon juice in large
bowl. Sprinkle with combined cornstarch
and Equal® and toss to coat. Let stand
30 minutes.

• Roll half of pastry on lightly floured
surface into circle 1 inch larger than
inverted 9 inch pie pan. Ease pastry into
pan; trim within 1 inch of edge of pan. Roll
remaining pastry to ⅛-inch thickness; cut
into 10 to 12 strips, ½ inch wide.

• Pour blueberry mixture into pastry.
Arrange pastry strips over filling and weave
into lattice design. Trim ends of lattice
strips; fold edge of lower crust over ends of
lattice strips. Seal and flute edge.

• Bake in preheated 425°F oven until crust is
browned and filling is bubbly, about 1 hour.
Cover edge of crust with aluminum foil if
browning too quickly. Cool on wire rack;
refrigerate leftovers.   *Makes 8 servings*

Nutrients per Serving: Calories: 345, Fat: 12 g,
Protein: 5 g, Carbohydrate: 55 g,
Cholesterol: 0 mg, Sodium: 143 mg

Dietary Exchanges: 2 Starch/Bread, 1½ Fruit,
2½ Fat

REDUCED-FAT PIE PASTRY
1¼ cups all-purpose flour
    1 teaspoon EQUAL® MEASURE™ or
        3 packets EQUAL® sweetener or
        2 tablespoons EQUAL® SPOONFUL™
    ¼ teaspoon salt
    4 tablespoons cold margarine, cut into
        pieces
    5 to 5½ tablespoons ice water

• Combine flour, Equal® and salt in medium
bowl; cut in margarine with pastry blender
until mixture resembles coarse crumbs. Mix
in water, 1 tablespoon at a time, stirring
lightly with fork after each addition until
dough is formed. Wrap and refrigerate until
ready to use.

• For prebaked crust, roll pastry on lightly
floured surface into circle 1 inch larger than
inverted 9-inch pie pan. Ease pastry into
pan; trim and flute edge. Pierce bottom and
side of pastry with fork. Bake in preheated
425°F oven until pastry is browned, 10 to
15 minutes. Cool on wire rack.
               Makes pastry for 9-inch pie
                         (8 servings)

TIP: Double recipe for double-crust or lattice
pies.

Nutrients per Serving: Calories: 123, Fat: 6 g,
Protein: 2 g, Carbohydrate: 15 g,
Cholesterol: 0 mg, Sodium: 134 mg

Dietary Exchanges: 1 Starch/Bread, 1 Fat

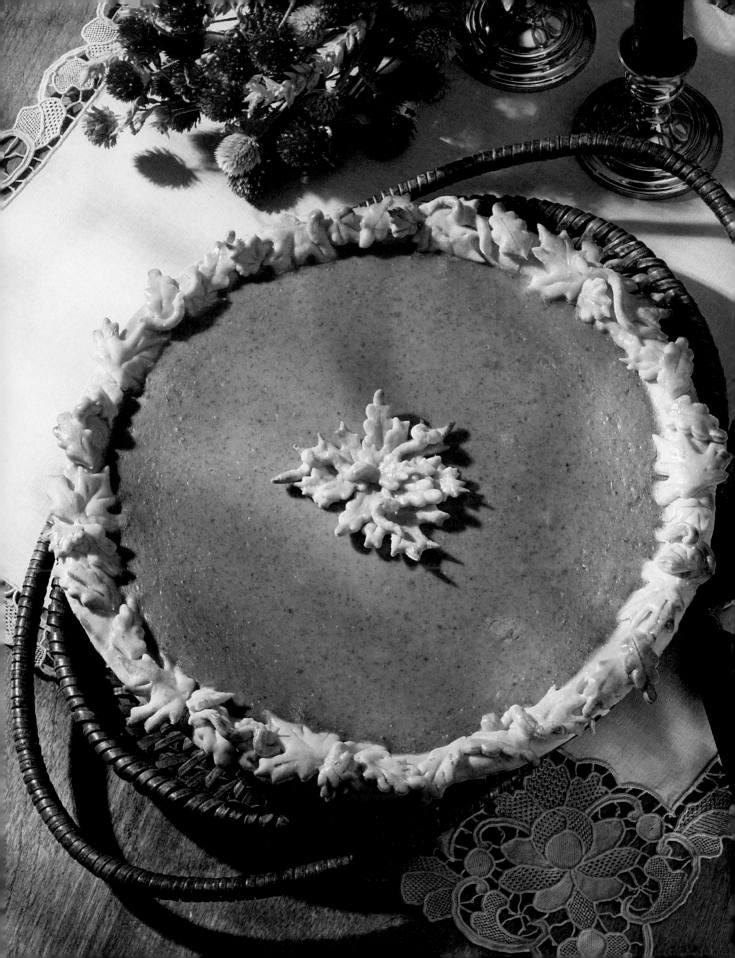

HEAVENLY DESSERTS

325 CHOCOLATE CREAM PIE

Reduced-Fat Pie Pastry (page 289) or
favorite pastry for 9-inch pie
⅓ cup cornstarch
¼ to ⅓ cup European or Dutch-process
cocoa
10¾ teaspoons EQUAL® MEASURE™ or
36 packets EQUAL® sweetener or
1½ cups EQUAL® SPOONFUL™
⅛ teaspoon salt
3 cups skim milk
2 eggs
2 egg whites
1 teaspoon vanilla
8 tablespoons thawed frozen light
whipped topping
Chocolate leaves (optional)

• Roll pastry on lightly floured surface into circle 1 inch larger than inverted 9-inch pie pan. Ease pastry into pan; trim and flute edge. Pierce bottom and side of pastry with fork. Bake in preheated 425°F oven until crust is browned, 10 to 15 minutes. Cool on wire rack.

• Combine cornstarch, cocoa, Equal® and salt in medium saucepan; stir in milk. Heat to boiling over medium-high heat, whisking constantly. Boil until thickened, about 1 minute.

• Beat eggs and egg whites in small bowl; whisk about 1 cup chocolate mixture into eggs. Whisk egg mixture into chocolate mixture in saucepan. Cook over very low heat, whisking constantly, 30 to 60 seconds. Remove from heat; stir in vanilla.

• Spread hot filling in baked crust; refrigerate until chilled and set, about 6 hours. Cut into wedges and place on serving plates; garnish each serving with dollop of whipped topping and chocolate leaves, if desired.   *Makes 8 servings*

Nutrients per Serving: Calories: 234, Fat: 8 g, Protein: 8 g, Carbohydrate: 32 g, Cholesterol: 55 mg, Sodium: 245 mg

Dietary Exchanges: 1½ Starch/Bread, ½ Milk, 1½ Fat

326 SPICED PUMPKIN PIE

Reduced-Fat Pie Pastry (page 289) or
favorite pastry for 9-inch pie
1 can (16 ounces) pumpkin
1 can (12 ounces) evaporated skim milk
3 eggs
5½ teaspoons EQUAL® MEASURE™ or
18 packets EQUAL® sweetener or
¾ cup EQUAL® SPOONFUL™
¼ teaspoon salt
1 teaspoon ground cinnamon
½ teaspoon ground ginger
¼ teaspoon ground nutmeg
⅛ teaspoon ground cloves

• Roll pastry on floured surface into circle 1 inch larger than inverted 9-inch pie pan. Ease into pan; trim and flute edge.

• Beat pumpkin, evaporated milk and eggs in medium bowl; beat in remaining ingredients. Pour into pastry shell. Bake in preheated 425°F oven 15 minutes; reduce heat to 350°F and bake until knife inserted near center comes out clean, about 40 minutes. Cool on wire rack.   *Makes 8 servings*

Nutrients per Serving: Calories: 219, Fat: 8 g, Protein: 9 g, Carbohydrate: 28 g, Cholesterol: 81 mg, Sodium: 282 mg

Dietary Exchanges: 2 Starch/Bread, 1½ Fat

Spiced Pumpkin Pie

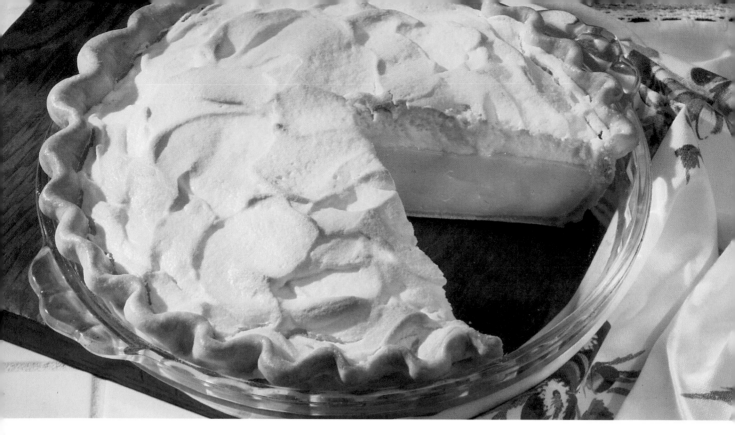

Mom's Lemon Meringue Pie

327 MOM'S LEMON MERINGUE PIE

Reduced-Fat Pie Pastry (page 289) or
favorite pastry for 9-inch pie
2¼ cups water
½ cup lemon juice
10¾ teaspoons EQUAL® MEASURE™ or
    36 packets EQUAL® sweetener or
    1½ cups EQUAL® SPOONFUL™
⅓ cup plus 2 tablespoons cornstarch
2 eggs
2 egg whites
1 teaspoon finely grated lemon peel
    (optional)
2 tablespoons margarine
1 to 2 drops yellow food color (optional)
3 egg whites
¼ teaspoon cream of tartar
3½ teaspoons EQUAL® MEASURE™ or
    12 packets EQUAL® sweetener*

EQUAL® SPOONFUL™ cannot be used in meringue recipes.

• Roll pastry on lightly floured surface into circle 1 inch larger than inverted 9-inch pie pan. Ease pastry into pan; trim and flute edge. Pierce bottom and side of pastry with fork. Bake in preheated 425°F oven until pastry is browned, 10 to 15 minutes. Cool on wire rack.

• Mix water, lemon juice, 10¾ teaspoons Equal® Measure™ or 36 packets Equal® sweetener or 1½ cups Equal® Spoonful™ and cornstarch in medium saucepan. Heat to boiling over medium-high heat, stirring constantly; boil and stir 1 minute. Beat eggs and 2 egg whites in small bowl; stir in about half of hot cornstarch mixture. Stir egg mixture back into remaining cornstarch mixture in saucepan; cook and stir over low heat 1 minute. Remove from heat; add margarine, stirring until melted. Stir in food color, if desired. Pour mixture into baked pie shell.

• Beat 3 egg whites in medium bowl with electric mixer until foamy; add cream of

HEAVENLY DESSERTS

tartar and beat to soft peaks. Gradually beat in 3½ teaspoons Equal® Measure™ *or* 12 packets Equal® sweetener, beating until stiff peaks form. Spread meringue over hot lemon filling, carefully sealing to edge of crust to prevent shrinking or weeping.

• Bake pie in preheated 425°F oven until meringue is browned, about 5 minutes. Cool completely on wire rack before cutting.

Makes 8 servings

Nutrients per Serving: Calories: 233, Fat: 10 g, Protein: 6 g, Carbohydrate: 29 g, Cholesterol: 53 mg, Sodium: 223 mg

Dietary Exchanges: 2 Starch/Bread, 2 Fat

328 COCONUT CUSTARD PIE

Reduced-Fat Pie Pastry (page 289) or favorite pastry for 9-inch pie
4 eggs
¼ teaspoon salt
2 cups skim milk
5½ teaspoons EQUAL® MEASURE™ or
   18 packets EQUAL® sweetener or
   ¾ cup EQUAL® SPOONFUL™
2 teaspoons coconut extract
½ cup flaked coconut

• Roll pastry on floured surface into circle 1 inch larger than inverted 9-inch pie pan. Ease into pan; trim and flute edge.

• Beat eggs and salt in large bowl until thick and lemon-colored, about 5 minutes. Mix in milk and remaining ingredients. Pour mixture into pastry shell.

• Bake pie in preheated 425°F oven 15 minutes. Reduce temperature to 350°F and bake until sharp knife inserted halfway between center and edge of pie comes out clean, 20 to 25 minutes. Cool on wire rack.

Serve at room temperature, or refrigerate and serve chilled. *Makes 8 servings*

Nutrients per Serving: Calories: 213, Fat: 10 g, Protein: 7 g, Carbohydrate: 23 g, Cholesterol: 107 mg, Sodium: 275 mg

Dietary Exchanges: ½ Bread, 1 Milk, 2 Fat

329 NECTARINE AND BERRY PIE

Reduced-Fat Pie Pastry (page 289) or favorite pastry for 9-inch pie
5 cups sliced nectarines (about 5 medium)
1 cup raspberries or sliced strawberries
1 cup fresh or frozen blueberries, partially thawed
2 teaspoons lemon juice
3 tablespoons cornstarch
7¼ teaspoons EQUAL® MEASURE™ or
   24 packets EQUAL® sweetener or
   1 cup EQUAL® SPOONFUL™
1 teaspoon grated lemon peel
¼ teaspoon ground allspice

• Roll pastry on floured surface into 12-inch circle; transfer to ungreased cookie sheet.

• Toss nectarines and berries with lemon juice in large bowl; sprinkle fruit with combined cornstarch, Equal®, lemon peel and allspice and toss to coat. Arrange fruit over pastry, leaving 2-inch border around edge of pastry. Bring edge of pastry toward center, overlapping as necessary. Bake pie in preheated 425°F oven until pastry is golden and fruit is tender, 35 to 40 minutes. Cool on wire rack. *Makes 8 servings*

Nutrients per Serving: Calories: 216, Fat: 7 g, Protein: 3 g, Carbohydrate: 38 g, Cholesterol: 0 mg, Sodium: 138 mg

Dietary Exchanges: 1 Bread, 1½ Fruit, 1½ Fat

HEAVENLY DESSERTS

330 APPLE–RAISIN SOUR CREAM PIE

1½ cups graham cracker crumbs
⅓ cup margarine, melted
1¾ teaspoons EQUAL® MEASURE™ or
        6 packets EQUAL® sweetener or
        ¼ cup EQUAL® SPOONFUL™
4 cups sliced, cored, peeled Granny Smith
        or other baking apples
        (4 to 6 medium)
2 teaspoons lemon juice
¼ cup dark raisins
½ cup reduced-fat sour cream
1 egg white, beaten
3½ teaspoons EQUAL® MEASURE™ or
        12 packets EQUAL® sweetener or
        ½ cup EQUAL® SPOONFUL™
1 tablespoon all-purpose flour
¼ teaspoon ground cinnamon
⅛ teaspoon ground nutmeg

• Mix graham cracker crumbs, margarine, and 1¾ teaspoons Equal® Measure™ *or* 6 packets Equal® sweetener *or* ¼ cup Equal® Spoonful™ in bottom of 9-inch springform pan. Reserve ¼ cup mixture; press remaining mixture firmly on bottom and 1 inch up side of pan. Bake in preheated 350°F oven until lightly browned, 5 to 8 minutes. Cool on wire rack.

• Toss apples with lemon juice in large bowl; add raisins. Combine sour cream and remaining ingredients; spoon mixture over apples, mixing until apples are coated.

• Spoon apple mixture into crust; sprinkle with reserved ¼ cup crumb mixture.

• Bake pie in 350°F oven until apples are tender, about 55 minutes. Cool on wire rack. Remove side of pan; place pie on serving plate.   *Makes 8 servings*

Nutrients per Serving: Calories: 245, Fat: 12 g, Protein: 3 g, Carbohydrate: 33 g, Cholesterol: 6 mg, Sodium: 239 mg

Dietary Exchanges: 1 Starch/Bread, 1 Fruit, 2½ Fat

331 MILE–HIGH APPLE PIE

Reduced-Fat Pie Pastry (2 recipes for
        double crust) (page 289) or favorite
        pastry for double crust 9-inch pie
3 tablespoons cornstarch
7¼ teaspoons EQUAL® MEASURE™ or
        24 packets EQUAL® sweetener or
        1 cup EQUAL® SPOONFUL™
¾ teaspoon ground cinnamon
¼ teaspoon ground nutmeg
¼ teaspoon salt
8 cups sliced, cored, peeled Granny Smith
        or other baking apples (about
        8 medium)

• Roll half the pastry on floured surface into circle 1 inch larger than inverted 9-inch pie pan. Ease pastry into pan.

• Combine cornstarch, Equal®, cinnamon, nutmeg and salt; sprinkle over apples in large bowl and toss. Arrange apple mixture in pie crust.

• Roll remaining pastry into circle large enough to fit top of pie. Cut out hearts from pastry with cookie cutters. Place remaining pastry on pie; seal edges, trim and flute. Press heart cut-outs on pastry. Bake in preheated 425°F oven until pastry is golden and apples are tender, 40 to 50 minutes. Cool on wire rack.   *Makes 8 servings*

Nutrients per Serving: Calories: 334, Fat: 12 g, Protein: 4 g, Carbohydrate: 53 g, Cholesterol: 0 mg, Sodium: 335 mg

Dietary Exchanges: 2½ Starch/Bread, 1 Fruit, 2½ Fat

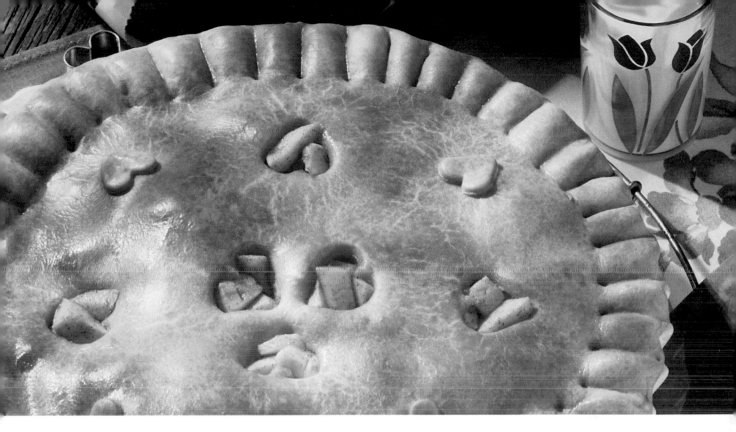

Mile-High Apple Pie

332 RHUBARB–STRAWBERRY PIE

Reduced-Fat Pie Pastry (page 289) or
   favorite pastry for 9-inch pie
3 cups 1-inch rhubarb pieces or
   1 package (16 ounces) frozen
   unsweetened rhubarb, thawed,
   undrained
¾ cup water
¼ cup all-purpose flour
3 tablespoons cornstarch
2 tablespoons lemon juice
3 cups sliced strawberries
12¼ teaspoons EQUAL® MEASURE™ or
   40 packets EQUAL® sweetener or
   1⅔ cups EQUAL® SPOONFUL™
¼ teaspoon ground nutmeg

• Roll pastry on lightly floured surface into circle 1 inch larger than inverted 9-inch pie pan. Ease pastry into pan; trim and flute edge. Pierce bottom and side of pastry with fork. Bake in preheated 425°F oven until pastry is browned, 10 to 15 minutes. Cool on wire rack.

• Cook rhubarb in large covered saucepan over medium heat until rhubarb releases liquid, about 5 minutes. Combine water, flour, cornstarch and lemon juice; stir into rhubarb and heat to boiling. Reduce heat and simmer, uncovered, until mixture is thickened and rhubarb is almost tender, 3 to 5 minutes, stirring frequently. Stir in strawberries and cook 2 to 3 minutes longer.

• Stir Equal® and nutmeg into fruit mixture; spoon into baked crust, spreading evenly. Bake in 350°F oven until bubbly, about 40 minutes. Cover edge of crust with aluminum foil if browning too quickly. Cool briefly on wire rack; serve warm.

Makes 8 servings

Nutrient per Serving: Calories: 199, Fat: 6 g, Protein: 3 g, Carbohydrate: 33 g, Cholesterol: 0 mg, Sodium: 138 mg

Dietary Exchanges: 1 Starch/Bread, 1 Fruit, 1 Fat

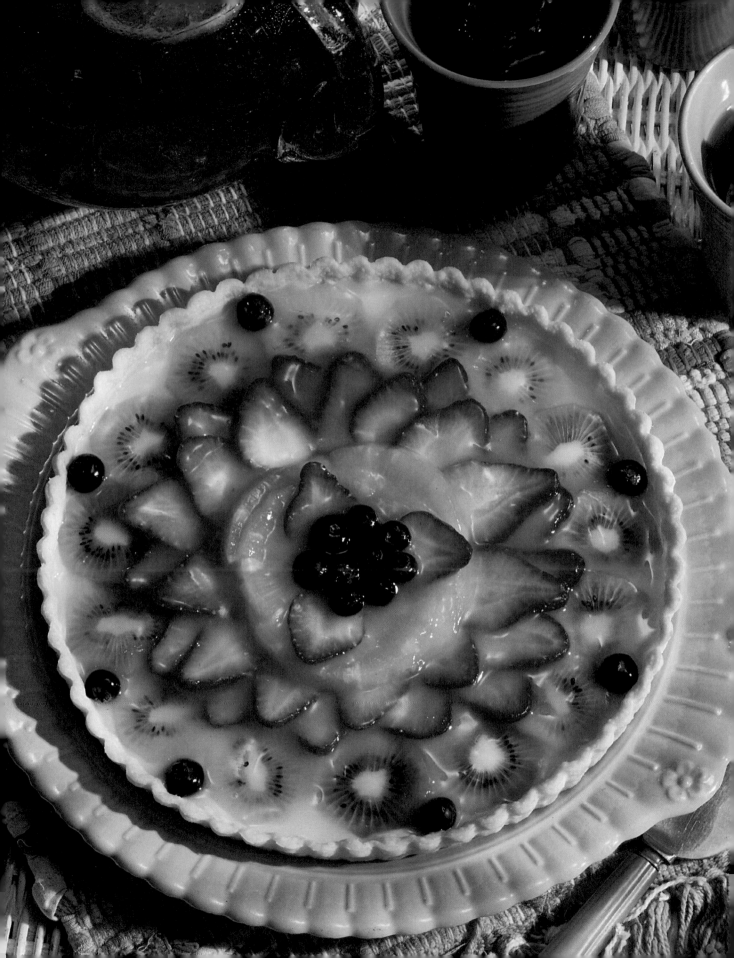

HEAVENLY DESSERTS

333 SUMMER FRUIT TART

1¼ **cups all-purpose flour**
¼ **teaspoon salt**
⅓ **cup shortening**
3 **to 4 tablespoons cold water**
¼ **cup plain nonfat yogurt**
¼ **cup reduced-fat dairy sour cream**
½ **teaspoon EQUAL® MEASURE™ or**
  2 packets EQUAL® sweetener or
  4 teaspoons EQUAL® SPOONFUL™
¼ **teaspoon almond extract**
4 **cups assorted fresh fruit**
¾ **cup pineapple juice**
1 **tablespoon lemon juice**
2 **teaspoons cornstarch**
1 **teaspoon EQUAL® MEASURE™ or**
  3 packets EQUAL® sweetener or
  2 tablespoons EQUAL® SPOONFUL™

• Combine flour and salt; cut in shortening. Sprinkle water over mixture; toss with fork until moistened. Form into a ball.

• Roll pastry on lightly floured surface into 10- or 11-inch circle and place in 9- or 10-inch tart pan with removable bottom. Press pastry up side; trim excess. Prick with fork. Line with foil. Bake in preheated 450°F oven 8 minutes. Remove foil; bake until golden, 5 to 6 minutes. Cool on wire rack.

• Combine yogurt, sour cream, ½ teaspoon Equal® Measure™ or 2 packets Equal® sweetener or 4 teaspoons Equal® Spoonful™ and almond extract. Spread over cooled crust. Arrange fruit on top.

• Combine pineapple juice, lemon juice and cornstarch in small saucepan. Cook and stir until thickened and bubbly. Cook and stir 2 minutes more. Remove from heat; stir in

1 teaspoon Equal® Measure™ *or* 3 packets Equal® sweetener *or* 2 tablespoons Equal® Spoonful™. Cool. Spoon over fruit; cover and chill. *Makes 10 servings*

Nutrients per Serving: Calories: 166, Fat: 8 g, Protein: 3 g, Carbohydrate: 22 g, Cholesterol: 1 mg, Sodium: 65 mg

Dietary Exchanges: 1 Starch/Bread, ½ Fruit, 1½ Fat

334 COUNTRY PEACH TART

Reduced-Fat Pie Pastry (page 289) or
  favorite pastry for 9-inch pie
1 **tablespoon all-purpose flour**
2½ **teaspoons EQUAL® MEASURE™ or**
  8 packets EQUAL® sweetener or
  ⅓ **cup EQUAL® SPOONFUL™**
4 **cups sliced, pitted, peeled fresh peaches**
  (about 4 medium) or frozen peaches,
  thawed
  Ground nutmeg

• Roll pastry on floured surface into 12-inch circle; transfer to ungreased cookie sheet. Combine flour and Equal®; sprinkle over peaches. Toss to coat. Arrange peaches over pastry, leaving 2-inch border around edge. Sprinkle lightly with nutmeg. Bring pastry edge toward center, overlapping as necessary. Bake tart in preheated 425°F oven until crust is browned and fruit is tender, 25 to 30 minutes. *Makes 8 servings*

Nutrients per Serving: Calories: 168, Fat: 6 g, Protein: 3 g, Carbohydrate: 27 g, Cholesterol: 0 mg, Sodium: 134 mg

Dietary Exchanges: 1½ Starch/Bread, ½ Fruit, 1 Fat

Summer Fruit Tart

HEAVENLY DESSERTS

335 APPLE–CRANBERRY TART

Tart Dough (recipe follows)
$^1/_3$ cup dried cranberries
$^1/_2$ cup boiling water
$^3/_4$ cup sugar
 1 teaspoon ground cinnamon
 2 tablespoons cornstarch
 4 medium baking apples
Vanilla frozen yogurt (optional)

1. Prepare Tart Dough.

2. Preheat oven to 425°F. Combine cranberries and boiling water in small bowl; let stand 20 minutes or until softened.

3. Roll out Tart Dough on floured surface to $^1/_8$-inch thickness; cut into 11-inch circle. (If leftover dough remains, use scraps for decorating top of tart.) Ease dough into 10-inch tart pan with removable bottom, leaving $^1/_4$ inch of dough above rim of pan. Prick bottom and sides of dough with tines of fork; bake 12 minutes or until dough begins to brown. Cool on wire rack. *Reduce oven temperature to 375°F.*

4. Combine sugar and cinnamon in large bowl; mix well. Reserve 1 teaspoon mixture for sprinkling over top of tart. Add cornstarch to bowl; mix well. Peel, core and thinly slice apples, adding pieces to bowl as they are sliced; toss well. Drain cranberries. Add to apple mixture; toss well.

5. Arrange apple mixture attractively over dough. Sprinkle reserved 1 teaspoon sugar mixture evenly over top of tart. Place tart on baking sheet; bake 30 to 35 minutes or until apples are tender and crust is golden brown. Cool on wire rack. Remove side of pan; place tart on serving plate. Serve warm or at room temperature with frozen yogurt, if desired. *Makes 8 servings*

TART DOUGH
$1^1/_3$ cups all-purpose flour
 1 tablespoon sugar
 $^1/_4$ teaspoon salt
 2 tablespoons vegetable shortening
 2 tablespoons margarine
 4 to 5 tablespoons ice water

1. Combine flour, sugar and salt in medium bowl; cut in shortening and margarine with pastry blender or two knives until mixture forms coarse crumbs. Mix in ice water, 1 tablespoon at a time, until mixture comes together and forms a soft dough. Wrap in plastic wrap; refrigerate 30 minutes.

Nutrients per Serving: Calories: 263 (22% Calories from Fat), Total Fat: 6 g, Saturated Fat: 2 g, Protein: 2 g, Carbohydrate: 50 g, Cholesterol: 0 mg, Sodium: 68 mg, Fiber: 2 g, Sugar: 29 g

Dietary Exchanges: $1^1/_2$ Starch/Bread, $1^1/_2$ Fruit, $1^1/_2$ Fat

336 KEY LIME TARTS

$^3/_4$ cup skim milk
 6 tablespoons fresh lime juice
 2 tablespoons cornstarch
 $^1/_2$ cup cholesterol-free egg substitute
 $^1/_2$ cup reduced-fat sour cream
 12 packages artificial sweetener *or* equivalent of $^1/_2$ cup sugar
 4 sheets phyllo dough*
Butter-flavored nonstick cooking spray
 $^3/_4$ cup thawed fat-free nondairy whipped topping

Cover with damp kitchen towel to prevent dough from drying out.

1. Whisk together milk, lime juice and cornstarch in medium saucepan. Cook over medium heat 2 to 3 minutes, stirring constantly until thick. Remove from heat.

HEAVENLY DESSERTS

2. Add egg substitute; whisk constantly for 30 seconds to allow egg substitute to cook. Stir in sour cream and artificial sweetener; cover and refrigerate until cool.

3. Preheat oven to 350°F. Spray 8 (2½-inch) muffin cups with cooking spray; set aside.

4. Place 1 sheet of phyllo dough on cutting board; spray with cooking spray. Top with second sheet of phyllo dough; spray with cooking spray. Top with third sheet of phyllo dough; spray with cooking spray. Top with last sheet; spray with cooking spray.

5. Cut stack of phyllo dough into 8 squares. Gently fit each stacked square into prepared muffin cups; press firmly against bottom and side. Bake 8 to 10 minutes or until golden brown. Carefully remove from muffin cups; cool on wire rack.

6. Divide lime mixture evenly among phyllo cups; top with whipped topping. Garnish with fresh raspberries and lime slices, if desired. *Makes 8 servings*

Nutrients per Serving: Calories: 82 (17% Calories from Fat), Total Fat: 1 g, Saturated Fat: trace, Protein: 3 g, Carbohydrate: 13 g, Cholesterol: 5 mg, Sodium: 88 mg, Fiber: trace, Sugar: 2 g

Dietary Exchanges: 1 Starch/Bread

Key Lime Tart

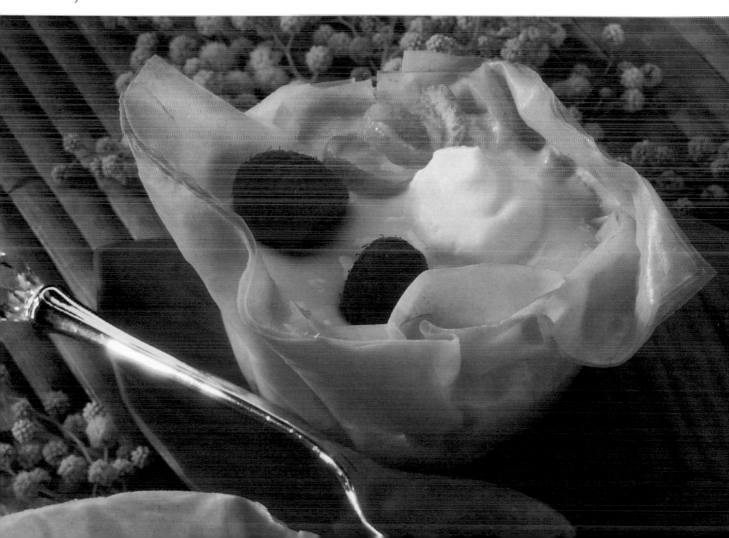

HEAVENLY DESSERTS

337 FRESH PLUM COBBLER

½ cup water
5½ teaspoons EQUAL® MEASURE™ or
    18 packets EQUAL® sweetener or
    ¾ cup EQUAL® SPOONFUL™
1½ tablespoons cornstarch
1 teaspoon lemon juice
4 cups sliced pitted plums
¼ teaspoon ground nutmeg
¼ teaspoon ground allspice
1 cup all-purpose flour
1½ teaspoons baking powder
1¾ teaspoons EQUAL® MEASURE™ or
    6 packets EQUAL® sweetener or
    ¼ cup EQUAL® SPOONFUL™
½ teaspoon salt
3 tablespoons cold margarine, cubed
½ cup skim milk

• Combine water, 5½ teaspoons Equal® Measure™ *or* 18 packets Equal® sweetener *or* ¾ cup Equal® Spoonful™, cornstarch and lemon juice in large saucepan; add plums and heat to boiling. Boil, stirring constantly, until thickened, about 1 minute. Stir in nutmeg and ⅛ teaspoon allspice. Pour mixture into ungreased 1½-quart casserole.

• Combine flour, baking powder, 1¾ teaspoons Equal® Measure™ *or* 6 packets Equal® sweetener *or* ¼ cup Equal® Spoonful™, salt and remaining ⅛ teaspoon allspice in medium bowl; cut in margarine with pastry blender until mixture resembles coarse crumbs. Stir in milk, forming dough. Spoon dough into 6 mounds on fruit.

• Bake cobbler, uncovered, in preheated 400°F oven until topping is golden brown, about 25 minutes. Serve warm.

Makes 6 servings

Nutrients per Serving: Calories: 195, Fat: 6 g, Protein: 3 g, Carbohydrate: 32 g, Cholesterol: 0 mg, Sodium: 378 mg

Dietary Exchanges: 1 Bread, 1 Fruit, 1 Fat

338 FRUIT BAKED APPLES

3½ teaspoons EQUAL® MEASURE™ or
    12 packets EQUAL® sweetener or
    ½ cup EQUAL® SPOONFUL™
1 tablespoon cornstarch
  Pinch ground cinnamon
  Pinch ground nutmeg
2 cups apple cider or juice
1 package (6 ounces) dried mixed fruit,
    chopped
1 tablespoon margarine
8 tart baking apples

• Combine Equal®, cornstarch, cinnamon and nutmeg in medium saucepan; stir in cider. Add dried fruit; heat to boiling. Reduce heat and simmer, uncovered, until fruit is tender and cider mixture is reduced to about 1 cup, 10 to 15 minutes. Add margarine and stir until melted.

• Remove cores from apples, cutting to but not through bottoms. Peel 1 inch around tops. Place apples in greased baking pan. Fill centers with fruit; spoon remaining cider mixture over apples.

• Bake, uncovered, in preheated 350°F oven until fork-tender, about 45 minutes.

Makes 8 servings

Nutrients per Serving: Calories: 176, Fat: 2 g, Protein: 1 g, Carbohydrate: 42 g, Cholesterol: 0 mg, Sodium: 22 mg

Dietary Exchanges: 2½ Fruit, ½ Fat

Fresh Plum Cobbler

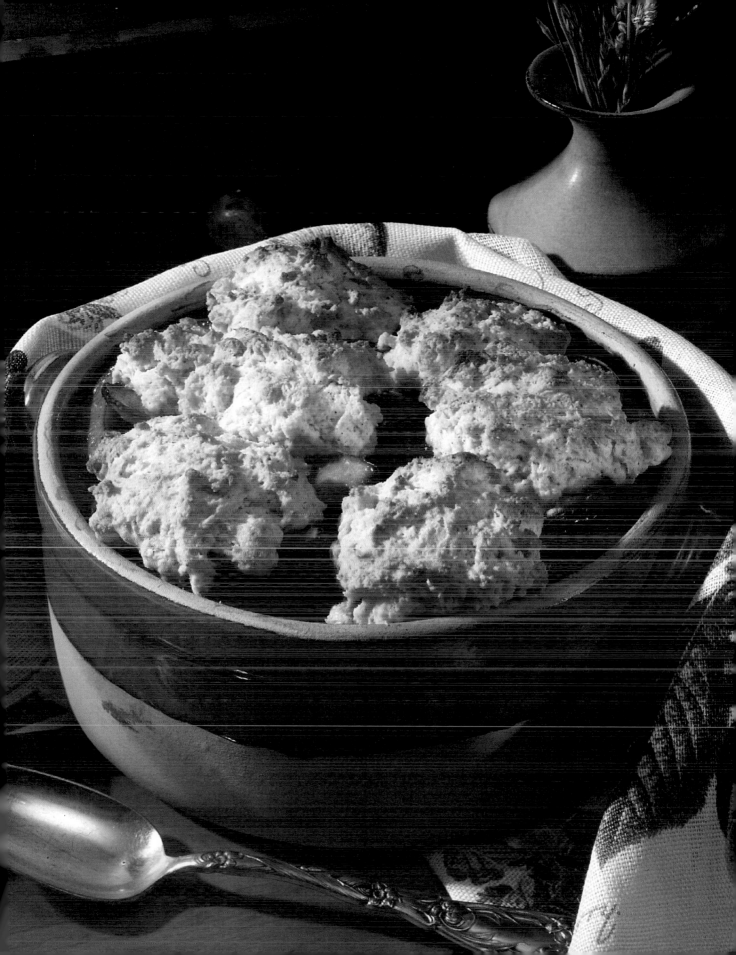

HEAVENLY DESSERTS

339 APPLE–CHERRY CRISP

1 pound Granny Smith apples, peeled,
    cored and sliced ¼ inch thick
1 can (16 ounces) tart pie cherries packed
    in water, drained
1 can (16 ounces) dark sweet pitted
    cherries in heavy syrup, drained
2 teaspoons vanilla
1 teaspoon cinnamon
1 cup fruit-juice-sweetened granola
    without raisins*
⅓ cup sliced almonds
1 quart fat-free vanilla ice cream or frozen
    yogurt

Available in the health food section of supermarkets.

1. Preheat oven to 350°F. Spray an 11×7-inch glass baking dish with nonstick cooking spray; set aside.

2. Combine apples, cherries, vanilla and cinnamon in large bowl; stir until well blended. Spoon into prepared baking dish. Cover with foil; bake 30 minutes.

3. Remove from oven; stir to distribute juices. Sprinkle granola and almonds evenly over fruit. Bake, uncovered, 15 minutes more or until juice is bubbling and almonds are golden; serve warm or at room temperature topped with ice cream.

Makes 8 servings

Nutrients per Serving: Calories: 296 (15% Calories from Fat), Total Fat: 5 g, Saturated Fat: 2 g, Protein: 7 g, Carbohydrate: 59 g, Cholesterol: 0 mg, Sodium: 100 mg, Fiber: 3 g, Sugar: 28 g

Dietary Exchanges: 2 Starch/Bread, 2 Fruit, 1 Fat

Apple-Cherry Crisp

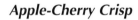

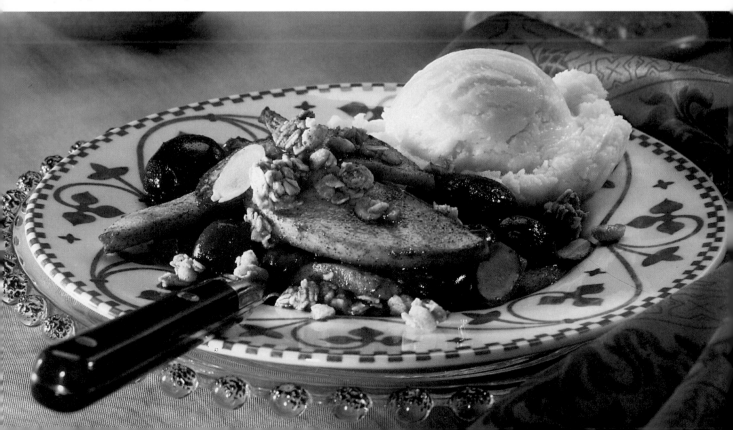

HEAVENLY DESSERTS

340 FRESH & FRUITY COBBLER

　　Biscuit Topping (recipe follows)
　5 teaspoons sugar, divided
　1 teaspoon cornstarch
　½ cup fresh or thawed frozen blueberries
　½ cup peeled nectarine slices
　½ cup strawberries, hulled and halved

1. Preheat oven to 350°F. Prepare Biscuit Topping.

2. Blend ¼ cup water, 3 teaspoons sugar and cornstarch in small saucepan; cook over medium heat 5 minutes or until mixture thickens, stirring constantly. Remove saucepan from heat; let stand 5 minutes.

3. Add fruit to sugar mixture; toss to coat. Spoon fruit mixture into 2 cup casserole; sprinkle with remaining 2 teaspoons sugar. Drop tablespoonfuls topping around edge of casserole.

4. Bake 20 minutes or until topping is browned. Serve immediately.

Makes 2 servings

BISCUIT TOPPING
　⅓ cup all-purpose flour
　1 tablespoon sugar
　¼ teaspoon baking powder
　⅛ teaspoon baking soda
　1 tablespoon plus 1 teaspoon
　　　reduced-calorie margarine
　3 tablespoons nonfat sour cream
　2 teaspoons cholesterol-free egg substitute
　¼ teaspoon vanilla

Combine flour, sugar, baking powder and baking soda in medium bowl; cut in margarine with pastry blender until mixture resembles coarse crumbs. Blend remaining ingredients in small bowl; stir into flour mixture just until dry ingredients are moistened.

Nutrients per Serving: Calories: 244, (16% Calories from Fat), Total Fat: 4 g, Saturated Fat: 1 g, Protein: 5 g, Carbohydrate: 48 g, Cholesterol: 0 mg, Sodium: 231 mg, Fiber: 3 g, Sugar: 24 g

Dietary Exchanges: 2 Starch/Bread, 1½ Fruit, ½ Fat

341 CHEESE–FILLED POACHED PEARS

　1½ quarts cranberry-raspberry juice cocktail
　2 ripe Bartlett pears with stems, peeled
　2 tablespoons Neufchâtel cheese
　2 teaspoons crumbled Gorgonzola cheese
　1 tablespoon chopped walnuts

1. Bring juice to a boil in medium saucepan over high heat. Add pears; reduce heat to medium-low. Simmer 15 minutes or until pears are tender, turning occasionally. Remove pears from saucepan; discard liquid. Let stand 10 minutes or until cool enough to handle.

2. Combine cheeses in small bowl until well blended. Cut thin slice off bottom of each pear so that pears stand evenly. Cut pears lengthwise in half, leaving stems intact. Scoop out seeds and membranes to form small hole in each pear half. Fill holes with cheese mixture; press halves together. Place nuts in large bowl; roll pears in nuts to coat. Cover; refrigerate until ready to serve.

Makes 2 servings

Nutrients per Serving: Calories: 240, (24% Calories from Fat), Total Fat: 7 g, Saturated Fat: 3 g, Protein: 4 g, Carbohydrate: 45 g, Cholesterol: 13 mg, Sodium: 98 mg, Fiber: 4 g, Sugar: 16 g

Dietary Exchanges: ½ Lean Meat, 3 Fruit, 1 Fat

HEAVENLY DESSERTS

342 BLUEBERRY TRIANGLES

1½ cups fresh or frozen blueberries, slightly
    thawed
3½ teaspoons EQUAL® MEASURE™ or
    12 packets EQUAL® sweetener or
    ½ cup EQUAL® SPOONFUL™
1½ teaspoons cornstarch
  2 to 4 teaspoons cold water
    Reduced-Fat Pie Pastry (page 289) or
    favorite pastry for 9-inch pie
    Skim milk
½ teaspoon EQUAL® MEASURE™ or
    1½ packets EQUAL® sweetener or
    1 tablespoon EQUAL® SPOONFUL™

• Rinse blueberries; drain slightly and place
in medium saucepan. Sprinkle berries with
3½ teaspoons Equal® Measure™ *or*
12 packets Equal® sweetener *or* ½ cup
Equal® Spoonful™ and cornstarch; toss to
coat. Cook over medium heat, stirring
constantly, until berries begin to release
juice and form small amount of thickened
sauce. (Add water, 1 teaspoon at a time, if
bottom of saucepan becomes dry.) Cool;
refrigerate until chilled.

• Roll pastry on floured surface to ⅛-inch
thickness; cut into 8 (5-inch) squares,
rerolling scraps as necessary. Place scant
2 tablespoons blueberry mixture on each
pastry square. Fold squares in half to form
triangles and press edges together to seal.
Flute edges of pastry or crimp with tines of
fork; pierce tops of pastries 3 or 4 times with
tip of knife.

• Brush tops of pastries lightly with milk
and sprinkle with ½ teaspoon Equal®
Measure™ *or* 1½ packets Equal® sweetener
or 1 tablespoon Equal® Spoonful™. Bake on
foil- or parchment-lined cookie sheet in
preheated 400°F oven until pastries are
browned, about 25 minutes.

Makes 8 servings

Nutrients per Serving: Calories: 147, Fat: 6 g,
Protein: 2 g, Carbohydrate: 21 g,
Cholesterol: 0 mg, Sodium: 134 mg

Dietary Exchanges: 1 Bread, ½ Fruit, 1 Fat

343 CHEESY CHERRY TURNOVERS

1 package (8 ounces) Neufchâtel cheese
1 cup 1% low-fat cottage cheese
½ cup sugar, divided
1 teaspoon vanilla
1 can (16½ ounces) dark sweet pitted
    cherries, rinsed and drained
8 sheets frozen phyllo dough, thawed
1 cup whole wheat bread crumbs
1 teaspoon ground cinnamon

1. Preheat oven to 350°F. Spray baking sheet
with butter-flavored cooking spray; set aside.
Combine cheeses, ¼ cup sugar and vanilla in
medium bowl; beat at medium speed until
well blended. Stir in cherries.

2. Spray 1 phyllo dough sheet with cooking
spray; fold sheet crosswise in half to form
rectangle. Sprinkle with 2 tablespoons bread
crumbs. Drop ⅓-cupful cheese mixture onto
upper left corner of sheet; fold left corner
over mixture to form triangle. Continue
folding triangle, right to left, until end of
dough. Repeat with remaining ingredients.
Place turnovers on prepared baking sheet.
Combine remaining ¼ cup sugar with
cinnamon; sprinkle over turnovers. Bake
12 to 15 minutes or until turnovers are crisp
and golden brown. *Makes 8 servings*

Nutrients per Serving: Calories: 170,
(29% Calories from Fat), Total Fat: 6 g,
Saturated Fat: 3 g, Protein: 8 g,
Carbohydrate: 24 g, Cholesterol: 11 mg,
Sodium: 314 mg, Fiber: 1 g, Sugar: 18 g

Dietary Exchanges: 1 Starch/Bread,
½ Lean Meat, ½ Fruit, 1 Fat

HEAVENLY DESSERTS

344 PEACH & BLACKBERRY SHORTCAKES

¾ cup plain low-fat yogurt, divided
5 teaspoons sugar, divided
1 tablespoon all-fruit blackberry preserves
½ cup coarsely chopped peeled peach
½ cup fresh or frozen blackberries, thawed
½ cup all-purpose flour
¼ teaspoon baking powder
⅛ teaspoon baking soda
2 tablespoons reduced-calorie margarine
½ teaspoon vanilla

1. Place cheesecloth or coffee filter in large sieve or strainer. Spoon yogurt into sieve; place over large bowl. Refrigerate 20 minutes. Remove yogurt from sieve; discard liquid. Measure ¼ cup yogurt; blend remaining yogurt, 2 teaspoons sugar and preserves in small bowl. Refrigerate.

2. Meanwhile, combine peach, blackberries and ½ teaspoon sugar in medium bowl.

3. Preheat oven to 425°F. Combine flour, baking powder, baking soda and remaining 2½ teaspoons sugar in small bowl; cut in margarine with pastry blender until mixture resembles coarse crumbs. Combine reserved ¼ cup yogurt with vanilla; stir into flour mixture just until dry ingredients are moistened. Shape dough into a ball.

4. Place dough on lightly floured surface; knead dough gently 8 times. Divide dough in half; roll out each half into 3-inch circle with lightly floured rolling pin. Place circles on ungreased baking sheet.

5. Bake 12 to 15 minutes or until lightly browned. Immediately remove from baking sheet; cool on wire rack 10 minutes.

6. Cut shortcakes in half; top bottom halves with fruit mixture, yogurt and remaining halves. *Makes 2 servings*

Nutrients per Serving: Calories: 327 (21% Calories from Fat), Total Fat: 8 g, Saturated Fat: 2 g, Protein: 8 g, Carbohydrate: 57 g, Cholesterol: 5 mg, Sodium: 311 mg, Fiber: 4 g, Sugar: 28 g

Dietary Exchanges: 2½ Starch/Bread, ½ Milk, 1 Fruit, 1 Fat

345 BAKED VANILLA CUSTARD

1 quart skim milk
6 eggs
6¼ teaspoons EQUAL® MEASURE™ or
  21 packets EQUAL® sweetener or
  ¾ cup plus 2 tablespoons EQUAL® SPOONFUL™
2 teaspoons vanilla
¼ teaspoon salt
  Ground nutmeg

• Heat milk just to boiling in medium saucepan; let cool 5 minutes.

• Beat eggs, Equal®, vanilla and salt in large bowl until smooth; gradually beat in hot milk. Pour mixture into 10 custard cups or 1½-quart glass casserole; sprinkle generously with nutmeg. Place custard cups or casserole in roasting pan; add 1 inch hot water to roasting pan.

• Bake, uncovered, in preheated 325°F oven until sharp knife inserted halfway between center and edge of custard comes out clean, 45 to 60 minutes. Remove custard dishes from roasting pan; cool on wire rack. Refrigerate until chilled.
  Makes 10 (½-cup) servings

Nutrients per Serving: Calories: 90, Fat: 3 g, Protein: 7 g, Carbohydrate: 8 g, Cholesterol: 129 mg, Sodium: 142 mg

Dietary Exchanges: ½ Milk, ½ Lean Meat

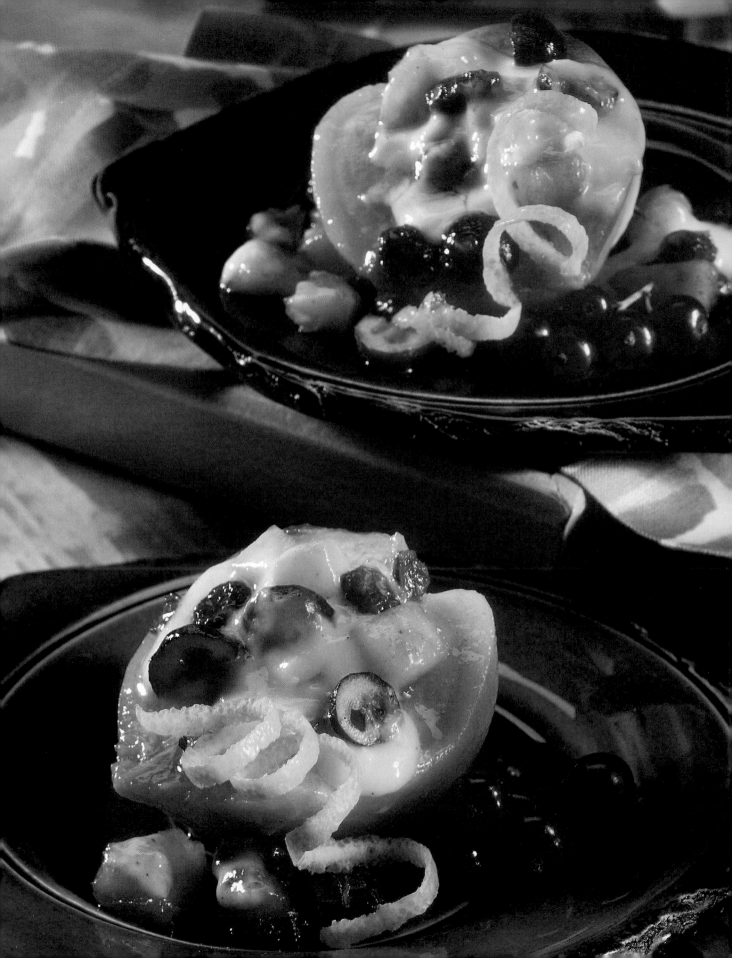

HEAVENLY DESSERTS

346 SHERRY–POACHED PEACHES WITH GINGERED FRUIT AND CUSTARD SAUCE

4 large ripe peaches, peeled, pitted and halved *or* 2 cans (16 ounces each) peach halves packed in juice, drained
⅓ cup dry sherry
1 cup assorted chopped mixed dried or fresh fruit (such as apples, golden raisins, prunes, peaches, apricots, pineapple, raisins and cranberries)
¼ cup water
½ teaspoon fresh minced ginger or
    ¼ teaspoon ground ginger
½ teaspoon grated orange peel
¼ cup all-fruit apricot preserves
1 cup skim milk
½ vanilla bean*
1 egg yolk
3 packages artificial sweetener or
    equivalent of 2 tablespoons of sugar
2½ teaspoons cornstarch

1½ teaspoons vanilla extract may be substituted for vanilla bean. Stir into cooked custard before serving.

1. Combine peaches and sherry in medium saucepan. Simmer, covered, over low heat for 8 to 15 minutes, stirring often, until peaches are tender. (Cooking time will vary based on ripeness of fruit.) Remove peaches from sherry; cool to room temperature.

2. Combine dried fruit, water, ginger and orange peel in medium microwavable bowl. Cover; microwave at HIGH for 2 to 3 minutes or until fruit is soft. Stir in preserves; cool to room temperature.

3. Pour milk into small saucepan. Cut vanilla bean in half lengthwise; scrape seeds into saucepan. Add bean halves to saucepan. Heat over medium heat just until milk begins to boil; remove from heat. Remove bean halves from milk; discard.

4. Combine egg yolk, artificial sweetener and cornstarch in medium bowl. Beat mixture with wire whisk until thick and lemon colored. Continue whisking mixture while very slowly pouring in hot milk mixture.

5. Slowly pour egg mixture back into saucepan. Cook over medium-low heat, stirring constantly until mixture thickens and coats metal spoon. *Do not boil.* Remove from heat.

6. Divide peach halves and fruit mixture among 4 plates. Top each serving with 2 tablespoons of custard sauce.

Makes 4 servings

Nutrients per Serving: Calories: 290 (5% Calories from Fat), Total Fat: 1 g, Saturated Fat: trace, Protein: 5 g, Carbohydrate: 59 g, Cholesterol: 54 mg, Sodium: 102 mg, Fiber: 4 g, Sugar: 34 g

Dietary Exchanges: 4 Fruit

Sherry-Poached Peaches with Gingered Fruit and Custard Sauce

HEAVENLY DESSERTS

347 CHOCOLATE ANGEL FRUIT TORTE

1 package chocolate angel food cake mix
2 bananas, thinly sliced
1½ teaspoons lemon juice
1 can (12 ounces) evaporated skim milk, divided
⅓ cup sugar
¼ cup cornstarch
⅓ cup cholesterol-free egg substitute
3 tablespoons nonfat sour cream
3 teaspoons vanilla
3 large kiwis, peeled and thinly sliced
1 can (11 ounces) mandarin orange segments, rinsed and drained

1. Prepare cake according to package directions; cool completely. Cut horizontally in half to form 2 layers; set aside.

2. Place banana slices in medium bowl. Add lemon juice; toss to coat. Set aside.

3. Combine ¼ cup milk, sugar and cornstarch in small saucepan; whisk until smooth. Whisk in remaining milk; bring to a boil over high heat, stirring constantly. Boil 1 minute or until mixture thickens, stirring constantly. Reduce heat to medium-low.

4. Blend ⅓ cup hot milk mixture and egg substitute in small bowl; add to saucepan. Cook 2 minutes, stirring constantly. Remove saucepan from heat; let stand 10 minutes, stirring frequently. Add sour cream and vanilla; blend well.

5. Place bottom half of cake on serving plate. Spread with half of milk mixture. Arrange half of banana slices, kiwi slices and mandarin orange segments on milk mixture. Place remaining half of cake, cut-side down, over fruit. Top with remaining milk mixture and fruit. *Makes 12 servings*

Nutrients per Serving: Calories: 233 (1% Calories from Fat), Total Fat: trace, Saturated Fat: trace, Protein: 7 g, Carbohydrate: 52 g, Cholesterol: 1 mg, Sodium: 306 mg, Fiber: 1 g, Sugar: 10 g

Dietary Exchanges: 2½ Starch/Bread, 1 Fruit

348 CHOCOLATE–STRAWBERRY CRÊPES

CRÊPES
⅔ cup all-purpose flour
6 packages artificial sweetener *or* equivalent of ¼ cup sugar
2 tablespoons unsweetened cocoa powder
¼ teaspoon salt
1¼ cups skim milk
½ cup cholesterol-free egg substitute
1 tablespoon margarine, melted
1 teaspoon vanilla
Nonstick cooking spray

FILLING AND TOPPING
4 ounces fat-free cream cheese, softened
1 package (1.3 ounces) chocolate-fudge-flavored sugar-free instant pudding mix
1½ cups skim milk
¼ cup all-fruit strawberry preserves
2 tablespoons water
2 cups fresh hulled and quartered strawberries

1. To prepare crêpes, combine flour, artificial sweetener, cocoa and salt in food processor; process to blend. Add milk, egg substitute, margarine and vanilla; process until smooth. Let stand at room temperature 30 minutes.

2. Spray 7-inch nonstick skillet with cooking spray; heat over medium-high heat. Pour 2 tablespoons crêpe batter into hot pan. Immediately rotate pan back and forth to swirl batter over entire surface of pan. Cook

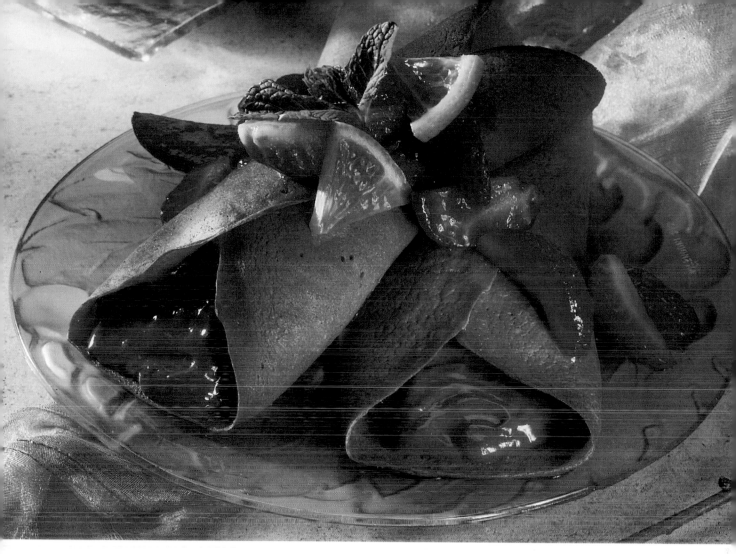

Chocolate-Strawberry Crêpes

1 to 2 minutes or until crêpe is brown around edge and top is dry. Carefully turn crêpe with spatula and cook 30 seconds more. Transfer crêpe to waxed paper to cool. Repeat with remaining batter, spraying pan with cooking spray as needed. Separate crepes with sheets of waxed paper.

3. To prepare chocolate filling, beat cream cheese in medium bowl with electric mixer at high speed until smooth; set aside. Prepare chocolate pudding with skim milk according to package directions. Gradually add pudding to cream cheese mixture; beat at high speed for 3 minutes.

4. To prepare strawberry topping, combine preserves and water in large bowl until smooth. Add strawberries; toss to coat.

5. Spread 2 tablespoons chocolate filling evenly over surface of crêpe; roll tightly. Repeat with remaining crêpes. Place two crêpes on each plate. Spoon ¼ cup strawberry topping over each serving. Serve immediately.

Makes 8 servings (2 crêpes each)

Nutrients per Serving: Calories: 161 (13% Calories from Fat), Total Fat: 2 g, Saturated Fat: trace, Protein: 8 g, Carbohydrate: 27 g, Cholesterol: 1 mg, Sodium: 374 mg, Fiber: 1 g, Sugar: 6 g

Dietary Exchanges: 1 Lean Meat, 2 Fruit

HEAVENLY DESSERTS

349 LEMON RASPBERRY TIRAMISU

2 packages (8 ounces each) fat-free cream cheese, softened

6 packages artificial sweetener *or* equivalent of ¼ cup sugar

1 teaspoon vanilla

⅓ cup water

1 package (0.3 ounce) sugar-free lemon-flavored gelatin

2 cups thawed fat-free nondairy whipped topping

½ cup all-fruit red raspberry preserves

¼ cup water

2 tablespoons marsala wine

2 packages (3 ounces each) ladyfingers

1 pint fresh raspberries or frozen unsweetened raspberries, thawed

1. Combine cream cheese, artificial sweetener and vanilla in large bowl. Beat with electric mixer at high speed until smooth; set aside.

2. Combine water and gelatin in small microwavable bowl; microwave at HIGH 30 seconds to 1 minute or until water is boiling and gelatin is dissolved. Cool slightly.

3. Add gelatin mixture to cheese mixture; beat 1 minute. Add whipped topping; beat 1 minute more, scraping sides of bowl. Set aside.

4. Whisk together preserves, water and marsala in small bowl until well blended. Reserve 2 tablespoons of preserves mixture; set aside. Spread ⅓ cup of preserves mixture evenly over bottom of 11×7-inch glass baking dish.

Lemon Raspberry Tiramisu

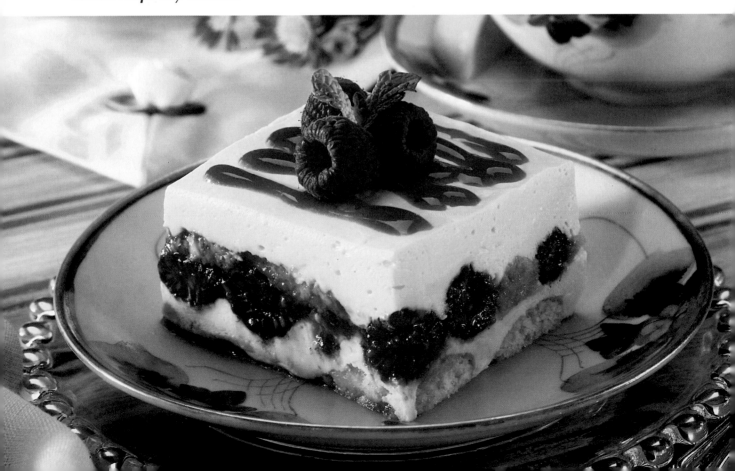

HEAVENLY DESSERTS

5. Split ladyfingers in half; place half in bottom of baking dish. Spread ½ of cheese mixture evenly over ladyfingers; sprinkle 1 cup of raspberries evenly over cheese mixture. Top with remaining ladyfingers; spread remaining preserves mixture over ladyfingers. Top with remaining cheese mixture. Cover; refrigerate for at least 2 hours. Sprinkle with remaining raspberries and drizzle with reserved 2 tablespoons of preserves mixture before serving.

Makes 12 servings

Nutrients per Serving: Calories: 158 (9% Calories from Fat), Total Fat: 1 g, Saturated Fat: trace, Protein: 7 g, Carbohydrate: 26 g, Cholesterol: 52 mg, Sodium: 272 mg, Fiber: 1 g, Sugar: 3 g

Dietary Exchanges: 2 Starch/Bread

350 TRIPLE FRUIT TRIFLE

    2 ripe pears, peeled, cored and coarsely
        chopped
    2 ripe bananas, thinly sliced
    1 tablespoon lemon juice
    2 cups fresh or frozen raspberries, thawed
    ¼ cup reduced-calorie margarine
    1 cup graham cracker crumbs
    1 can (12 ounces) evaporated skim milk,
        divided
    ⅓ cup sugar
    ¼ cup cornstarch
    ⅓ cup cholesterol-free egg substitute
    2 tablespoons nonfat sour cream
 1½ teaspoons vanilla
    3 tablespoons all-fruit apricot preserves

1. Combine pears, bananas, lemon juice and raspberries in large bowl; set aside.

2. Melt margarine in small saucepan over medium heat; stir in graham cracker crumbs until well blended. Remove saucepan from heat; set aside.

3. Blend ¼ cup milk, sugar and cornstarch in another small saucepan; whisk in remaining milk. Bring to a boil over medium heat, stirring constantly. Boil 1 minute or until mixture thickens, stirring constantly. Reduce heat to medium-low.

4. Blend ⅓ cup hot milk mixture and egg substitute in small bowl; add to milk mixture. Cook 2 minutes, stirring constantly. Remove saucepan from heat; let stand 10 minutes, stirring frequently. Stir in sour cream and vanilla; blend well.

5. Spoon half of milk mixture into trifle dish or medium straight-sided glass serving bowl. Layer half of fruit mixture and ½ cup graham cracker crumb mixture over milk mixture. Repeat layers, ending with graham cracker crumb mixture. Blend preserves and 1 teaspoon water until smooth; drizzle over trifle. Garnish with additional fresh fruit, if desired. *Makes 12 servings*

Nutrients per Serving: Calories: 181 (17% Calories from Fat), Total Fat: 3 g, Saturated Fat: trace, Protein: 5 g, Carbohydrate: 34 g, Cholesterol: 1 mg, Sodium: 151 mg, Fiber: 2 g, Sugar: 16 g

Dietary Exchanges: ½ Starch/Bread, ½ Milk, 1½ Fruit, ½ Fat

HEAVENLY DESSERTS

351 RASPBERRY–ALMOND BARS

2 cups all-purpose flour
3½ teaspoons EQUAL® MEASURE™ or
    12 packets EQUAL® sweetener or
    ½ cup EQUAL® SPOONFUL™
⅛ teaspoon salt
8 tablespoons cold margarine, cut into
    pieces
1 egg
1 tablespoon skim milk or water
2 teaspoons grated lemon peel
⅔ cup seedless raspberry spreadable fruit
1 teaspoon cornstarch
½ cup chopped toasted almonds, walnuts
    or pecans

• Combine flour, Equal® and salt in medium bowl, cut in margarine with pastry blender until mixture resembles coarse crumbs. Mix in egg, milk and lemon peel. (Mixture will be crumbly.)

• Press mixture evenly into bottom of greased 11×7-inch baking dish. Bake in preheated 400°F oven until edges of crust are browned, about 15 minutes. Cool on wire rack.

• Mix spreadable fruit and cornstarch in small saucepan; heat to boiling. Boil until thickened, stirring constantly, 1 minute; cool slightly. Spread mixture evenly over cooled crust; sprinkle with almonds. Bake in preheated 400°F oven until spreadable fruit is thick and bubbly, about 15 minutes. Cool on wire rack; cut into squares.

Makes 2 dozen bars

Nutrients per Serving: (1 bar), Calories: 116, Fat: 6 g, Protein: 2 g, Carbohydrate: 15 g, Cholesterol: 9 mg, Sodium: 59 mg

Dietary Exchanges: 1 Starch/Bread, 1 Fat

352 NO–GUILT CHOCOLATE BROWNIES

1 cup semisweet chocolate chips
¼ cup packed brown sugar
2 tablespoons granulated sugar
½ teaspoon baking powder
¼ teaspoon salt
½ cup cholesterol-free egg substitute
1 jar (2½ ounces) first-stage baby food
    prunes
1 teaspoon vanilla
1 cup uncooked rolled oats
⅓ cup nonfat dry milk solids
¼ cup wheat germ
2 teaspoons powdered sugar

1. Preheat oven to 350°F. Spray 8-inch square baking pan with nonstick cooking spray; set aside. Melt chips in top of double boiler over simmering water. Set aside.

2. Combine brown and granulated sugars, baking powder and salt in large bowl with electric mixer. Add egg substitute, prunes and vanilla; beat at medium speed until well blended. Stir in oats, milk solids, wheat germ and chocolate.

3. Pour batter into prepared pan. Bake 30 minutes or until wooden pick inserted in center comes out clean. Cool completely. Cut into 2-inch squares. Dust with powdered sugar before serving. *Makes 16 servings*

Nutrients per Serving: Calories: 124 (30% Calories from Fat), Total Fat: 5 g, Saturated Fat: trace, Protein: 3 g, Carbohydrate: 21 g, Cholesterol: trace, Sodium: 65 mg, Fiber: trace, Sugar: 10 g

Dietary Exchanges: 1 Starch/Bread, 1 Fat

Raspberry-Almond Bars

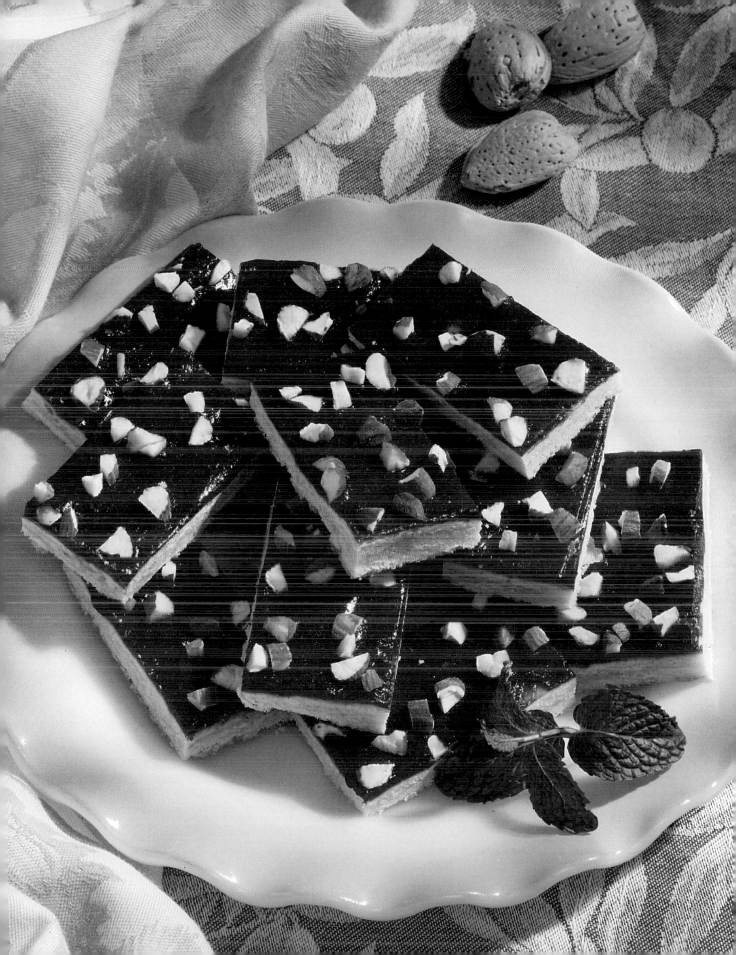

HEAVENLY DESSERTS

353 CHEWY COCONUT BARS

2 eggs
7¼ teaspoons EQUAL® MEASURE™ or
    24 packets EQUAL® sweetener or
    1 cup EQUAL® SPOONFUL™
¼ teaspoon maple flavoring
½ cup margarine, melted
1 teaspoon vanilla
½ cup all-purpose flour
1 teaspoon baking powder
¼ teaspoon salt
1 cup unsweetened coconut,* finely
    chopped
½ cup chopped walnuts (optional)
½ cup raisins

Unsweetened coconut can be purchased in health food stores. Or, substitute sweetened coconut and decrease amount of EQUAL® to 5¼ teaspoons EQUAL® MEASURE™ or 18 packets EQUAL® sweetener or ¾ cup EQUAL® SPOONFUL™.

• Beat eggs, Equal® and maple flavoring in medium bowl; mix in margarine and vanilla. Combine flour, baking powder and salt in small bowl; stir into egg mixture. Mix in coconut, walnuts and raisins. Spread batter evenly in greased 8-inch square baking pan.

• Bake in preheated 350°F oven until browned and toothpick inserted in center comes out clean, about 20 minutes. Cool in pan on wire rack; cut into squares.

Makes 16 bars

Nutrients per Serving: (1 bar), Calories: 126, Fat: 9 g, Protein: 2 g, Carbohydrate: 10 g, Cholesterol: 27 mg, Sodium: 141 mg

Dietary Exchanges: ½ Starch/Bread, 2 Fat

354 COCOA HAZELNUT MACAROONS

⅓ cup hazelnuts
¾ cup quick oats
⅓ cup packed brown sugar
6 tablespoons unsweetened cocoa powder
2 tablespoons all-purpose flour
4 egg whites
1 teaspoon vanilla
½ teaspoon salt
⅓ cup plus 1 tablespoon granulated sugar

1. Preheat oven to 375°F. Place hazelnuts on baking sheet; bake 8 minutes or until lightly browned. Quickly transfer nuts to dry dish towel. Fold towel; rub vigorously to remove as much of the skins as possible. Finely chop hazelnuts using food processor. Combine with oats, brown sugar, cocoa and flour in medium bowl; mix well. Set aside.

2. *Reduce oven temperature to 325°F.* Combine egg whites, vanilla and salt in clean dry medium mixing bowl. Beat with electric mixer on high until soft peaks form. Gradually add granulated sugar, continuing to beat on high until stiff peaks form. Gently fold in hazelnut mixture with rubber spatula.

3. Drop level measuring tablespoonfuls of dough onto cookie sheet. Bake 15 to 17 minutes or until tops of cookies no longer appear wet. Transfer to cooling rack. Store in loosely covered container.

Makes 3 dozen cookies

Nutrients per Serving: (3 cookies), Calories: 104 (24% Calories from Fat), Total Fat: 3 g, Saturated Fat: trace, Protein: 3 g, Carbohydrate: 18 g, Cholesterol: 0 mg, Sodium: 112 mg, Fiber: 1 g, Sugar: 6 g

Dietary Exchanges: 1 Starch/Bread, ½ Fat

Cocoa Hazelnut Macaroons

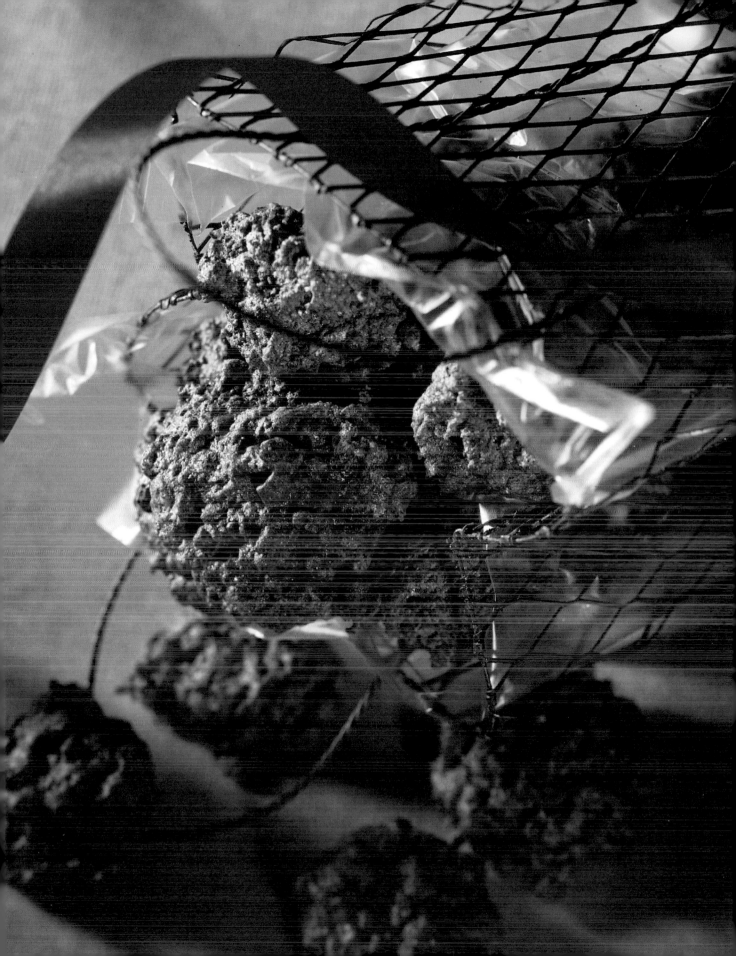

HEAVENLY DESSERTS

355 CREAM CHEESE AND JELLY COOKIES

¾ cup margarine, softened
1 package (8 ounces) reduced-fat cream cheese, softened
2½ teaspoons EQUAL® MEASURE™ or 8 packets EQUAL® sweetener or ⅓ cup EQUAL® SPOONFUL™
2 cups all-purpose flour
¼ teaspoon salt
¼ cup black cherry or seedless raspberry spreadable fruit

• Beat margarine, cream cheese and Equal® in medium bowl until fluffy; mix in flour and salt to form a soft dough. Cover and refrigerate until dough is firm, about 3 hours.

• Roll dough on lightly floured surface into circle ⅛ inch thick; cut into rounds with 3-inch cutter. Place rounded ¼ teaspoon spreadable fruit in center of each round; fold rounds into halves and crimp edges firmly with tines of fork. Pierce tops of cookies with tip of sharp knife. Bake cookies on greased cookie sheets in preheated 350°F oven until lightly browned, about 10 minutes. Cool on wire racks.

Makes about 3 dozen

Nutrients per Serving: (1 cookie), Calories: 80, Fat: 5 g, Protein: 1 g, Carbohydrate: 7 g, Cholesterol: 4 mg, Sodium: 78 mg

Dietary Exchanges: ½ Starch/Bread, 1 Fat

356 OATMEAL RAISIN COOKIES

¼ cup margarine, softened
3 tablespoons granulated sugar *or* 1¼ teaspoons EQUAL® MEASURE™ *(5 packets)* or 2 tablespoons fructose
¼ cup egg substitute *or* 2 egg whites
¾ cup unsweetened applesauce
¼ cup frozen unsweetened apple juice concentrate, thawed
1 teaspoon vanilla
1 cup all-purpose flour
1 teaspoon baking soda
½ teaspoon ground cinnamon
1½ cups QUAKER® Oats (quick or old fashioned, uncooked)
⅓ cup raisins, chopped

Heat oven to 350°F. Lightly spray cookie sheet with vegetable oil cooking spray. Beat together margarine and sugar until creamy. Beat in egg substitute. Add applesauce, apple juice concentrate and vanilla; beat well. Blend in combined flour, soda, and cinnamon. Stir in oats and chopped raisins. Drop by rounded teaspoonsful onto prepared cookie sheet. Bake 15 to 17 minutes or until cookies are lightly browned. Cool 1 minute on cookie sheet; remove to wire rack. Cool completely. Store in air-tight container.

Makes about 3 dozen

Nutrients per Serving: 2 cookies (made with granulated sugar, Equal® or fructose), Calories: 110 (27% Calories from Fat), Total Fat 3: g, Saturated Fat: 1 g, Cholesterol: 0 mg, Sodium: 40 mg, Fiber: 1 g, Protein: 2 g, Sugar: 6 g, Carbohydrate: 17 g, Made with Equal®: 15 g, Made with fructose: 16 g

Dietary Exchanges: 1 Starch/Bread, ½ Fat

HEAVENLY DESSERTS

357 MOCHA CRINKLES

1¾ cups all-purpose flour
¾ cup unsweetened cocoa powder
2 teaspoons instant espresso or coffee granules
1 teaspoon baking soda
¼ teaspoon salt
⅛ teaspoon ground black pepper
1⅓ cups packed light brown sugar
½ cup vegetable oil
¼ cup low-fat sour cream
1 egg
1 teaspoon vanilla
½ cup powdered sugar

1. Mix flour, cocoa, espresso, baking soda, salt and pepper in medium bowl; set aside.

2. Beat brown sugar and oil in another medium bowl with electric mixer at medium speed until well blended. Beat in sour cream, egg and vanilla.

3. Beat in flour mixture until soft dough forms. Form dough into disc; cover. Refrigerate dough until firm, 3 to 4 hours.

4. Preheat oven to 350°F. Place powdered sugar in shallow bowl. Cut dough into 1-inch pieces; roll into balls. Coat with powdered sugar. Place on ungreased cookie sheets.

5. Bake 10 to 12 minutes or until tops of cookies are firm to the touch. *Do not overbake.* Cool cookies completely on wire racks.   *Makes 6 dozen cookies*

Nutrients per Serving: (1 cookie), Calories: 44 (30% Calories from Fat), Total Fat: 1 g, Saturated Fat: trace, Protein: 0 g, Carbohydrate: 7 g, Cholesterol: 3 mg, Sodium: 28 mg, Fiber: 0 g, Sugar: trace

Dietary Exchanges: ½ Starch/Bread

Mocha Crinkles

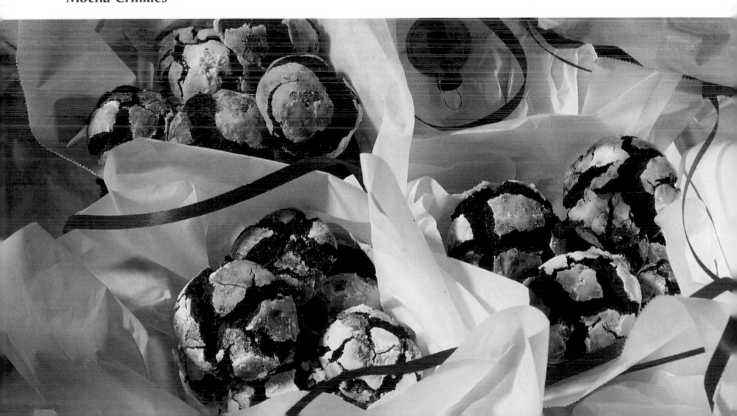

HEAVENLY DESSERTS

358 MAPLE CARAMEL BREAD PUDDING

8 slices cinnamon raisin bread
2 whole eggs
1 egg white
⅓ cup sugar
1½ cups 2% low-fat milk
½ cup maple syrup
½ teaspoon cinnamon
¼ teaspoon ground nutmeg
¼ teaspoon salt
6 tablespoons fat-free caramel ice cream topping

1. Preheat oven to 350°F. Spray 8×8-inch baking dish with nonstick cooking spray. Cut bread into ¾-inch cubes; arrange in prepared dish.

2. Beat whole eggs, egg white and sugar in medium bowl. Beat in milk, syrup, cinnamon, nutmeg and salt; pour evenly over bread. Toss gently to coat.

3. Bake 45 minutes or until center is set. Transfer dish to wire cooling rack; let stand 20 minutes before serving. Serve warm with caramel topping. *Makes 8 servings*

Nutrients per Serving: Calories: 235 (12% Calories from Fat), Total Fat: 3 g, Saturated Fat: 1 g, Protein: 6 g, Carbohydrate: 47 g, Cholesterol: 57 mg, Sodium: 228 mg, Fiber: trace, Sugar: 31 g

Dietary Exchanges: 3 Starch/Bread, ½ Fat

Maple Caramel Bread Pudding

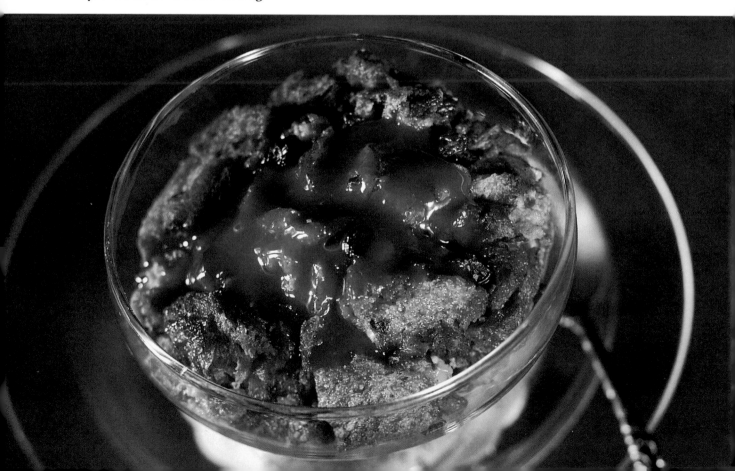

HEAVENLY DESSERTS

359 TROPICAL BREAD PUDDING WITH PIÑA COLADA SAUCE

BREAD PUDDING
- **6 cups cubed day-old French bread**
- **1 cup skim milk**
- **1 cup frozen orange-pineapple-banana juice concentrate, thawed**
- **½ cup cholesterol-free egg substitute**
- **2 teaspoons vanilla**
- **½ teaspoon butter-flavored extract**
- **1 can (8 ounces) crushed pineapple in juice, undrained**
- **½ cup golden raisins**

PIÑA COLADA SAUCE
- **¾ cup all-fruit pineapple preserves**
- **⅓ cup shredded unsweetened coconut, toasted**
- **1 teaspoon rum or ⅛ teaspoon rum extract**

1. To prepare bread pudding, preheat oven to 350°F. Spray 11×7-inch glass baking dish with nonstick cooking spray. Place cubed bread in large bowl; set aside.

2. Combine milk, juice concentrate, egg substitute, vanilla and butter-flavored extract in another large bowl; mix until smooth. Drain pineapple; reserve juice. Add milk mixture, pineapple and raisins to bread; gently mix with large spoon. Spoon bread mixture evenly into prepared baking dish and flatten slightly; bake, uncovered, 40 minutes. Cool slightly.

3. To prepare Piña Colada Sauce, add water to reserved pineapple juice to equal ¼ cup. Combine juice, preserves, coconut and rum in microwavable bowl. Microwave at HIGH 2 to 3 minutes or until sauce is hot and bubbling; cool to room temperature.

4. Divide pudding among 8 plates; top each serving with 2 tablespoons of Piña Colada Sauce. *Makes 8 servings*

Nutrients per Serving: Calories: 280 (6% Calories from Fat), Total Fat: 2 g, Saturated Fat: 1 g, Protein: 6 g, Carbohydrate: 61 g, Cholesterol: 1 mg, Sodium: 178 mg, Fiber: 1 g, Sugar: 12 g

Dietary Exchanges: 1 Starch/Bread, 3 Fruit, ½ Fat

360 CREAMY TAPIOCA PUDDING

- **2 cups skim milk**
- **3 tablespoons quick-cooking tapioca**
- **1 egg**
- **⅛ teaspoon salt**
- **3½ teaspoons EQUAL® MEASURE™ or 12 packets EQUAL® sweetener or ½ cup EQUAL® SPOONFUL™**
- **1 to 2 teaspoons vanilla**
- **Ground cinnamon and nutmeg**

• Combine milk, tapioca, egg and salt in medium saucepan. Let stand 5 minutes. Cook over medium-high heat, stirring constantly, until boiling. Remove from heat; stir in Equal® and vanilla.

• Spoon mixture into serving dishes; sprinkle lightly with cinnamon and nutmeg. Serve warm, or refrigerate and serve chilled. *Makes 4 (⅔-cup) servings*

Nutrients per Serving: Calories: 101, Fat: 1 g, Protein: 6 g, Carbohydrate: 16 g, Cholesterol: 55 mg, Sodium: 146 mg

Dietary Exchanges: 1 Starch/Bread, ½ Milk

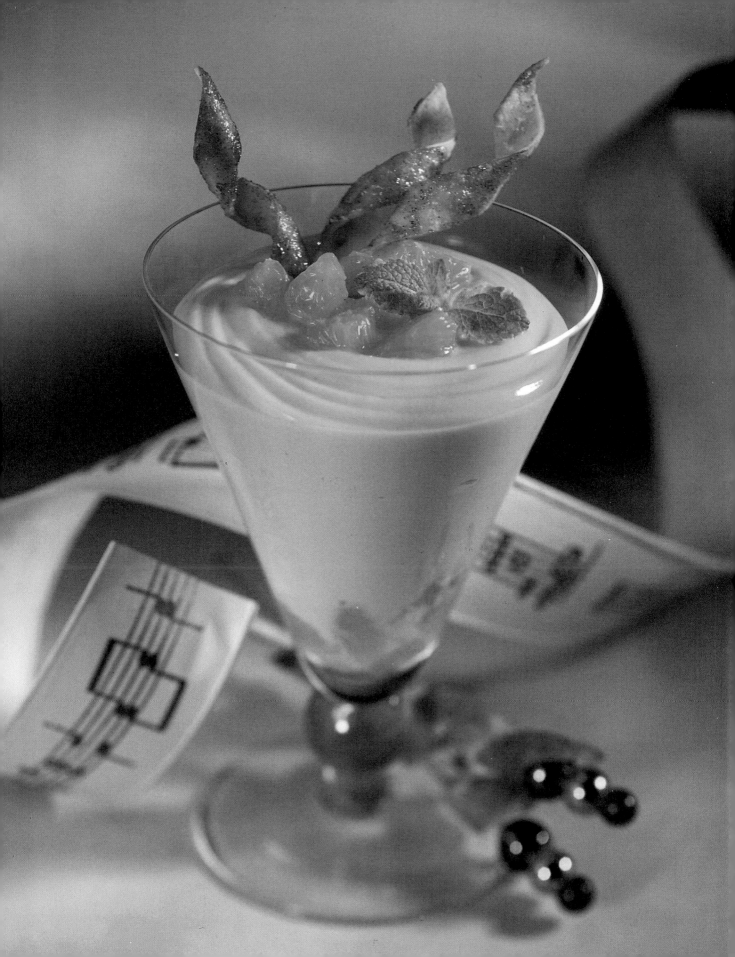

HEAVENLY DESSERTS

361 FRENCH VANILLA FREEZE

10¾ teaspoons EQUAL® MEASURE™ or
    36 packets EQUAL® sweetener or
    1½ cups EQUAL® SPOONFUL™
2 tablespoons cornstarch
1 piece vanilla bean (2 inches)
⅛ teaspoon salt
2 cups skim milk
2 tablespoons margarine
1 cup real liquid egg product
1 teaspoon vanilla

• Combine Equal®, cornstarch, vanilla bean and salt in medium saucepan; stir in milk and margarine. Heat to boiling over medium-high heat, whisking constantly. Boil until thickened, whisking constantly, about 1 minute.

• Whisk about 1 cup milk mixture into egg product in small bowl; whisk egg mixture back into milk mixture in saucepan. Cook over very low heat, whisking constantly, 30 to 60 seconds. Remove from heat and stir in vanilla. Let cool; remove vanilla bean. Refrigerate until chilled, about 1 hour.

• Freeze mixture in ice cream maker according to manufacturer's directions. Pack into freezer container and freeze until firm, 8 hours or overnight. Before serving, let stand at room temperature until slightly softened, about 15 minutes.

Makes 6 (½-cup) servings

Nutrients per Serving: Calories: 134, Fat: 5 g, Protein: 8 g, Carbohydrate: 13 g, Cholesterol: 2 mg, Sodium: 205 mg

Dietary Exchanges: 1 Milk, 1 Fat

Tropical Fruit Cream Parfait

362 TROPICAL FRUIT CREAM PARFAITS

1 cup 2% low-fat milk
1 package (4-serving size) sugar-free vanilla instant pudding mix
½ cup mango nectar
  Cinnamon-Ginger Tortilla Sticks (recipe follows)
1 large orange, peeled, chopped

1. Pour milk into medium bowl. Add pudding mix; whisk 1 minute or until smooth and thickened. Stir in mango nectar; chill.

2. Prepare Cinnamon-Ginger Tortilla Sticks. Reserve 10 sticks; divide remaining sticks equally in 5 parfait dishes or small glasses. Top each with pudding mixture, orange and two reserved tortilla sticks.

Makes 5 servings

CINNAMON–GINGER TORTILLA STICKS
3 tablespoons brown sugar
2 tablespoons margarine
½ teaspoon ground ginger
½ teaspoon ground cinnamon
4 (6-inch) flour tortillas, cut into ½-inch strips

1. Preheat oven to 375°F. Combine sugar, margarine, ginger and cinnamon in small microwavable bowl; microwave at HIGH 1 minute or until smooth when stirred.

2. Twist tortillas into spirals and arrange on baking sheet sprayed with nonstick cooking spray. Brush each with brown sugar mixture; bake 10 to 12 minutes or until edges are lightly browned. Cool. *Makes 5 servings*

Nutrients per Serving: Calories: 277 (22% Calories from Fat), Total Fat: 7 g, Saturated Fat: 4 g, Protein: 4 g, Carbohydrate: 51 g, Cholesterol: 16 mg, Sodium: 357 mg, Fiber: 1 g, Sugar: 5 g

Dietary Exchanges: ½ Milk, 3 Fruit, 1 Fat

HEAVENLY DESSERTS

363 CREAMY RICE PUDDING

2 cups water
1 cinnamon stick, broken into pieces
1 cup converted rice
4 cups skim milk
¼ teaspoon salt
7¼ teaspoons EQUAL® MEASURE™ or
    24 packets EQUAL® sweetener or
    1 cup EQUAL® SPOONFUL™
3 egg yolks
2 egg whites
1 teaspoon vanilla
¼ cup raisins
    Ground cinnamon and nutmeg

• Heat water and cinnamon stick to boiling in large saucepan; stir in rice. Reduce heat and simmer, covered, until rice is tender and water is absorbed, 20 to 25 minutes. Discard cinnamon stick.

• Stir in milk and salt; heat to boiling. Reduce heat and simmer, covered, until mixture starts to thicken, about 15 to 20 minutes, stirring frequently. (Milk will not be absorbed and pudding will thicken when it cools.) Remove from heat and cool 1 to 2 minutes; stir in Equal®.

• Beat egg yolks, egg whites and vanilla in small bowl until blended. Stir about ½ cup rice mixture into egg mixture; stir back into saucepan. Cook over low heat, stirring constantly, 1 to 2 minutes. Stir in raisins.

• Spoon pudding into serving bowl; sprinkle with cinnamon and nutmeg. Serve warm or at room temperature.

Makes 6 (⅔-cup) servings

Nutrients per Serving: Calories: 244, Fat: 3 g, Protein: 11 g, Carbohydrate: 43 g, Cholesterol: 109 mg, Sodium: 200 mg

Dietary Exchanges: 2 Starch/Bread, 1 Milk, ½ Fat

364 MOCHA SAUCE

1 cup skim milk
4 teaspoons unsweetened cocoa
2 teaspoons cornstarch
1 teaspoon instant coffee crystals
1 teaspoon vanilla
1¼ teaspoons EQUAL® MEASURE™ or
    4 packets EQUAL® sweetener or
    3 tablespoons EQUAL® SPOONFUL™

• Combine milk, cocoa, cornstarch and coffee crystals in small saucepan. Cook and stir until thickened and bubbly. Cook and stir 2 minutes more. Remove from heat; stir in vanilla and Equal®. Cool. Cover and chill.

Makes about 1 cup

Nutrients per Serving: (1 tablespoon), Calories: 10, Protein: 1 g, Fat: 0 g, Carbohydrate: 2 g, Cholesterol: 0 mg, Sodium: 8 mg

Dietary Exchanges: Free Food

365 RASPBERRY SAUCE

2 cups fresh raspberries or thawed frozen
    unsweetened raspberries
1 tablespoon orange juice
1¼ teaspoons EQUAL® MEASURE™ or
    4 packets EQUAL® sweetener or
    3 tablespoons EQUAL® SPOONFUL™
½ teaspoon finely grated orange peel

• Place raspberries in blender container; blend until smooth. Strain through sieve; discard seeds. Stir orange juice, Equal® and orange peel into puréed berries.

Makes 1 cup

Nutrients per Serving: (¼ cup), Calories: 35, Protein: 1 g, Fat: 0 g, Carbohydrate: 9 g, Cholesterol: 0 mg, Sodium: 0 mg

Dietary Exchanges: ½ Fruit

ACKNOWLEDGMENTS

The publisher would like to thank the companies and organizations listed below for the use of their recipes in this publication.

Equal® sweetener

California Prune Board

EGG BEATERS® Healthy Real Egg Substitute

FLEISCHMANN'S® Spread

GREY POUPON® Mustard

Guiltless Gourmet®

Healthy Choice®

The Quaker® Kitchens

INDEX

INDEX

INDEX

INDEX

INDEX

INDEX

INDEX

INDEX

INDEX

INDEX

INDEX

METRIC CONVERSION CHART

VOLUME MEASUREMENTS (dry)

¹/₈ teaspoon = 0.5 mL
¹/₄ teaspoon = 1 mL
¹/₂ teaspoon = 2 mL
³/₄ teaspoon = 4 mL
1 teaspoon = 5 mL
1 tablespoon = 15 mL
2 tablespoons = 30 mL
¹/₄ cup = 60 mL
¹/₃ cup = 75 mL
¹/₂ cup = 125 mL
²/₃ cup = 150 mL
³/₄ cup = 175 mL
1 cup = 250 mL
2 cups = 1 pint = 500 mL
3 cups = 750 mL
4 cups = 1 quart = 1 L

VOLUME MEASUREMENTS (fluid)

1 fluid ounce (2 tablespoons) = 30 mL
4 fluid ounces (¹/₂ cup) = 125 mL
8 fluid ounces (1 cup) = 250 mL
12 fluid ounces (1¹/₂ cups) = 375 mL
16 fluid ounces (2 cups) = 500 mL

WEIGHTS (mass)

¹/₂ ounce = 15 g
1 ounce = 30 g
3 ounces = 90 g
4 ounces = 120 g
8 ounces = 225 g
10 ounces = 285 g
12 ounces = 360 g
16 ounces = 1 pound = 450 g

DIMENSIONS

¹/₁₆ inch = 2 mm
¹/₈ inch = 3 mm
¹/₄ inch = 6 mm
¹/₂ inch = 1.5 cm
³/₄ inch = 2 cm
1 inch = 2.5 cm

OVEN TEMPERATURES

250°F = 120°C
275°F = 140°C
300°F = 150°C
325°F = 160°C
350°F = 180°C
375°F = 190°C
400°F = 200°C
425°F = 220°C
450°F = 230°C

BAKING PAN SIZES

Utensil	Size in Inches/Quarts	Metric Volume	Size in Centimeters
Baking or Cake Pan (square or rectangular)	8×8×2	2 L	20×20×5
	9×9×2	2.5 L	23×23×5
	12×8×2	3 L	30×20×5
	13×9×2	3.5 L	33×23×5
Loaf Pan	8×4×3	1.5 L	20×10×7
	9×5×3	2 L	23×13×7
Round Layer Cake Pan	8×1½	1.2 L	20×4
	9×1½	1.5 L	23×4
Pie Plate	8×1¼	750 mL	20×3
	9×1¼	1 L	23×3
Baking Dish or Casserole	1 quart	1 L	—
	1½ quart	1.5 L	—
	2 quart	2 L	—

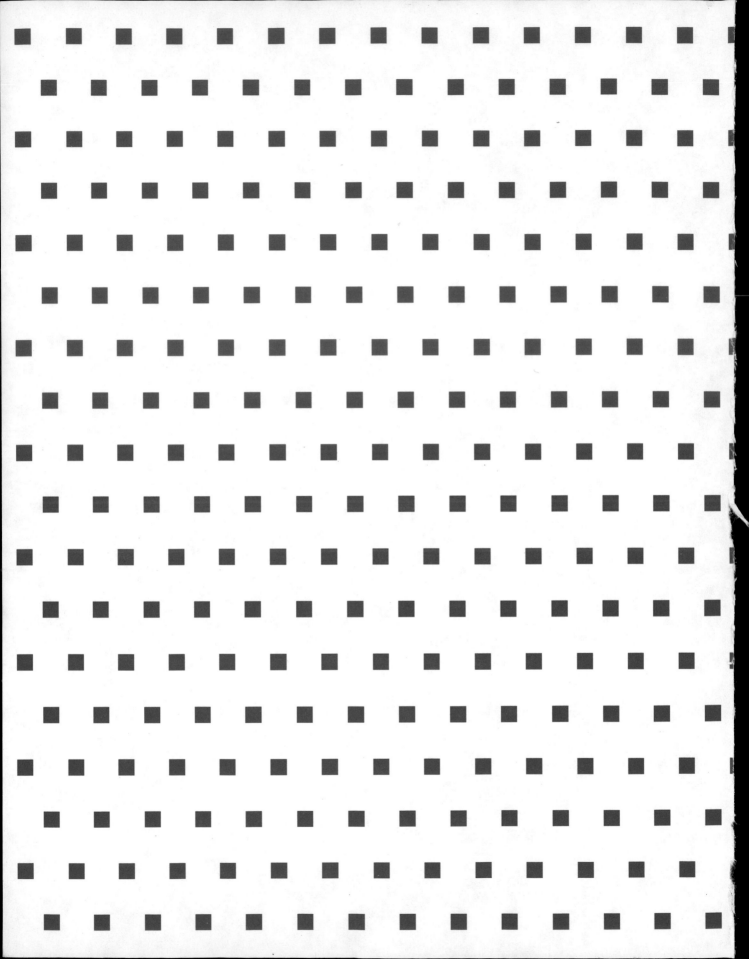